# THE DNP PROFESSIONAL

TRANSLATING VALUE FROM CLASSROOM TO PRACTICE

# THE DNP PROFESSIONAL

### TRANSLATING VALUE FROM CLASSROOM TO PRACTICE

Editor

## *Linda A. Benson, DNP, ACNP-BC, CPHQ*
### *Tampa, Florida*

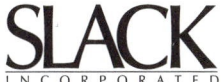

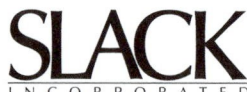

SLACK Incorporated
6900 Grove Road
Thorofare, NJ 08086 USA
856-848-1000   Fax: 856-848-6091
www.slackbooks.com
© 2021 by SLACK Incorporated

Senior Vice President: Stephanie Arasim Portnoy
Vice President, Editorial: Jennifer Kilpatrick
Vice President, Marketing: Mary Sasso
Acquisitions Editor: Julia Dolinger
Director of Editorial Operations: Jennifer Cahill
Vice President/Creative Director: Thomas Cavallaro
Cover Artist: Amarie Mitchell
Project Editor: Joseph Lowery

The procedures and practices described in this publication should be implemented in a manner consistent with the professional standards set for the circumstances that apply in each specific situation. Every effort has been made to confirm the accuracy of the information presented and to correctly relate generally accepted practices. The authors, editors, and publisher cannot accept responsibility for errors or exclusions or for the outcome of the material presented herein. There is no expressed or implied warranty of this book or information imparted by it. Care has been taken to ensure that drug selection and dosages are in accordance with currently accepted/recommended practice. Off-label uses of drugs may be discussed. Due to continuing research, changes in government policy and regulations, and various effects of drug reactions and interactions, it is recommended that the reader carefully review all materials and literature provided for each drug, especially those that are new or not frequently used. Some drugs or devices in this publication have clearance for use in a restricted research setting by the Food and Drug and Administration or FDA. Each professional should determine the FDA status of any drug or device prior to use in their practice.

Any review or mention of specific companies or products is not intended as an endorsement by the author or publisher.

SLACK Incorporated uses a review process to evaluate submitted material. Prior to publication, educators or clinicians provide important feedback on the content that we publish. We welcome feedback on this work.

Library of Congress Cataloging-in-Publication Data

Names: Benson, Linda A., DNP, editor.
Title: The DNP professional : translating value from classroom to practice
  / editor, Linda A. Benson.
Other titles: Doctor of nursing practice professional
Description: Thorofare, NJ : SLACK Incorporated, [2021] | Includes
  bibliographical references and index.
Identifiers: LCCN 2020055901 (print) | LCCN 2020055902 (ebook) | ISBN
  9781630917111 (paperback) | ISBN 9781630917128 (epub) | ISBN
  9781630917135
Subjects: MESH: Advanced Practice Nursing | Education, Nursing, Graduate |
  Evidence-Based Nursing | United States
Classification: LCC RT41  (print) | LCC RT41  (ebook) | NLM WY 128 | DDC
  610.73--dc23
LC record available at https://lccn.loc.gov/2020055901
LC ebook record available at https://lccn.loc.gov/2020055902

For permission to reprint material in another publication, contact SLACK Incorporated. Authorization to photocopy items for internal, personal, or academic use is granted by SLACK Incorporated provided that the appropriate fee is paid directly to Copyright Clearance Center. Prior to photocopying items, please contact the Copyright Clearance Center at 222 Rosewood Drive, Danvers, MA 01923 USA; phone: 978-750-8400; website: www.copyright.com; email: info@copyright.com

Printed in the United States of America.

Last digit is print number: 10   9   8   7   6   5   4   3   2   1

# DEDICATION

This book is dedicated to all DNP students and practicing DNPs who have been enriched by their education and seek to apply the DNP Essentials, quantify successful DNP-prepared practitioner outcomes, and describe the overall impact of the nursing practice doctorate.

*—Linda*

# CONTENTS

# Acknowledgments

This book would not have become a reality without the contributing authors who shared their DNP journeys and expertise in incorporating the DNP Essentials into a variety of roles and settings. I am grateful for their willingness to provide their contributions on the impact of the DNP degree and disseminate their successes. My successes as the nursing clinical quality specialist have been made possible only through the total assistance and support of my role provided by the Tampa General Hospital nurse executive team, nurse managers, and nursing quality champions. Most importantly, I would be remiss not to mention my family, particularly my husband, Frank, who has supported me during this writing journey and allowed me to devote my time to this chapter and to this book as well.

# ABOUT THE EDITOR

*Linda A. Benson, DNP, ACNP-BC, CPHQ* has been a nurse for more than 40 years working in acute care and critical care settings. She has held a variety of positions including staff nurse, charge nurse, clinical preceptor, unit-based clinical instructor, critical care clinical nurse specialist, acute care nurse practitioner, and clinical quality specialist for various departments of nursing. Her education has consisted of a Bachelor of Science and Master of Science in Adult Health from the State University of New York at Buffalo (SUNYAB). This was followed by a post-master's certificate from the University of Rochester and ended in the terminal nursing degree of the DNP from Madonna University. Her DNP capstone project concentrated on the impact of a nurse practitioner rapid response team on sepsis outcomes. After obtaining her DNP degree, she focused on performance improvement as a clinical quality specialist for Tampa General Hospital Department of Nursing. She has held adjunct faculty positions at SUNYAB and Western Michigan University teaching Bachelor of Science in Nursing and Master of Science in Nursing students. She has disseminated new knowledge and creative solutions through more than 35 podium presentations at regional and national levels as well as 10 poster presentations. In addition, she has published in multiple peer-reviewed journals predominantly as the primary author. Throughout her career she has chosen to give back to her profession having precepted and mentored numerous nurses at all degree levels.

# Contributing Authors

*Mallory Andrzejak, DNP, FNP-BC (Chapter 19)*
Neighborhood Health Center
Buffalo, New York

*Tammy Austin-Ketch, PhD, FNP-BC, FAANP (Chapter 19)*
Dean and Professor
College of Nursing
SUNY Upstate Medical University
Syracuse, New York

*Debbie Barber, DNP, CRNA (Chapter 9)*
Owner
Triple Crown Anesthesia
Louisville, Kentucky
Adjunct Assistant Clinical Professor
Northern Kentucky University
Highland Heights, Kentucky

*Rebecca A. Bates, DNP, APRN, FNP-C, PMP (Chapter 1)*
ADAMS Compassionate Healthcare Network
Chantilly, Virginia

*Garry Brydges, PhD, DNP, MBA, APRN, CRNA, ACNP-BC, FAAN (Chapter 8)*
President
American Association of Nurse Anesthetists
Cleveland, Ohio
Chief Nurse Anesthetist
The University of Texas MD Anderson Cancer Center
Houston, Texas

*Debra A. Burke, RN, DNP, MBA, NEA-BC (Chapter 16)*
Senior Vice President
Patient Care Services
Chief Nurse
Jeanette Ives and Paul Erickson Chair in Nursing
Massachusetts General Hospital
Boston, Massachusetts

*Deborah Chasco, DNP, CCRN, APRN, CNS (Chapter 22)*
Director Nursing Informatics
University Medical Center of El Paso
El Paso, Texas

*Ileen Craven, DNP, CNS, MSN, RN-BC (Chapter 6)*
Clinical Nurse Specialist
Vidant Medical Center
Greenville, North Carolina

*Janet Hunt Davis, DNP, RN, NE-BC, CPHQ (Chapter 14)*
Senior Vice President
Chief Nursing Officer
Tampa General Hospital
Tampa, Florida

*Michelle M. Davis, DNP, RNC-OB, NNP, CNM (Chapter 12)*
Associate Clinical Professor
Medical OB/GYN
University of Arizona
Tucson, Arizona
Maricopa Obstetrics and Gynecology Associates
Banner University Medical Center Phoenix
Phoenix, Arizona

*Melinda Earle, DNP, RN, NEA-BC, FACHE (Chapter 18)*
Program Director
Transformative Leadership DNP: Systems Program
Assistant Professor
Health Systems Management
College of Nursing and College of Health Sciences
Rush University
Chicago, Illinois

*Carol Essenmacher, DNP, PMHCNS-BC, NCTTP (Chapter 7)*
Tobacco Treatment Coordinator
Battle Creek VA Medical Center
Battle Creek, Michigan

*Mary Field, DNP, MBA, RN, CPHON (Chapter 23)*
Clinical Practice Manager
Cancer Care Unit
Seattle Children's Hospital
Seattle, Washington

*Kelly Hancock, DNP, RN, NE-BC, FAAN (Chapter 15)*
Executive Chief Nurse
Cleveland Clinic Medical Center
Cleveland, Ohio

*Marcia Johansson, DNP, APRN, ACNP-BC (Chapter 21)*
Assistant Professor
College of Nursing
University of South Florida
Tampa, Florida

*Mary C. Loughran, DNP, RN, MHA (Chapter 17)*
Clinical Assistant Professor
Director
DNP Program Coordinator
School of Nursing
Duquesne University
Pittsburgh, Pennsylvania

*Robert Metzger, DNP, APRN, FNP-BC (Chapter 24)*
Director of Advanced Practice
Parkland Health and Hospital System
Dallas, Texas
Graduate Studies Adjunct Professor
Texas Woman's University
Denton, Texas
Administrator
The North Texas Nurse Practitioners
Immediate Past President
Nomination Council Chair
American Association of Nurse Practitioners
Austin, Texas

*Tracie L. Moore, DNP, FNP, ACNP, ACNS-BC (Chapter 3)*
Family and Acute Care Nurse Practitioner
Nurse Educator/Adult Health Clinical Nurse Specialist
Hospitalist Nurse Practitioner
Methodist North Hospital
Memphis, Tennessee

*Kara Morgan, DNP, APRN, CPNP-BC, CGC (Chapter 2)*
Nurse Practitioner
Department of Pediatrics
Division of Genetics and Metabolism
University of South Florida
Tampa, Florida

*Maria Teresa Palleschi, RN, DNP, ACNP-BC, CCRN (Chapter 4)*
Director of Patient Care Services
Sepsis and Magnet Programs
DMC Harper Hospital
Detroit, Michigan

*Pamela Paplham, DNP, AOCNP, FNP-BC, FAANP (Chapter 19)*
Assistant Dean
MS/DNP Programs
Clinical Professor
Family Nurse Practitioner Program Coordinator
State University of New York at Buffalo
Buffalo, New York

*Courtney Pladsen, DNP, FNP-BC, RN (Chapter 20)*
Director of Clinical and Quality Improvement
National Health Care for the Homeless Council
Nashville, Tennessee
Fellow
Robert Wood Johnson Culture of Health Leaders
Princeton, New Jersey

*Dixie Shaheen Rasmussen, DNP, MSN-Ed, CNM (Chapter 13)*
Mountain Utah Family Medicine
Richfield, Utah

*Nancy Renn-Bugai, DNP, MSN, CNM (Chapter 11)*
Maternal Fetal Medicine
Spectrum Health
Grand Rapids, Michigan

*Carol Shade, DNP, MS, RN, CPHIMS, FHIMSS (Chapter 23)*
Director of Nursing Informatics, Training, and Technology
Seattle Children's Hospital
Seattle, Washington

*Susanna Sirianni, RN, DNP, ACNP-BC, ANP-BC, CCRN (Chapter 4)*
Sinai Grace Hospital
Detroit, Michigan
Madonna University
Livonia, Michigan

*Jorge A. Valdes, DNP, CRNA, APRN (Chapter 10)*
Interim Chair
Clinical Associate Professor
Florida International University
Miami, Florida

Note: Affiliations given are those at the time of writing.

# PREFACE

Every year, the number of Doctor of Nursing Practice (DNP) graduates continues to increase. According to the American Association of Colleges of Nursing, the number of DNPs graduated from 2017 to 2018 increased from 6090 to 7039 and is expected to continue on an upward climb.[1] More nurses who have their bachelor's or master's degree are recognizing the value of the DNP skill set. The DNP Essentials emphasize organizational and systems leadership for quality improvement and systems thinking. The DNP graduate is keenly positioned to promote evidence-based practice as it affects population health and to utilize data-mining techniques to optimize patient outcomes. This is extremely valuable as health care has become quality oriented with zero tolerance for hospital-acquired conditions. Consumers have become savvy in the search for optimal health care outcomes, which the DNP can be uniquely positioned to provide.

However, many recent graduates have found themselves unable to transition into a position that allows them to utilize their newly developed skills from their education or to even apply the valuable performance improvement and quality tools into their existing advanced practice nursing roles. This can lead to role frustration as nursing leadership may not always understand what the DNP degree has to offer. The price tag on hiring a DNP graduate may be a deterrent for either creation of a new position or even a salary increase in an existing role. The onus does rest with the DNP graduate to be able to articulate what they bring to the table as a return on investment and to establish an accompanying business plan for doing so. With exemplars from across the continuum of practice sites and roles, *The DNP Professional: Translating Value From Classroom to Practice* enables both students and DNP graduates to optimize the curricular Essentials in the practice setting.

## Reference

1. DNP Fact Sheet. American Association of Colleges of Nurses. Accessed October 19, 2019. https://www.aacnnursing.org/News-Information/Fact-Sheets/DNP-Fact-Sheet

# INTRODUCTION

## Purpose

In the subsequent pages, multiple DNP authors will present how they successfully operationalized the skill set post-graduation and implemented the DNP Essentials. The typical advanced practice nursing roles of nurse practitioner, clinical nurse specialist, certified nurse anesthetist, and nurse-midwife will be presented with a focus on how the DNP Essentials were implemented for each. A variety of practice settings are presented, including inpatient, outpatient, and mobile settings. Both adult and pediatric patient populations are depicted. Academic settings that have not only DNP professors but DNP program directors as well are portrayed. Nurse executives who have obtained their DNPs are uniquely positioned to not only understand how the DNP can affect clinical, satisfaction, and cost outcomes, but can also provide preceptorship and mentoring. Examples of DNP involvement in population health, informatics, and legislative activity will also be featured.

All chapters will have a similar content template. The authors present exemplars on how they individually implemented the DNP Essentials on a daily basis, implemented evidence-based practice, utilized data to drive practice, demonstrated a return on investment, and promoted professional nursing practice.

All first authors are exclusively graduates of DNP programs. An effort has been made to select authors from across the country with regional diversity. Author recruitment for the text took place over a 2- to 3-month period. Authors were recruited using a variety of methods. Some authors were recruited from presentations at national conferences. Others were selected based on involvement and leadership roles in their respective professional organizations. Some authors have received either state or national awards in their advanced practice roles. Certain authors have received American Association of Colleges of Nursing DNP capstone writing awards.

Each DNP author will describe their practice setting in detail. The DNP Essentials are the common core curriculum elements in all DNP educational programs and serve as the structure or foundation for DNP practice. The Essentials will serve as the commonality and linking thread between the various DNP chapter authors. Page space will be devoted to how the chapter author created the role or expanded on their existing role to incorporate the DNP Essentials. Business plans that were utilized for role or position creation and/or delineation are incorporated into chapters as appropriate. Cost savings or revenue generation, whichever can be demonstrated, will be described. The DNP authors demonstrated how they have incorporated evidence into practice and how data mining has driven outcomes. Each author describes clinical, cost, functional, and satisfaction outcomes that they have achieved in the role. Promotion of the nursing profession is incorporated into each chapter but will look different for each of the roles. Each author was asked to share any possible pearls that they may have for those DNP graduates who wish to follow in their footsteps. Most importantly, each exemplar author will summarize the impact that the DNP degree has had on their professional role.

This text should serve as a resource for both DNP graduates and students. As they embark on their practicum experiences, DNP students will find this text useful throughout their education, particularly as they embark on practicum experiences. The text provides examples of DNP Essentials implementation that would be pertinent for students designing practicum experiences. Likewise, graduate DNPs will find the text useful in providing examples of incorporation of the DNP Essentials into practice. The text could assist in providing methods to either enhance a current practice or to establish a completely new practice.

## Objectives

At the completion of each chapter exemplar, the reader will be able to:

- Describe the chapter author's transition from DNP graduate to their current role. Discuss if the current role was a newly created position or an expansion of an existing one.
- Describe the author's current practice setting.
- Elaborate on how the DNP Essentials were integrated into the individual professional roles. List strategies that have enabled the authors to utilize the DNP Essentials.
- List any successes, barriers, or opportunities each author may have discussed in operationalizing their role and in incorporating the DNP Essentials.
- Discuss implementation of evidence into practice by the DNP-prepared professionals. List specific examples of gap analysis and how evidence was incorporated into practice.
- Describe data-mining techniques employed by the DNP-prepared professionals. Describe how the authors have implemented data-mining techniques to leverage data and drive practice or population outcomes.

- List practice and population outcomes as described by the chapter authors. This may be inclusive of, but not limited to, clinical, functional, cost, and satisfaction outcomes. Describe any performance improvement tools that have been utilized to measure processes or outcomes.
- Discuss how individual chapter authors have utilized their DNP skill set to collaborate with other professionals to evoke system change.
- Describe how the DNP-prepared nurses have furthered their professional growth and promoted the nursing profession since obtaining their DNP degrees.
- Describe the impact that the DNP degree has had for the various chapter authors in the multitude of professional roles presented in this text.

# SECTION I

## NURSE PRACTITIONER EXEMPLARS

# CHAPTER 1

# DNP Translated Practice Innovations for a Nurse Practitioner–Managed Free Clinic

*Rebecca A. Bates, DNP, APRN, FNP-C, PMP*

## Introduction

This chapter describes my journey as a Doctor of Nursing Practice (DNP) graduate and the transformation in my professional practice as a result of undertaking this journey. After graduating with my DNP in 2015, I made a conscious decision to leave private practice to work in free clinics. This chapter will focus on how the DNP Essentials helped with role development, the return on investment, evidence-based practice, identifying gaps in care, using information technology to improve health care, interprofessional education, and professional leadership. Many of the examples in this chapter come from my work as a primary care provider in a free clinic and additional opportunities that have arisen because of my unique skill set as a nurse practitioner and DNP graduate. Most of these new roles I hold were not part of my personal strategic plan, but they have expanded my work outside the walls of the one clinic to create positive impacts on the health of patients throughout the world.

Prior to becoming a family nurse practitioner (FNP), I worked in oncology and recognized that the majority of the patients I cared for had preventable cancers and comorbid chronic diseases that could be better prevented or mitigated through primary and secondary prevention. This realization motivated me to become a nurse practitioner so I could directly impact the health care patients and families received. After working for a few years as an FNP, I understood the need for a broader understanding of the health care system and how I could work to improve health care access, treatment, and outcomes. I decided to pursue the DNP degree at Old Dominion University while working full-time in a private primary care practice. My goal in pursuing the DNP degree was to learn as much as possible about translating evidence into practice and creating new models of care to improve health care outcomes for the most vulnerable populations. The journey was so much more than I anticipated. The knowledge and experiences I gained from my DNP education, as well as the network connections and new skills, enabled me to develop new models of care, create new workforce development opportunities, reach a broad audience with health policy advocacy, and branch out into project management.

Shortly after completing my DNP, I left private practice to work part-time in 2 different free clinics. One was a grant-funded academic-community partnership of a local university that created a grant-funded bridge care program through a series of weekly clinics at various sites. In this position, I provided primary care services for people living with serious

Benson LA, ed. *The DNP Professional:*
*Translating Value From Classroom to Practice* (pp 3-18).

mental illness and/or substance use disorders and precepted Advanced Practice Registered Nurse (APRN) students. The second position was with Adams Compassionate Healthcare Network (ACHN) clinic. ACHN is a free clinic that was started about 18 months prior to my hiring by a small group of people who believed a free clinic was needed to meet the needs of those in the community who were uninsured. It is in northern Virginia, less than an hour from Washington, DC. The clinic is in an industrial park in a rented space that houses a mosque. The mosque provides the clinic space and charges a nominal fee. Through this partnership, the clinic was provided with 4 exam rooms, a private office, waiting room, and front desk space. The clinic accepts any patient who has no health care insurance and lives 200% or below the federal poverty limit. The majority of our patients are adults from Muslim-majority countries and who are immigrants, refugees, or asylum seekers. However, we see anyone of any age who meets the eligibility criteria regardless of geographic location, age, gender, or religion.

There are more than 1400 free clinics in the United States. In 2018, these clinics provided services for 2 million individuals for a total of 6.3 million patient visits. Free clinics typically provide about $5 worth of services for every $1 spent and most operate on a yearly budget of less than $250 000 per year.[1] ACHN has almost 1000 active patients with a yearly budget of less than $200 000 that covers employee salaries, clinic expenses, and clinic supplies. Patients pay a significantly reduced price for laboratory tests. Those who qualify are eligible to receive medications through a local pharmacy that works with free clinics in northern Virginia. Patients pay $5 per prescription for a 30- to 90-day supply of the medication depending on drug availability.

Many of our patients have not had access to safe and reliable health care services and many live with chronic diseases such as diabetes, hypertension, hyperlipidemia, and obesity. A significant number of our patients also live with depression, anxiety, or other mental health disorders, often as a result of internal displacement in their home countries, fleeing persecution, or violence and oppression. Many have family members who still live in their countries of origin with whom they have limited contact and worry about since many of these countries are in the midst of war and conflict.

Originally, the clinic was staffed only on Saturday mornings by volunteer physicians and personnel. I was hired as the only employed provider with an office manager and an administrative assistant as the only other employees. We now have 4 employees as we recently added a social worker. The social worker was a former student at ACHN a few years ago. I am in the clinic for 3 days during the week for a total of 17 hours per week. The clinic remains open on Saturdays and is staffed by volunteer staff and providers then. Currently, we have 48 medical volunteers and assistants, including 32 specialists who see patients in their own offices, and many interdisciplinary health care students who rotate through the clinic each semester.

Prior to taking a position at ACHN, I worked in private practice in another state, for a free clinic in another state, and volunteered at a different free clinic in northern Virginia. Part of my Master of Science in Nursing-Family Nurse Practitioner (MSN-FNP) education was in a federally qualified health care center in rural upstate New York that provided health care for children. This experience transformed the way I thought about health care and solidified my passion for working with underserved and vulnerable populations. Consequently, I have actively sought opportunities to work with the population I currently serve.

# DNP ESSENTIALS AND ROLE DEVELOPMENT

When I completed the DNP degree, I made a conscious decision to leave private practice and to work for ACHN as a primary care provider where I could expand my role to fully utilize the DNP Essentials[2] and to practice primary care the way I was educated and trained to do without restrictions from insurance payors. I believe everyone has a right to health care that is high-quality, evidence-based, accessible, and affordable. One of my frustrations in private practice was being limited in the frequency and method of contact with patients because of reimbursement restrictions. My collaborating physicians further impacted my ability to practice autonomously because of incident-to billing, clinic policies and procedures, and legislative restrictions. Virginia, where I live and work, is a restricted practice state for nurse practitioners. Until January 2019, a licensed nurse practitioner was required to have a collaborative agreement with a licensed physician. Currently, in order to practice autonomously, a nurse practitioner must have a collaborative agreement with a licensed physician unless they attest that they have at least 9000 hours of practice as an nurse practitioner. Additionally, nurse practitioners in Virginia are regulated by a joint board of nursing and medicine. This arrangement allows another profession, medicine, to regulate the profession of nursing. At ACHN, my collaborating physician is the medical director who has his own private practice. He has never practiced in the clinic with me. As of 2019, I no longer require a collaborating physician to be able to practice in Virginia.

When I was hired at ACHN, one of the conditions of employment that I required was the ability to precept students in the clinic. This was important to me as professional development and clinical placement opportunities for students are limited and many private practices have very short appointment times that limit experiential learning and critical thinking. As many of our patients have complicated health histories, speak various languages, and need care navigation, an interdisciplinary team of students helps to fill the needs of our patients. Some of our students are also from other countries and are able to speak to patients in their preferred language. Other students learn how to provide care navigation services. And of course, we have APRN students who learn how to provide health care services for this population.

Experience gained during my DNP education, through meeting competencies based on the DNP Essentials, set me apart from other candidates. In my private practice, I had created and implemented a successful, shared-medical appointments for diabetes program. The Organizational and Systems Leadership for Quality Improvement and Systems Thinking Essential provided the foundation needed to start and implement an evidence-based program. After overcoming resistance from colleagues and administration, the program resulted in improved outcomes for patients living with diabetes and contributed to a National Committee for Quality Assurance (NCQA) recognition for the practice.

Through my DNP program, I also learned about telehealth and how to incorporate telehealth into my primary care practice to improve access to care. Prior to graduation, I had spent time learning more about telehealth and attending state and regional telehealth conferences where I was exposed to innovative and cost-effective models of care using telehealth as a tool. While in private practice, my employer was unwilling to consider using telehealth. In the past few years, telehealth has had a significant impact in the care I am able to offer my patients. Telehealth tools have enabled us to expand the reach to our patients. For example, many of our patients lack reliable transportation and therefore miss appointments. Through a mini-grant from my local nurse practitioner organization, I was able to purchase a computer, wireless printer, rolling bag, and hot spot. I can send teams of 2 students to patients' homes to complete a health care visit for chronic disease management. As they do in the clinic, students report to me and we develop a treatment plan with the patient's input and agreement. I can then order labs or other tests, refill medications, and see my patients via video-teleconferencing provided through a state telehealth program. Some of our patients do not speak English well and need translation services. We can use a telehealth platform to bring translators into the office visit to facilitate communication between the provider and patient. Without telehealth, we could not offer the frequent visits every 2 weeks that allow us to support our patients in chronic disease self-management efforts.

Focusing on population health, including prevention at all levels, is an integral part of health care. Using technology such as an electronic health record and patient registry allows me to focus on population health to evaluate clinic outcomes and to better understand the health of our patients.[3] This also allows me to consider what interventions may best meet the needs of our patients.

During the last 2 semesters of my doctoral program, I was selected as one of the first 2 students accepted into the Virginia Nurse Advocate Health Policy Fellowship. This fellowship was separate from the degree requirements and offered the opportunity to gain competency in health policy advocacy at the state level. Working with a nurse lobbyist who only works with nonprofit health groups, I spent time before and after the Virginia General Assembly session meeting with stakeholders, participating in legislative advocacy groups, sitting in and listening to hours of legislative sessions, and meeting with legislators. This experience helped me understand the power of health policy advocacy to impact health care on a population health level. I also became active in advocacy at the national level for health care issues related to nurse practitioner practice, global health, and health care reform.

As you may imagine, a practice that serves a mainly immigrant population has to be aware of not only the local and national political issues, but also the global political issues and policies that affect patients we care for at ACHN. Being well-versed in health policy advocacy has been a wonderful asset as we seek to find community resources for our patients and advocate for health care resources for our uninsured population. My experience in health policy also helped me to secure the position at ACHN. During my 2 interviews, I was asked specifically about my advocacy experience. ACHN holds a health fair once per year for the community. We have had the governor and many local and state politicians attend these events which helps boost our visibility in the community and gives our population a voice in the political discourse.

Interprofessional collaboration was also a significant part of my education and training during my MSN-FNP and DNP programs. One of the sites I trained in during my master's program was an interprofessional pediatric Federally Qualified Health Center (FQHC) in rural upstate New York. After graduation, I worked in a free clinic for the homeless as a primary care provider with other service providers (social work, community health workers, substance use treatment programs), and volunteered in a local free clinic as a primary care provider. Along with translators, specialty providers, and behavioral health therapists, this free clinic provided integrated services for uninsured adults. This experiential learning solidified my passion for working with underserved and vulnerable populations and supported my understanding that high-quality, cost-effective, evidence-based primary health care is one of the keys to driving down costs and significantly improving outcomes for patients and families.

# SWOT Analysis: Adams Compassionate Healthcare Network Clinic Challenges and Successes

At ACHN, we focus on primary and secondary prevention in the primary care outpatient setting. Approaching health care with a population health focus helps me recognize the needs of our patients and to help plan evidence-based programs that benefit our patients. This is frequently done through masters and doctoral student projects. I precept a group of students each semester who each bring a different skill set. In 2018, we had 25 students rotate through the clinic from 10 different universities. As a preceptor, I work with students to identify a need in our population and help design an appropriate intervention. For example, a master's level community health nursing student created a disaster preparedness plan for the clinic and provided education for the clinic staff, providers, and the connected mosque. Another student completing a Master of Public Health (MPH) degree created our patient care registry to track patients living with chronic diseases such as diabetes, hypertension, hyperlipidemia, and obesity. Identifying sub-populations in my patient panel that would benefit from additional interventions is vitally important to targeting individuals who could benefit from high touch care to improve outcomes.

A recent DNP student focused on medication reconciliation. This student provided patient and provider education about the importance of bringing all medications to every appointment and reviewing them as part of the health care visit. Patients were provided with a medication bag to help them remember the importance of bringing their medication to every office visit. Other students have provided diabetes self-management education through individual and group education delivered via telehealth. These focused projects directly benefit patients and clinical outcomes. Student work and clinic support of their work has become an integral part of the identity of ACHN to the point where when students are not in the clinic during semester breaks, patients ask if the students are coming back!

ACHN has had many challenges over the past 5 years, including creating a strategic plan, creating a business plan, fundraising, and creating community partnerships and support. There have been a number of successes along the way also (Table 1-1). In the past 4 years, we have increased the number of hours the clinic is open each week from 3 hours on Saturday, to a total of 20 hours per week over 4 days. We have also received 4 telehealth grants. One of these grants was obtained through an academic-community partnership, 2 were from our local nurse practitioner organization, and 1 through a state-funded pilot program. In addition, ACHN has agreements with multiple universities to precept health care students as previously described. We have successfully increased our volunteer network. Many of our volunteers are college students and recent college graduates who plan to pursue a career in health care and spend time volunteering with us to gain some experience before applying to graduate programs. Other volunteers have been APRNs, physician assistants, and physicians who are new to the area and volunteer with us while they seek paid employment. ACHN also has a partnership with a local laboratory for low-cost labs. While we cannot order anything possible, the majority of the labs we need to order are significantly cheaper for our patients than if they paid the cash-pay rate at a private clinic. A local nonprofit collaborative pharmacy offers low-cost, chronic disease and life-saving medications for our patients and processes some of the patient assistance program

applications for our patients. These community partners and volunteers are the key to providing the health care services and care navigation our patients need.

Over the past few years, we have welcomed a number of other volunteer providers. Our volunteer physicians offer specialty care either at ACHN or in their private practice settings at no cost for the first visit. Pain management provided by an anesthesiologist who comes to ACHN once a month has been particularly beneficial to many of our patients who suffer from chronic pain. His interventions include joint injections and acupuncture rather than pills and patches. A retired gastroenterologist has also offered his services once per week at ACHN for the past few years. Many of our patients present with symptoms of reflux, constipation, diarrhea, and abdominal pain and meet criteria for gastroesophageal reflux disease and irritable bowel syndrome. Our gastroenterologist's expertise has assisted us in navigating patients into the most appropriate diagnostic evaluations, treatment, and follow-up care. We have additional volunteer physicians and a physician's assistant who volunteer regularly, often staffing the patient appointment slots on Saturday mornings.

Other volunteers provide specialty care off-site for our patients who need cardiology, dermatology, sleep medicine, otolaryngology, and allergy/asthma care. A local hospital provides a mobile mammography unit every other month. The *Mammovan* provides screening mammography for asymptomatic patients with no prior history of breast cancer. There is no charge for patients who are uninsured and meet the income criteria. Another local hospital provided a tablet we can use for some language translation for a year.

ACHN is in the Washington, DC metro area and the National Institutes of Health (NIH) is less than an hour's drive from the clinic. The NIH National Institute of Diabetes and Digestive and Kidney Diseases (NIDDK) provides esophagogastroduodenoscopies (EGDs) and colonoscopies for our patients for either screening or diagnostic purposes. Over the years, they have successfully removed polyps from many of our patients, diagnosed early stage colon cancer, and diagnosed and treated multiple cases of *Helicobacter pylori*- and other infections.

For the past 2 years, we have been able to offer free influenza vaccines that are provided through the state association for free and charitable clinics. These are the only immunizations we offer at ACHN. All other routine immunizations are available through the local health departments for a fee. While ACHN is able to offer gynecology exams, the cost of a Pap smear is prohibitive for most of our patients. One of the local hospital systems has a monthly subscription program for basic primary care services. Through this program, our patients may have a Pap smear for the $40 monthly fee that also covers office visits, basic labs, and Pap smear. Our laboratory fee for a Pap smear is almost double that cost. Free clinics often have a policy that patients must choose one clinic in which to receive services. This hospital-based program is not a free clinic and is available to anyone in the community, not only to uninsured individuals.

**Table 1-1**

## STRENGTHS, WEAKNESSES, OPPORTUNITIES, THREATS ANALYSIS

| STRENGTHS | WEAKNESSES |
|---|---|
| • Students (interprofessional care) | • Lack of effective communication channels |
| • Programs (eg, DEEEP impact, hotspotting,* medication reconciliation) | • Lack of outreach to local community (non-Muslims; non-immigrants) |
| • Amazing patients | • Lack of volunteers (weekdays) |
| • Low-cost clinic space | • Marketing challenges |
| • Coordination of care/care navigation | • Lack of partnerships with health systems |
| • Outcomes research | • Lack of partnerships with hospitals |
| • Screening for social determinants of health | • Lack of collaboration with other free clinics |
| | • No free labs or imaging |
| **OPPORTUNITIES** | **THREATS** |
| • Encourage community partners | • Lack of strategic plan |
| • Academic-community partnerships | • Lack of consistent leadership |
| • Increase volunteers | • Lack of stable funding strategy |
| • Grant funding | |

Abbreviation: DEEEP Impact = diabetes education exercise eating plan
*Identifying high-risk patients to provide high-touch interventions

# A POSITIVE RETURN ON INVESTMENT: DNP IMPACT

When I was hired, there was no business plan for the clinic. The clinic was started by a small group of community members and the local mosque provided space for the clinic in a business park. The founders were clear that their mission was to ensure every uninsured, low-income individual had access to primary care and preventative services. Unlike most free clinics, we provide care regardless of county and state lines. When ACHN started, patients were only seen on Saturdays for 3 hours. After I was hired, patients were seen on 3 additional days for a total of 20 hours per week. We currently have almost 1000 active patients with 61% female and 39% male. The majority of our patients are more than 50 years of age and live with at least 1 chronic disease.

When the clinic started, equipment and supplies, including exam tables, were donated by a local physician who was closing her practice and by other practices who had extra supplies they were willing to donate as they updated their equipment. Additional funding came from a donor who provided capital funds that covered most of the expenses for the first 3 years. The space where the clinic started is still used today. There have been a few updates such as a bathroom just for the clinic, instead of having to share the mosque's bathroom, and a multipurpose room that we use for lunch, conversation, learning, and student charting space. After I was hired, I created a business plan and forwarded it to the Board of Directors (BOD). The business plan provides the framework for our day-to-day operations (Appendix A).

In the past 5 years, ACHN has provided more than $1.5 million in direct goods and services and cared for more than 2000 unique patients. This cost of care does not include the physical space the clinic occupies, which is provided for a very low rental fee of $1 per month. It also does not include the value of the student or volunteer hours providing direct and indirect services that facilitate the care patients receive. Services included in this cost of care are: primary care visits, low cost laboratory studies, low cost medications provided through a pharmacy partnership, free mammograms provided by the local *Mammovan*, an on-site eye clinic that was operating once a month, telehealth visits, and specialty care visits with volunteer providers. The free and low-cost services ACHN provides for uninsured individuals, with significant help from students and volunteers as well as our community partners, alleviates the burden of disease and potential worsening outcomes related to lack of access to adequate primary health care.

# EVIDENCE-BASED PRACTICE

At ACHN clinic, we follow the most recent guidelines and recommendations for screening, diagnosis, and treatment of hypertension, hyperlipidemia, diabetes, and other conditions as well as primary prevention screening and interventions. When students start their rotation at the clinic, they are provided with a new student packet that includes what is expected of them while they are in the clinic, a list of resources available at the clinic, smart phone based applications I use for clinical decision making, a student information form, and a requirement to complete at least 1 module of Smiles for Life.[4] This last requirement is particularly important as many of our patients have never had any oral health care services and have very poor dentition and oral health. I expect my students to know and use the evidence-based guidelines when creating a treatment plan to offer patients. I also expect them to use clinical judgement and partner with patients to provide evidence-based care that is accessible and affordable. This means that when a lower cost medication is available with similar efficacy, we choose that medication. When a patient needs diagnostic studies, we help them to find the lowest cost option. If a patient is food insecure or lacks adequate housing, we help find resources to meet those needs.

Focusing on the social determinants of health that support patients' basic needs is part of holistic health care. Our intake form asks questions about the living situation, marital status, preferred language, education level, abuse history, substance use, depression screen, and family history. The registration form contains information about their economic status, family size, resident status, and employment. During the first office visit, we review the initial history form with each patient and ask about their ability to afford a safe place to live, access to food, if they are job seeking, and we again ask about personal safety and substance use. With the patient's permission, the students and I help find the resources a patient needs. With the addition of our social worker, she has taken on many of these linkages to care, but the students also learn about the complexity of navigating the system. The social worker also helps patients apply for Supplemental Nutrition Assistance Program (SNAP) benefits, Medicaid, Medicare, or private insurance if they are eligible. With the recent announcement of the public charge rule by the presidents' administration, many of our patients have been afraid to apply for some of these programs as they believe it will prevent them from qualifying for a green card and eventually citizenship. When patients have adequate housing and food, they are able to engage in treatment plans such as improved diabetes self-management. Without stable housing, access to food, or fear for their personal safety, engaging in healthy behaviors to support improved health goals is not possible.

Creating an interdisciplinary team of students each semester takes time and creativity. I usually interview students before I accept them in the clinic to ensure they have a good understanding of the patient population, the model we use to care for patients, and the time we take to provide holistic care. There are some students who do not have an interest in working with this population, working in a free clinic, or taking a holistic view of health care. However, the student workforce that has worked with us has brought new insight and ideas to ACHN as we work to improve patient outcomes. Student DNP projects are theory- and evidence-based and translate evidence into a unique practice setting with varying success. Part of the DNP project requires identifying a gap in care and designing an intervention to fill that gap. As some students have learned, the most thoughtfully designed interventions are sometimes not well received because of other barriers such as time, distance to travel, or language barriers. The more successful student projects have considered how to reduce or mitigate these barriers.

As a primary care clinician, recognizing the need for preventive services and the lack of comprehensive primary care services available to this population has driven creative programs and partnerships. One of the challenges in providing primary care to an uninsured population that is also a largely immigrant population, is the inability to provide all recommended preventive services such as cervical and breast cancer screenings, colonoscopies, diabetic retinopathy exams, and recommended immunizations. I have a professional responsibility to my patients to offer evidence-based care and services to improve health outcomes. However, individuals are not always ready or willing to accept the offered intervention particularly if it is unaffordable and therefore unattainable. For example, for a woman who is 65 years old, normal weight, a non-smoker, sexually active, and has no significant personal or family history, the United States Preventive Services Taskforce (USPSTF) recommends she have cervical cancer screening, colorectal cancer screening, breast cancer screening, hypertension screening, and depression screening.[5] Many of my patients have never had a health care visit that most patients and providers in the United States would consider a "wellness" exam focused on primary prevention strategies. Therefore, when recommending a pelvic exam, colonoscopy, or mammogram, some patients do not understand the purpose of screening for potential conditions when they "feel fine." In my experience with this particular population, a number of individuals have witnessed family members die from cancer or other preventable or treatable conditions because there were no available or affordable treatment options in their countries of origin and do not realize that screening can help detect problems such as cancer before symptoms start. Part of our patient education includes discussions of what screenings are available, to whom, and why these are recommended at various ages. Additionally, many patients are not able to afford the cost of receiving these recommended screenings and immunizations and are ineligible for programs aimed at uninsured individuals because they are not US citizens. Consequently, the disease burden and the burden of treatment is high in this population.

Disease burden is the impact of disease on an individual measured in disability adjusted life years, quality of life years, and health adjusted life years.[6] In a recent publication from Kaiser Permanente that compares the impact of social determinants of health on health care outcomes in the United States and 11 other comparable countries, the United States has poor outcomes. In this study, the United States has the lowest rate of individuals who are insured and those who are uninsured are more likely to forego medical treatment because of cost. Additionally, the incidence of obesity is higher among individuals who are low income. By definition this includes individuals who live below 400% of the federal poverty limit.[7]

The United States spends almost twice as much per person as 10 other high-income countries and our life expectancy is the lowest.[8] Primary prevention strategies cost considerably less than secondary and tertiary prevention and improve individual patient outcomes by preventing disease or mitigating the burden of disease. At ACHN, we focus on primary prevention and offer secondary and tertiary prevention when needed. Because we are not limited by insurance reimbursement rules, we are able to create and test new models of care to provide interventions that improve patient outcomes.

# EVIDENCE INTO PRACTICE: TELEHEALTH

Telehealth is a tool that we use to connect with patients and to connect patients to care. In 2016, I was asked by my colleagues at Old Dominion University, where I am adjunct faculty, if I would like to participate in a telehealth program. APN-PLACE was a grant-funded program created to support a preceptor telehealth education program, facilitate student preceptor placement, and to connect faculty to students at their clinical sites.[9] Through this program, ACHN received a telehealth cart with peripherals including: electronic stethoscope, otoscope, and dermoscope. As a preceptor, I received access to training modules focused on precepting and telehealth.

In 2017, we were able to start an on-site eye clinic, staffed by a volunteer optometrist, to screen patients for eye disease such as retinopathy from diabetes and hypertension. Offering screening for eye diseases in the clinic reduced the number of referrals we needed to make to outside providers for screening, reduced the cost to patients, and helped us triage those who needed urgent referrals vs systematic screening. Unfortunately, our optometrist left the area to attend medical school to become an ophthalmologist. Therefore, we needed a new solution. As adjunct faculty at Old Dominion University, I heard a DNP presentation by a student whose project focused on screening for retinopathy using a new device called D-EYE (www.d-eyecare.com). This device

was created for providers to be able to complete a screening ophthalmologic exam in the primary care or emergency care settings. This low-cost solution includes an attachment for an iPhone (Apple) that allows the provider to examine the un-dilated eye and take photographs or a video of the exam. For this solution, I applied for and received a small grant from our regional nurse practitioner organization. This allowed me to purchase the product and a used iPhone so we can evaluate the use of this device in this particular setting. One of our ophthalmology volunteers will be available to review images that are stored and forwarded through a Health Information Technology for Economic and Clinical Health (HITECH) and Health Insurance Portability and Accountability Act (HIPAA) compliant application and to help with triage and follow up as needed.

Another telehealth program we have is called *hotspotting*. This program was based on the Camden Coalition model of targeting the highest-risk patients to provide high-touch interventions with a goal of improving outcomes.[10] This is a home-visit model that we have adapted to provide improved access to care for patients who have transportation challenges. We can send a student dyad to the patient's home with a rolling bag that contains a laptop computer, wireless printer, telehealth peripherals, blood pressure cuff, scale, pulse oximeter, and thermometer. The students are able to complete the history and pertinent physical exam in the patient's home and then use the telehealth platform to connect with me at the clinic. If needed, the peripherals, a dermoscope, electronic stethoscope, and otoscope can be attached to the computer so I can visualize or hear the pertinent exam. I am also able to conduct a virtual visit with the patient and order labs, other diagnostics, and medications as needed. We can also bring in an interpreter via telehealth if needed. This model is used only for established patients who live less than 30 minutes from the clinic.

Through my health policy advocacy work, I have been part of our state nurse practitioner organization and have advocated for removal of restrictions to nurse practitioner practice. In 2016, a bill was introduced in Virginia that would have removed many of the barriers to autonomous practice for nurse practitioners. However, it was substituted at the last moment and the bill that was passed provided funding for a pilot study. The reasoning for the substitute submitted by organized medicine, was that nurse practitioners have repeatedly made the argument that it is often hard to find a collaborating physician if you are not part of a large medical group or hospital system. Organized medicine's proposal was to create a pilot project, funded by taxpayers, that would help to connect nurse practitioners who needed a collaborating physician with physicians who were willing to enter into a collaborative agreement with a nurse practitioner. There was no funding provided to pay these collaborating physicians. However, $390 000 in funding was made available over a 2-year period to provide telehealth equipment and training for interested nurse practitioners and physicians so they could establish collaborative partnerships.[11] I volunteered

ACHN as a participating site. We already had the necessary equipment, a laptop with video-teleconferencing capabilities, but we needed a telehealth platform to connect with patients and the pilot program provided access to the telehealth platform. I also volunteered to be on the data subcommittee to help evaluate how this program was working. Over the past 3 years, we have been working to accrue participating providers and health care sites, collect data, and evaluate the outcomes. The final report was due to the Virginia General Assembly in the Fall of 2019.

# EVIDENCE BASED PRACTICE: ANALYSIS OF GAPS IN CARE

Our gap in care continues to be mental and behavioral health care. Although we screen for depression and substance use, we struggle to find appropriate psychotherapy resources or care for those with serious mental illness who need care that is outside the scope of primary care. Local mental health resources are already under-resourced and wait times can be long unless the patient is in crisis. Some of the community-based services are not available to those who are not US residents. For those patients living with serious mental illness or who have moderate to severe depression or anxiety, we do have a community walk-in screening option close to the clinic where we refer patients for non-emergent psychiatric evaluations.

Additional gaps in care are identified through social determinants of health screening. For example, a patient living with diabetes who has trouble making rent payments and buying adequate food is not able to adequately focus on diabetes self-management through regular blood glucose monitoring, eating a diet rich in vegetables and lean proteins, and exercising daily. Diabetes is a disease with long-term consequences. Lack of housing and food are immediate needs that must be addressed. Therefore, we spend time and resources (often using our social worker, students, or volunteers) to help navigate patients through the confusing system of social services. However, as many of our patients are immigrants and refugees, many of the services are not available to them. Over the years, we have identified other nonprofit agencies, such as our clinic, who do not use government resources and therefore do not have the same residency or citizenship requirements. The current administration has repeatedly stated it will deny a path to citizenship for those who have ever used any public welfare programs. This proposed policy enforcement creates a fear among our patients that if they use services available to them, they will lose their ability to become US citizens. This further reduces access to care for the most vulnerable in our communities who are trying to start a new life in a country that purports to offer opportunities and safety.

# MINING AND INFORMATION TECHNOLOGY TO IMPROVE HEALTH CARE

The most important tool for data mining is to have a functional electronic health record (EHR) with these capabilities. As a free clinic, we use Athena Health that offers a free version for free clinics. This means some of the functionality of the full-priced version is not available to us, but data-mining capabilities are available. Using the EHR, we can run reports to evaluate our current active patient population, see how many people we have with different diagnoses, what medications are prescribed, lab analyte values, etc. This also allows us to create a patient care registry. A patient care registry is a valuable tool for monitoring the health of the population and identifying patients who may need a change in interventions and an updated care plan. Patient registries have been used in many forms as a population health tool to evaluate patient outcomes or track disease progression or for quality improvement.[3] For the past 2 years, we have had a patient care registry that is updated quarterly.

Using the registry, currently an Excel spreadsheet, we can sort patient data, run detailed analyses of patient outcomes and the trajectory of their disease, and target those patients whose diseases are uncontrolled. For example, instead of looking at each patient's EHR record individually, I can look at our population overall and also look at each patient's care over time to screen for rising hemoglobin A1c values, for example. Using the registry, a group of patients who are identified as having uncontrolled diabetes, for example, can then be offered telehealth appointments or home visits for high-touch care with a goal of reducing their A1cs and their disease burden. Of note, a fully functioning EHR may have this population health capability without the added burden of downloading individual data to a spreadsheet to evaluate outside of the EHR. We store the reports in a HIPAA compliant and password protected database. The database was created by me and DNP, MPH, and community health students who have helped with updating the database regularly. As with other clinical activities and interventions, students are a valuable part of our clinical and administrative team.

# INTERDISCIPLINARY COLLABORATION

The consistent care team includes the primary care provider (me), the administrative assistant, the manager, and the social worker. The administrative assistant, who is a physician from Ethiopia and provides Amharic translation, is responsible for the daily clinic function including patient registration, appointment scheduling, check-in and check-out, telephone calls, and all patient-related documents that come into the clinic. Check-out includes discharge instructions, including referral information for our specialty providers and local resource information for low-cost services for dental care, labs, and radiology. The manager, who is a physician from Pakistan, also helps with Urdu translation, patient eligibility/registration, care navigation, and establishing community partnerships in addition to fundraising and communication with the board. He is also responsible for the daily clinic management including bills and reports, coordinating volunteers, and other administrative tasks. The medical social worker is our newest employee. She was a former student who is now employed with us and provides the majority of care navigation, help with accessing food, housing, social services, and other resources that support our patients' needs to optimize their health and wellness. Our social worker also provides Spanish language translation as needed and attends local social services conferences and meetings as ACHN's representative. She is an Army veteran who has experience working with veterans who have returned from recent military deployments and are living with mental health needs. In some respects, many of the psychosocial issues our military veterans have are similar to the needs of our patient population at ACHN who largely come from Iraq, Afghanistan, Somalia, Nigeria, Syria, and other countries where our military have been in the past 2 decades.

During the semesters, we have an array of interdisciplinary students, many of whom are also immigrants or first-generation US citizens, who provide constant collaboration opportunities with the volunteer providers, staff, and with each other. Some of our students also provide translation services for additional languages. Many of our students have worked in other fields before nursing and bring their knowledge and experience from these disciplines into their work with us as well such as information technology, nutrition sciences, or grant writing. Students and volunteers are screened and interviewed before we accept them into our team. We try to ensure the mix of students and volunteers will meet their education and professional objectives but also the needs of the clinic. This also provides an extra level of assurance that we have individuals who are passionate about caring for this particular population in a thoughtful, effective, and compassionate manner.

Interprofessional collaboration is not always easy. One of the secrets to creating effective interprofessional teams is to have open and honest communication. At ACHN, we have signs on each exam room door with the name of the licensed provider who is using that room. There is one exam room I use consistently, but our volunteers sometimes use it or one of the other exam rooms when they are in clinic and their title and name is put on the door. When I started at the clinic and my name was put on the exam room door as Dr. Rebecca Bates, Nurse Practitioner, one of the ACHN board members complained that I was calling myself "Doctor." This was an opportunity to educate the BOD about what a DNP degree means and the fact that the holder of any earned doctorate may use the title, "Doctor." Once this information was clearly conveyed, no one else has challenged the use of my earned academic degree title. I am careful to refer to my colleagues by their professional designations when talking about them as well. For example, I will say "my physician colleague" or "my public health colleague" to be clear about each of our roles.

We also have collaborations with our specialty and community partners. On a daily basis, we send and receive information about patient care, community events, collaboration opportunities, and funding opportunities. The DNP degree is an asset to interprofessional collaboration as I now have a language, knowledge, and experience outside of nursing and health care to effectively communicate with patients and colleagues who have a different background. For example, when talking with a potential community partner about starting a satellite site, I am able to discuss external assessments, gap analyses, return on investment, data analysis, organizational leadership, health policy and advocacy, in addition to translational research, clinical practice, and population health. The skill set I developed through the DNP education and the experiential learning required to achieve competency in each of the 8 Essentials has been an asset to my current role at ACHN. The clinic has benefitted from having a DNP-educated nurse practitioner. I not only focus on the direct patient care but I also understand the importance of creating a health care environment that meets the needs of our patients and our staff. I have the tools and skills to create a new model of care that is safe, effective, and improves patient outcomes.

## PROFESSIONAL LEADERSHIP

The DNP degree provided me with the knowledge and skills necessary to be a leader. My leadership journey has taken various forms over the years. Beginning with the health policy fellowship, I realized one of the most impactful activities we can do for our patients and our profession is to be active in health policy advocacy. When I moved to Virginia, I joined our state nurse practitioner organization and started attending our regional meetings. During my DNP education I volunteered to be part of the government relations (GR) committee and helped organize the annual nurses' legislative reception. Eventually, I was asked to co-chair the GR committee. This organization provided opportunities to work with our state organization on policy issues such as full practice authority for nurse practitioners. As the years progressed, various bills were introduced and shepherded through the legislative process with varying degrees of success.

As I learned more about the political process in Virginia, I offered to lecture at various universities about health policy advocacy. I believe this is part of my professional duty to help nurses at all levels learn how the legislative process works and how to be an effective advocate. Our local nurse practitioner group organizes a nurses legislative reception each October.

We invite all nursing organizations to participate in the reception. Invitations go to all state legislators and candidates for our region as well as to students and faculty from the local university nursing programs. There are many local, state, and national opportunities for nurses to get a "seat at the table" and most of the time, simply volunteering for an open position is all that is required. When we use our collective voice to actively advocate for nurses to practice to the full extent of their education and training, our profession and our patients benefit. A colleague once said to me that nursing abdicated control of our profession to physicians many decades ago. Since then, we have struggled to regain control of the nursing profession by being able to practice with autonomy and to the fullest extent of our education and training.

My journey has led me to be elected as the regional president of the state nurse practitioner organization. Stepping into a leadership role in my profession has allowed me to challenge the status quo of our organization. We have since continued to move forward in promoting nurse practitioners as safe and effective practitioners of evidence-based care in our region. Our members are doing amazing things such as starting their own practices, leading practice change efforts in private practices and hospital systems, and creating new models of care that improve patient outcomes. The more we can highlight these professional opportunities, our students, colleagues, and other professions will begin to see the value of the DNP degree. This degree is relatively new. Those of us who were early adopters have a responsibility to demonstrate the impact we have had and will have on improving access to care, decreasing the cost of care, and improving patient outcomes.

As an educator, I have held adjunct faculty positions at various universities. Part of my professional obligation is to encourage students to pursue the DNP degree as a terminal degree. Achieving a terminal degree in any profession demonstrates a commitment to the profession and a level of knowledge mastery that elevates DNP-prepared nurses to the same level as other health professions that require a doctorate-level degree for entry into practice. The education and experiential learning gained through completing a DNP degree significantly improves our ability to be professional leaders who can change the health care trajectory through data and evidence-driven innovation. Helping students realize their passion and potential to be health care leaders is a rewarding process. Students often start their DNP journey with a goal of simply earning a terminal degree. Many are not aware that course requirements and experiences are a transformative process. They way DNPs think about health care, patient outcomes, policy, health systems, and collaboration, fundamentally alters our approach to working with individuals, families, and communities.

Precepting interdisciplinary students at the ACHN clinic creates an interprofessional opportunity for students to learn about each other's profession and to be able to articulate their own. For example, a public health nurse and a community health nurse have different roles. However, many students assume these are the same. While there is some overlap in roles they can fill, the education is different. An MPH student does not necessarily have experience working directly with patients. Including an MPH student as part of the clinic team has expanded the understanding of population health in our setting and allowed us to better understand some of the drivers of health and barriers to health in our population. These experiences and discussions have also helped our students and staff better understand the need for health policy advocacy to help improve the outcomes of our patients. For example, many of our patients are foreign born. Many have come from countries where infectious diseases such as diarrheal illness, pneumonia, polio, and measles continue to affect the families of these patients. Policy opportunities such as joining the United Nations Foundation Shot @ Life advocacy initiative is a powerful way for students to learn how to advocate for childhood immunizations in developing countries. The impact of improved immunization rates in the communities from which our patients come will have a positive effect on the health of the next generation.

Leadership also means sharing professional development and project outcomes so others can benefit from that knowledge. As part of this professional responsibility, I regularly submit abstracts for state, national, and international conferences. The innovations we have piloted and evaluated at the ACHN clinic have been well-received at all levels. Colleagues and students are able to learn about our creative approach to patient care and consider what elements or lessons they can take back to their practices. Sometimes, just sharing what you are doing even if you do not think it is innovative or remarkable is enough to generate conversation and to spark an idea for someone else.

One of the leadership opportunities that arose near the end of my DNP program was the opportunity to create a new state organization. The Virginia Association of Doctors of Nursing Practice (VADNP) was started by a small group of us in 2015 about 2 months after we graduated from Old Dominion University.[12] In the first year, our group of newly minted DNPs plus 2 of our former professors, created a state organization and organized and held our first conference. For the past 4 years, I have been the secretary of the VADNP. We recently concluded our fourth annual conference. The challenges and barriers we have encountered in this all volunteer organization over the past few years have been mitigated by the power of bringing together DNP students, faculty, and graduates from all over the state. We have had the opportunity to start new collaborations, share ideas and research, and to support each other as we start new jobs and implement new programs. When we started the organization, we used all of the knowledge and skills we learned through our DNP program to essentially start a new business and to successfully launch it. We did not do this in isolation although we were one of the first state DNP organizations in the country. When we started considering what our organization would look like, we consulted with Dr. David O'Dell who was a founding organizer of the Doctors of Nursing

Practice, the national DNP organization that holds a conference every year (https://www.doctorsofnursingpractice.org). The opportunity we had to start a new organization right after graduation required that we use all of our new knowledge and skills based in the DNP Essentials.

# DNP DEGREE: A TRANSFORMATIVE JOURNEY

One of my lessons learned as I transformed into a DNP is that understanding the DNP Essentials and being able to speak to my competency in each of these areas has helped me find new opportunities. For example, in addition to my work with the ACHN clinic, I also became a project manager for 2 federally funded grants. I had never considered what additional roles may be available to me outside of clinical care, even after completing my DNP degree. However, after working at the ACHN clinic and another free clinic where I provided primary care services for uninsured patients who accessed services for people living with substance use and or serious mental illness, I was asked to become project manager for a grant focused on collaborative care.[13]

In this role, I oversee the implementation of this well-established model at 5 different clinical locations, collect data, work with our evaluator to analyze the data, help write reports for the funding agency, and disseminate our findings through conferences and journal articles. This has been a truly enlightening experience to see how different clinics work, consider the workflow of each clinic and how this grant can be implemented in so many different settings, and learn more about the interprofessional collaboration required in each setting.

Recently, I was asked to become project manager for another large federally funded project working on primary, secondary, and tertiary prevention of adverse childhood events and opioid use and to mitigate the impacts of substance use on children, families, and the community. This initiative brings together multiple stakeholders to focus on not only treatment and prevention of opioid use as we currently think of these strategies, but also to consider the social determinants of health that create an environment where drug use thrives. The DNP Essentials along with additional experiences after graduation have provided me with the skills and knowledge needed to be able to oversee a complex community system change. The project management domains include initiation, planning, executing, monitoring and controlling, and closing.[14] Each of these domains and associated tasks closely mirror the nursing process. The DNP Essentials, especially organizational leadership, information systems, and interprofessional collaboration, provided a solid foundation for the complexity required for this work.

As described above, being able to clearly articulate how the DNP degree has equipped me to be, not only a health care leader, but an excellent clinician with additional knowledge and skills to impact individual, family, and population health has moved my career forward. I am in a unique position as a project manager and a clinician to understand the challenges, barriers, and needs of various stakeholders as well as the considerations of running a business with a focus on return on investment.

The journey to completing the DNP degree was challenging, especially while working full-time and raising an active family. I had the full support of my husband and 4 children as I started the program and despite the workload, long hours, adding on the health policy fellowship, and consideration of multiple scheduling challenges, I was able to graduate on time. However, I fully acknowledge that the sacrifices and support provided by my family and extended network helped me achieve this goal. As someone who is an introvert, I never considered that I would find a passion in working in the health policy arena as an advocate. I have worked with my state organization to prepare testimony for the state legislature and participated in multiple meetings with state senators and representatives to advocate for reducing restrictions on nurse practitioner practice. Being able to use my advocacy skills to talk with legislators and other stakeholders about the need for full practice authority for nurse practitioners or to advocate for lower prescription drug prices for my patients has been a huge learning curve, but it has also been worth the considerable effort as the long-term outcomes from this advocacy will impact health care outcomes.

My long-term plan never included becoming a leader in a professional organization or starting a new organization. Both have happened in the past few years and I attribute much of this to the foundation laid during my DNP program. The professional and personal networks that grew out of my DNP program experiences have continued to support my growth as a health care leader and change agent. As I focus my efforts on continuing to improve health outcomes for my patients, precepting and mentoring students and colleagues, and advocating for my patients and my profession, I know my work will leave a lasting legacy.

# CONCLUSION: IMPACT OF THE DNP DEGREE

As a result of obtaining my DNP degree, I have had many opportunities to work in areas I had not previously considered as a family nurse practitioner. The DNP has also become a conversation starter. As it is a relatively new degree, many people do not know the essential elements and competencies that must be demonstrated to earn the DNP. Embracing the DNP Essentials and being able to articulate how each of these Essentials makes me a better practitioner, researcher, manager, or educator has led to many more opportunities.

As a job candidate for the FNP position at ACHN, I talked about the DNP Essentials and how my knowledge and experience was not limited to clinical care. Working with vulnerable populations requires use of all of the Essentials on a daily basis to ensure the care offered is necessary, cost-effective, evidence-based, culturally appropriate, and timely. It is necessary to have a clear understanding of population health prevention practices and the use of innovative models of care to adequately address the needs of patients who have limited resources.

When I started the DNP journey I planned to earn the terminal degree in my profession. I was not prepared to graduate with a new appreciation for my profession, a new way of understanding problems in health care, and a robust toolkit of knowledge, resources, and experiences. The DNP toolkit has been invaluable as I embark upon new endeavors. It has changed how I approach health care, how I teach my students to offer high-quality, cost-effective care, and how I actively seek out interdisciplinary partners to improve health care delivery. The DNP-prepared nurse is ready to challenge the status quo in health care.

## ACKNOWLEDGMENTS

I want to thank the DNP faculty of Old Dominion University for instilling a deep knowledge and understanding of the DNP Essentials and for introducing me to telehealth: Drs. Carolyn Rutledge, Deborah Gray, Tina Gustin, Kathy Zimbro, and Dawn Adams. You pushed me to expand my comfort zone and to seek out experiences that allowed me to operationalize the Essentials and imagine new models of health care.

ACHN allowed me to share my knowledge and experiences with a wide variety of students and colleagues as we provided high-quality, evidence-based, cost-effective care for this vulnerable population. The ability to try new models of care and implement continuous quality improvement measures in a timely fashion was possible because of the synergistic relationship of our small but brilliant staff. Thank you Nabeel Hasan, Neima Surur, and Patricia Rhodes.

Finally, thank you to my husband, Chad, and my children, Caleb, Eliza, Silas, and Naomi, for supporting me through the DNP journey and for picking up the slack as I completed my coursework and practicum hours. You made this possible. I love you all.

## REFERENCES

1. Informational tools. National Association of Free & Charitable Clinics. https://www.nafcclinics.org/advocacy/tools

2. The essentials of doctoral education for advanced nursing practice. American Association of Colleges of Nursing. October 2006. https://www.aacnnursing.org/Portals/42/Publications/DNP Essentials.pdf

3. Gliklich RE, Dreyer NA, Leavy MB, Agency for Healthcare Research and Quality. Registries for evaluating patient outcomes: a user's guide. April 2014. Accessed September 4, 2019. https://www.ncbi.nlm.nih.gov/books/NBK208643/

4. Smiles for life: A national oral health curriculum. Smiles for Life. Accessed September 20, 2019. https://smilesforlifeoralhealth.org/buildcontent.aspx?tut=555&pagekey=62948&cbreceipt=0

5. Agency for Health Care Research and Quality. Electronic preventive services selector (ePSS). US Preventive Services Task Force. Accessed August 31, 2019. https://epss.ahrq.gov/ePSS/GetResults.do?method=search

6. More than just numbers: exploring the concept of burden of disease. National Collaborating Centre for Infectious Diseases. January 2016. https://nccid.ca/publications/exploring-the-concept-of-burden-of-disease/

7. Kamal R, Cox C, Blumenkranz E. What do we know about social determinants of health in the US and comparable countries? Peterson Center on Healthcare. November 2017. https://www.healthsystemtracker.org/chart-collection/know-social-determinants-health-u-s-comparable-countries/

8. Papanicolas I, Woskie LR, Jha AK. Health care spending in the united states and other high-income countries. *JAMA.* 2018;319(10):1024. doi:10.1001/jama.2018.1150

9. APN Place. Accessed September 20, 2019. https://www.apnplace.org/index.php

10. About. Camden Coalition of Healthcare Providers. Accessed September 20, 2019. https://www.camdenhealth.org/about/

11. 2016 uncodified acts. LIS. Accessed September 20, 2019. https://law.lis.virginia.gov/uncodifiedacts/2016/session1/chapter763/

12. Virginia association of doctors of nursing practice. EPN Network. Accessed September 20, 2019. https://vadnp.enpnetwork.com/

13. Collaborative care. AIMS Center. Accessed September 15, 2019. https://aims.uw.edu/collaborative-care

14. Project management professional: examination content outline. Project Management Institute. June 2015. https://www.pmi.org/-/media/pmi/documents/public/pdf/certifications/project-management-professional-exam-outline.pdf

# Appendix A
## Business Plan

## Executive Summary

Patients are at the center of everything we do. We know that chronic diseases are the most costly and preventable health problems in the United States today. The majority of all adults in the United States have 1 or more chronic diseases, and 80% of health care dollars are spent on chronic disease management for these individuals.[1] Cardiovascular disease, cancer, diabetes, obesity, arthritis, and asthma cost more than $1 trillion annually. The patients who access services have lived with undiagnosed or untreated chronic diseases for years. They may be from different cultures and have literacy and language barriers. Vulnerable populations that comprise 5% of our population utilize 50% of our health care expenditures.[2] Our patients are part of this vulnerable population and many live with chronic diseases that have been poorly managed. Disease progression occurs when patients lack education, resources, and empowerment to self-manage a chronic disease.[3]

This business proposal for improved care addresses these issues. These proposed changes will offer our patients an improved health care experience designed to help them optimize their health. The efforts to provide improved care coordination and collaboration through interprofessional and community partnerships will improve outcomes for our patients, improve their patient experience, and keep costs down for both the clinic and our community. This focus will also make us more competitive for grant funding and ensure our community partners that we have a legitimate and evidence-based practice that provides high-quality, cost-effective care for vulnerable populations.[4]

This small free clinic can provide a unique offering to improve health outcomes for our vulnerable patients (see Table 1-1 for SWOT analysis). The clinic can be a leader in innovative health care delivery by providing integrated and coordinated interprofessional care through maximizing our academic and community partnerships.

## Mission/Vision Statement

- Mission statement: Our mission is to ensure every uninsured, low-income individual has access to primary care and preventative services.
- Vision statement: The clinic envisions itself as a part of larger network of institutions addressing the health and

well-being of underserved and indigent individuals. It will cultivate a network of collaborative relationships with individuals and organizations in the community for the purpose of providing comprehensive health care.

## Background Information

We have the resources to offer coordinated care for our patients. With the chronic disease epidemic in the United States, the clinic can directly improve outcomes of our patients through improved coordination of care with our academic and community partners.

## Objectives

1. Survey 50 patients about current visits (patient satisfaction surveys).
2. Create a strategic plan for the clinic.
3. Present the business plan to the BOD.

## Capital Requirements

Capital requirements include office space rental, office supplies, and advertising. Clinic rental includes all utilities, telephone, and wireless internet service. Office supplies are budgeted per quarter. This includes printer paper, ink, and other office supplies such as pens, pads of paper, and staples.

Revenue will be generated from yearly fundraisers. Monthly donations are also sought. Community grants may be additional sources of revenue. Marketing efforts are also planned to raise funds for the clinic.

## Management Team

Our volunteer BOD and Executive Director need to be actively engaged in the clinic through helping to create these partnerships, attending meetings with the state association of free and charitable clinics and community partners, and exploring new funding mechanisms. The clinic staff must have input into the strategic plan and policies and procedures as this team has direct patient contact every day.

## Strategy

The clinic has the potential to leverage the knowledge, skills, and abilities of volunteers and students who rotate through the clinic to provide high-quality, cost-effective, evidence-based health care services. The students provide hours of service through direct patient care, care navigation, support for health fairs and other outreach programs. We need

to continue to intentionally include students and volunteers, including providers, and to recognize their significant contribution to the provision of care at the clinic. This needs to be undertaken in a systematic and thoughtful manner. A well, thought-out strategic plan will optimize our patient outcomes, increase patient satisfaction, keep costs lower, and foster our relationships with our student, volunteers, and community partners.

## Key Factors in Delivery of Service

Key factors distinguishing the clinic and contributing to its success are:

- Convenience: wait times of 1 week or less for a first appointment
- No residency restrictions (patients do not have to live in a specific geographic area)
- Service by the same provider: continuity of care
- Cost-effective: free office visits, low-cost labs, low-cost medications, care navigation
- Evidence-based care
- Provide self-management education for patients living with chronic diseases
- Care navigation services

## Definition of the Market

The market for ACHN patients should target all the areas of high poverty in our geographical catchment area. Using Census data, we have identified the areas of highest poverty in our county. In the area where the clinic is located, the poverty rate is 7.5%, which accounts for almost 8500 individuals living in poverty. Foreign-born individuals are more likely to live in poverty.[5] All segments of the catchment area should be included in the market.

## Analysis of the Market

Chronic diseases are the most costly and preventable health problems in the United States today. More than half of all adults in the United States have 1 or more chronic diseases and 80% of health care dollars are spent on chronic disease management for these individuals.[1] Heart disease and cancer account for more than 48% of all deaths and cost $472 billion yearly. Obesity affects one-third of our population and costs $147 billion yearly. Arthritis, the most common cause of disability costs $123 billion, and pre-diabetes and diabetes affects almost half of our adult population costing more than $245 billion annually. Asthma affects 1 in 11 children and 1 in 12 adults costing more than $245 billion annually.

**Table 1-2**

### PROJECTED OPERATING EXPENSES, MONTH BY MONTH ($)

| | JAN | FEB | MAR | APR | MAY | JUN | JULY | AUG | SEPT | OCT | NOV | DEC |
|---|---|---|---|---|---|---|---|---|---|---|---|---|
| *DNP-FNP* | | | | | | | | | | | | |
| *Clinic Manager* | | | | | | | | | | | | |
| *Administrative Assistant* | | | | | | | | | | | | |
| *Social Worker* | | | | | | | | | | | | |
| *Continuing Education/ Conference* | | | | | | | | | | | | |
| *Office Space Rental* | | | | | | | | | | | | |
| *Office Supplies* | | | | | | | | | | | | |
| *Advertising* | | | | | | | | | | | | |
| *Monthly Expenses* | | | | | | | | | | | | |
| *Year to Date Expenses* | | | | | | | | | | | | |

The clinic patient population includes hundreds of individuals living with chronic diseases who would benefit from targeted interventions and education as well as referrals to community partners to improve their outcomes and reduce health care costs significantly.

## COMPETITION

The clinic has a unique patient population which is largely immigrants and refugees. There are no geographical restrictions for patients who are visiting or in the area for a limited time. The clinic has an excellent reputation through our current patients. There are other free clinics that provide similar services, but their hours are limited and strict eligibility criteria including residency restrictions prevent access to care, and wait times are long to be seen for an initial visit.

## BUSINESS RISKS

The biggest risk is lack of regular funding sources, other than fundraisers and donations, that will result in the clinic not remaining viable. The clinic is also not on a bus route. This makes transportation challenging for our patients who lack personal transportation.

## PLAN FOR MARKETING

Marketing needs to be multifocal, specifically to social service agencies, coalitions, community partners, and other free clinics and FQHCs who may have long wait times. We could care for many of these patients at the clinic. Our initiatives need to be well publicized through social media, traditional print media, and word of mouth to increase participation in activities such as health fairs.

## FINANCIAL PLAN

Total operating expenses includes salaries, monies for staff education, office rental, office supplies, and advertising (Table 1-2).

Clinic employed staff includes 4 individuals:

1. DNP-FNP, 0.5 full-time employee (FTE)
   - Responsible for clinical care and care coordination
2. Clinic manager, 1.0 FTE
   - Responsible for the day-to-day operations and budget as well as community outreach, volunteer coordination, and fundraising
3. Administrative assistant, 0.5 FTE
   - Responsible for front-desk operations and eligibility screening
4. Social worker, 0.5 FTE
   - Responsible for community engagement, care navigation, and brief interventions.

In addition to staff salaries, monies are dedicated for continuing education for the nurse practitioner and for the staff to attend the annual conference of the state association of free and charitable clinics.

The clinic needs multiple funding streams to remain a viable business model. This will come from grants, community partnerships, donations, and sponsorships (Table 1-3).

**Table 1-3**

### PROJECTED INCOME, MONTH BY MONTH ($)

| | JAN | FEB | MAR | APR | MAY | JUN | JULY | AUG | SEPT | OCT | NOV | DEC |
|---|---|---|---|---|---|---|---|---|---|---|---|---|
| *Semi-Annual Fundraiser Dinners* | | | | | | | | | | | | |
| *Monthly Donations* | | | | | | | | | | | | |
| *Community Grant* | | | | | | | | | | | | |
| *Special Project Donations* | | | | | | | | | | | | |
| *Monthly Income* | | | | | | | | | | | | |

## REFERENCES

1. National Center for Chronic Disease Prevention and Health Promotion. Centers for Disease Control and Prevention. Accessed October 12, 2019. https://www.cdc.gov/chronicdisease/index.htm

2. Bell M. Why 5% of patients create 50% of health care costs. Forbes. Published January 10, 2013. Accessed October 12, 2019. https://www.forbes.com/sites/michaelbell/2013/01/10/why-5-of-patients-create-50-of-health-care-costs/

3. Heng J, Tham J, Eng NGY, Ling FW, Menon EB. Engaging patients in the management of chronic conditions in an outpatient clinic setting. *Singap Nurs J.* 2013;4(2):12-18.

4. Handmaker K. Building the IT infrastructure for population health and care management. *Psychology Today.* February 23, 2014. Accessed October 12, 2019. https://www.psychologytoday.com/us/blog/tech-support/201412/the-most-toxic-pattern-in-any-relationship

5. Poverty in Fairfax County and the cities of Fairfax and Falls Church, VA. Fairfax County. Accessed October 12, 2019. https://www.fairfaxcounty.gov/demographics/poverty

# CHAPTER 2

# THE DNP ESSENTIALS IN CLINICAL PRACTICE

## A PEDIATRIC NURSE PRACTITIONER'S EXPERIENCE IN MEDICAL GENETICS AND METABOLISM

*Kara Morgan, DNP, APRN, CPNP-BC, CGC*

## INTRODUCTION

The setting for my practice as a pediatric nurse practitioner is in a general and metabolic genetics clinical practice within a large academic health system. Examples of indications for general genetics clinic include developmental delays/intellectual disabilities, congenital anomalies, connective tissue disorders, neurodegenerative conditions, unexplained seizures, hearing loss, and family history of genetic disorders, among others. Examples of indications for metabolic genetics clinic include referrals from the state newborn screening program, inborn errors of metabolism, and mitochondrial disorders, among others. The process of a genetics clinical evaluation typically consists of extensive history gathering and records review, collection and analysis of family history information, dysmorphology physical exam, and laboratory and imaging studies. This diagnostic process is lengthy and typically takes place over the course of many appointments, often spanning months to years. When a diagnosis is reached, the therapeutic relationship continues with results disclosure, genetic counseling, and continued follow-up with recommendations for management and surveillance. Our team additionally provides inpatient consultation services to local hospitals for indications such

as those previously listed. We are also a site for patients enrolled in both observational and interventional clinical trials. The practice has grown into a team of physician medical geneticists, a nurse practitioner, genetic counselors, dieticians, nurses, and administrative support personnel.

Prior to entering the field of nursing, my experience as a health care professional was as a genetic counselor. Genetic counselors are professionals who have specialized education and training in genetics and counseling to provide personalized information, guidance, and support to patients and families as they make decisions about their genetic health. Genetic counselors help patients and families navigate topics such as how inherited conditions might affect them, how family and medical histories may impact the chance of disease occurrence or recurrence, informed decision making for genetic testing strategies, benefits and limitations of genetic testing, interpretation and evaluation of test results, psychosocial considerations, and potential courses of action.[1] After completion of my Master of Science in genetic counseling, I successfully became a certified genetic counselor (CGC) though the American Board of Genetic Counseling. Genetic counselors may work in many settings such as prenatal or maternal fetal medicine, pediatrics, oncology, cardiology, neurology, laboratory settings, and more. In my former role

Benson LA, ed. *The DNP Professional:*
*Translating Value From Classroom to Practice* (pp 19-26).

as a genetic counselor, I worked in both inpatient and outpatient pediatrics settings to help patients and families understand and cope with the medical, psychosocial, and familial implications of genetic disorders. I was also involved in the clinical aspects of state newborn screening programs for inborn errors of metabolism, cystic fibrosis, and congenital hearing loss. My work as a genetic counselor led me to realize that I desired to provide more hands-on patient care, and so I began my nursing education and set my final goal as obtaining a Doctor of Nursing Practice (DNP) degree. Like the field of genetic counseling, the nursing model of care combines evidence-based practice with the holistic and psychosocial aspects of health to provide the highest quality patient- and family-centered care.

## CREATION OF ROLE

Genetics is defined as "the study of individual genes and their impact on relatively rare single gene disorders."[2] Genomics is defined as "the study of all the genes in the human genome together, including their interactions with each other, the environment, and the influence of other psychosocial and cultural factors."[2] Advances in genetic and genomic science and technology are revolutionizing our understanding of health and illness. Nurses across roles and education levels are at the forefront of implementing these advances into patient care and health care systems. A unique opportunity to combine my education and training as a DNP-prepared advanced practice nurse with my knowledge, skills, and experience as a genetic counselor was identified, and my position was created as a new role. My clinically based role as a genetics nurse practitioner affords me a unique opportunity to use my DNP skill set as a practitioner, educator, consultant, researcher, and leader.

## INCORPORATION OF DNP ESSENTIALS IN GENETICS AND GENOMICS

In 2006, the American Association of Colleges of Nursing (AACN) published *The Essentials of Doctoral Education for Advanced Nursing Practice*.[3] There are many opportunities to integrate these Essentials into both the clinical and educational aspects of genetics and genomics in practice. As a DNP-prepared advanced practice nurse, I have experienced that *The Essentials of Doctoral Education for Advanced Nursing Practice* are a fundamental part of my practice, but there are certain Essentials that are especially pertinent to my day-to-day role as an advanced practice nurse in clinical genetics, as illustrated in this chapter.

## *DNP Essential: Scientific Underpinnings for Practice*

In *The Essentials of Doctoral Education for Advanced Nursing Practice*, DNP Essential I: Scientific Underpinnings for Practice, genomics is included as one of the foundational sciences that provide a basis for nursing practice. DNP Essential I also states that DNP graduates must be prepared to integrate the foundational sciences with ethical, biophysical, psychosocial, analytical, and organizational knowledge as the basis for the highest level of nursing practice.[3] The integration of genomics as one of the foundational sciences with physiologic, ethical, psychosocial, and organizational aspects of patient care is at the core of my daily practice. Although my clinical practice is quite specialized, the integration of genetics and genomics into practice is relevant and important to all DNP-prepared nurses.

Genetics has been identified as an educational need for nurses for more than 50 years.[4] In the 1990s through 2000s, the American Association of Colleges of Nursing, the American Nurses Association, the American Academy of Nursing, and the International Society of Nurses in Genetics each published competencies or position statements regarding the need for all nurses to become more knowledgeable about human genetics.[4] *The Essentials of Genetic and Genomic Nursing: Competencies, Curricula Guidelines, and Outcome Indicators* was originally published by the American Nurses Association in 2006 and revised in 2008.[2] The 25 competencies outlined in this publication establish the minimum genetic and genomic competencies expected of every registered nurse regardless of academic preparation, practice setting, role, or specialty.[2] In 2012, the American Nurses Association and the International Society of Nurses in Genetics expanded these competencies specifically for nurses with advanced degrees with the publication of the *Essential Genetic and Genomic Competencies for Nurses with Graduate Degrees*.[5] These 38 competencies are organized under categories of risk assessment and interpretation; genetic education; counseling; testing and results interpretation; clinical management; ethical, legal, and social implications; professional role; leadership; and research. They apply to all nurses prepared at the master's or doctoral level, including clinical nurse specialists, nurse practitioners, nurse educators, nurse administrators, and nurse scientists. They build on the original *Essentials of Genetic and Genomic Nursing* and presume that nurses pursuing graduate degrees have already achieved those competencies.[5] An increased demand for genetics and genomics services and a shortage of genetics specialists is moving provision of these services away from traditional medical genetics clinics and into primary care and other non-genetics specialties.[6] However, evidence shows that nurses trained at both the master's and doctoral levels feel unprepared to meet these needs.[7-9] The *Essentials of Genetic and Genomic*

*Nursing* and the *Essential Genetic and Genomic Competencies for Nurses with Graduate Degrees* have not been well disseminated, and both baccalaureate and graduate nursing faculty report that their programs do not fully meet the competencies therein.[4,7,9] The US Department of Health and Human Services Secretary's Advisory Committee on Genetics, Health, and Society recognized that inadequate education of health care providers plays a significant role in the challenge of integrating genetics and genomics into clinical care.[10] My prior experience as a genetics health care professional gave me a unique perspective as I progressed through my own graduate nursing program. I recognized limitations in the genetics and genomics curricular content and viewed them as an opportunity for improvement, planting the seeds of an idea for a curriculum quality improvement project as my capstone project. Virtually all diseases have a genetics or genomics component, and the genetics/genomics factors that influence common diseases such as cardiovascular disease, diabetes, and cancer are increasingly relevant in primary care as well as in non-genetics specialties.[9] Unfortunately, there is risk for patient harm when health care professionals are not sufficiently trained in genetics and genomics. Several studies have documented instances of negative patient outcomes due to services delivered by inadequately trained providers. These negative outcomes include adverse psychosocial effects, screening and testing errors, misinterpretation of results, medical mismanagement, and inappropriate use of health care resources.[11-14]

In short, essential genetics and genomics competencies have been recommended by several nursing and other health care organizations, but evidence shows that nurses across educational levels and professional roles are not demonstrating these competencies, and there is risk for patient harm when health care professionals are not adequately trained. Thus, it is necessary to provide graduate level nursing students with the knowledge needed to work toward competency in genetics and genomics. My capstone curriculum quality improvement project was a step toward achieving that goal within my institution. A literature search and gap analysis were conducted and found varied, good, and consistent evidence that nurses across all professional roles and education levels do not demonstrate the competencies needed to offer comprehensive care to people with or at risk for genetic conditions, nor are they familiar with the essential competencies outlined by the American Nurses Association and the International Society of Nurses in Genetics.[4,7,15] The overarching goal of my capstone curriculum quality improvement project was to advance genetic and genomic learning outcomes among graduate nurse practitioner students through development and integration of an educational module framed on the American Nurses Association and the International Society of Nurses in Genetics' *Essential Genetic and Genomic Competencies for Nurses with Graduate Degrees* with pre- and post-instructional assessments of knowledge using an objective, reliable, and validated instrument.[16] The instrument used was a concept inventory. Concept inventories are designed to measure difficult concepts and intentionally include common misconceptions in the response choices as incorrect responses.[17] Concept inventories are useful as both pre- and post-instructional knowledge assessments because they are designed to measure meaningful understanding of critical concepts rather than rote recall.[18] A small-scale pilot of an educational module with knowledge assessment using a pre- and post-test design was conducted.

Improved post-test scores were used as the primary outcome to gauge the success of the project. Scores were hypothesized to change after presentation of a genetics and genomics education module. In a group of n = 47 graduate level nurse practitioner students, total scores changed from mean (M) = 12.81 (SD = 3.66) before the module presentation to M = 15.91 (SD = 4.36) after the module presentation.[16] This change was statistically significant, $t(46) = -6.48$, $P = .00$. The scores changed in the positive direction, indicating a gain in knowledge.[16] The pre-test mean of 12.81 points translated to 41% correct which is consistent with the difficulty level associated with concept inventory-based testing.[16] The post-test mean of 15.91 points translated to 51% correct, so although the mean total score improvement was statistically significant, the mean post-test score represented participants answering still only about half of the survey items correctly.[16] My training program's grading standards required a minimal passing score of 74% for didactic coursework. So, neither the pre-test nor post-test average scores would have been within passing range. The highest score on the pre-test was 21 points (68% correct) with 0 participants achieving a score of 74% or above.[16] The highest score on the post-test was 23 points (74% correct), with 2 participants achieving that score.[16] This suggested that while implementation of an education module did contribute to knowledge gains, more genetics curricular content is needed to further increase knowledge. I further applied the Essential I foundational science of genomics to the education of future graduate prepared nurses through the creation and refinement of additional genetics and genomics educational modules for a nurse practitioner program didactic course, including the provision of resources for further independent individual education.

# DNP Essential: Organizational and Systems Leadership for Quality Improvement and Systems Thinking

Through the representation of DNP Essential II: Organizational and Systems Leadership for Quality Improvement and Systems Thinking in my DNP training program, I developed an increased understanding of how organizational and systems issues can affect direct patient care. My practice's involvement in my state's newborn screening program provides an example. The Secretary of the Department of Health and Human Services recommends a list of disorders for states to include in their newborn screening programs, called the Recommended Uniform Screening Panel.[19] Disorders on the Recommended Uniform Screening Panel are chosen based on the incidence of the condition, the burden of disease, the cost of treatment, the benefits of early identification and intervention, the technical aspects of screening for the condition (test availability, methodology, cost, availability of diagnostic confirmation, etc), and the availability of effective intervention or treatment.[19] In recent years, there have been rapid advancements in treatment for many genetic disorders. Thus, the Recommended Uniform Screening Panel is updated over time and many states continue to add new disorders to their screening panels. As new disorders are added, an understanding of complex organizational structures, health care systems, and policies at both the local and state level is crucial. My team participates in monthly conference calls with representatives from the state and stakeholders from other genetics referral centers across the state as we implement screening for new disorders and evaluate their effects on patient care and clinical practice.

## DNP Essential: Clinical Scholarship and Analytical Methods for Evidence-Based Practice

The tenets of DNP Essential III: Clinical Scholarship and Analytical Methods for Evidence-Based Practice are also integrated into my daily practice. In DNP Essential III, the concept of clinical scholarship includes that "scholars give meaning to isolated facts and make connections across disciplines through the scholarship of integration."[3] This concept is especially relevant to genetics and genomics clinical practice. Genetic conditions are often multisystemic disorders and the clinical genetics provider must move beyond thinking of body systems in isolation in order to link signs and symptoms that may not have an obvious connection. Also, as previously discussed, genetic conditions are often characterized by complex medical, psychosocial, and familial implications. Connections across disciplines must be made to other health care providers, therapists, social workers, family members, etc, to care for the patient as a whole person. Clinical scholarship also includes translation of research into practice through assessing and applying high-quality evidence. As the field of genetics and genomics rapidly evolves, the clinical genetics provider must continually use their critical appraisal skills to review recent literature and evidence in order to identify quality improvement opportunities and implement evidence-based patient care.

## DNP Essential: Information Systems/Technology and Patient Care Technology for the Improvement and Transformation of Health Care

As the science of genetics and genomics rapidly advances, its surrounding technologies rapidly advance as well. It is important for all providers, in both clinical genetics settings and other settings, to be able to assess the value of these technologies and incorporate them appropriately to patient care. One example of this in my practice is the use of a secure mobile device application that assists in the matching of facial features in patient photos to the phenotypes of genetic disorders. This is a tool that can be used to add objectivity and consistency to a dysmorphology physical exam. The information generated through the application can also be communicated to certain testing laboratories as part of the patient's clinical information, which allows refined analysis of the patient's genotypic data and may improve diagnostic yield.

In the modern age of the internet, there are countless sources of information that both patients and families and other professionals may encounter, but the quality of this information is highly variable. I also incorporate DNP Essential IV into my practice by critically evaluating information aimed at health care consumers and guiding patients and families toward sources that are patient-friendly, up-to-date, and accurate. I also serve as a resource for health care providers in other specialties and sub-specialties by providing recommendations for sources of information that they can use for their own learning as well as sources of information that they can provide to their patients.

## DNP Essential: Health Care Policy for Advocacy in Health Care

The phrase "health care policy" often evokes ideas of large scale political activism, but it can also be represented as small practice level changes. It is in this way that I apply DNP Essential V to my practice. As an example, after a recent study suggested a change in management for patients with a particular diagnosis, my team reviewed and discussed our guidelines and protocol for patients with this diagnosis and made a practice level policy decision to change our approach. Our new approach aims to improve delivery of services and support patients and families by streamlining care, reducing the number of clinic appointments, and reducing stress that may be experienced by the patient and family. We engage in monthly team meetings where we continually evaluate practice protocols and other care delivery issues such as equitable access to care and patient and practice financial concerns. On a larger scale, I have written my local congress member in support of national legislation to help my genetic counselor colleagues requesting co-sponsorship of the Access to Genetic Counselor Services Act, HR 3235, which would have the Centers for Medicare & Medicaid Services recognize genetic counselors as Medicare practitioners.[20] I am also involved in my state's genetic counselor professional organization, which is working toward state licensure for genetic counselors. Though I no longer practice as a genetic counselor, efforts made for the benefit of my colleagues elevate the entire field of clinical genetics and genomics.

## DNP Essential: Interprofessional Collaboration for Improving Patient and Population Health Outcomes

The ability to work as part of an interdisciplinary team is essential to clinical genetics practice, as in DNP Essential VI: Interprofessional Collaboration for Improving Patient and Population Health Outcomes. Our clinical division consists of physician medical geneticists, a genetics nurse practitioner, genetic counselors, metabolic registered dietitians, a genetic counseling assistant, a licensed practical nurse, and an office administrator. Each member provides their own unique and invaluable contribution to our team's mission to provide the highest quality patient care. Our team's model of outpatient clinical genetics visits is different from what most patients have experienced in primary care or even in other subspecialty visits. Our clinic model requires that preparation takes place before an appointment is even scheduled. For example, the unique heritable nature of our patients' indications for appointments often means the patient cannot be viewed as an isolated individual. If a patient is referred because they have an affected family member then our office administrator, licensed practical nurse, and/ or genetic counseling assistant work together to assist with obtaining said family member's records. Our clinical providers (genetic counselors, nurse practitioner, dietitians, and physicians) then review records and work to ensure we are proceeding with the most accurate, informative, and cost-effective diagnostic evaluation. For patients who are referred for individual indications, as opposed to family history, our administrative team members still work diligently to obtain all relevant records which are reviewed by the clinical providers prior to the patient's appointment. The clinic visits are staffed by both a genetic counselor and a nurse practitioner or physician provider. Prior to clinic, the genetic counselors and providers discuss the patients in order to establish a plan for evaluation and potential diagnostic testing, making the appointments themselves timelier and more efficient.

After diagnoses are established, the clinical providers work together to interpret results, conduct literature searches if needed, and provide disease-related education, counseling, and support to the patient and family. Our administrative team members and clinical team members also work together to coordinate future appointments, coordinate management and surveillance recommendations, and coordinate treatment needs (eg, prior authorizations, medication refills, referral requests, etc). For patients who have an inborn error of metabolism for which there is dietary management, our metabolic registered dietitians are especially involved in both outpatient clinic visits and management between visits for patient needs such as dietary management questions, procurement of medical foods and specialty formulas, and monitoring response to treatment. Our team is also fortunate to have access to a clinical psychologist who can provide developmental assessments and recommendations for patients who are at risk for learning or intellectual disabilities due to inborn errors of metabolism. Each team member's contribution is necessary to ensure that patients are triaged and scheduled appropriately, that appointments proceed efficiently, that diagnostic imaging or lab studies are done appropriately, and that patients and families receive education and support in navigating the rare disease journey.

Beyond recognizing the importance of our internal team relationships, I also collaborate frequently with physicians and advanced practice providers from primary care and from other sub-specialties, therapists, internal and external laboratory personnel, pharmacists, nurses, social workers, case managers, medical students, and families. In these collaborative relationships, I often serve as a subject matter expert, providing education and support to other members of the health care team as well as to patients and families. As an example, my interprofessional collaboration skills are important and impactful when providing inpatient consultation services in the neonatal intensive care unit. As a consultant, I provide recommendations for testing and management for the patient, along with information, counseling, and support for the families. Beyond this, I also provide resources and education for nurses, nurse practitioners, medical students, and physicians in the unit. Topics often include methodology, rationale, benefits, and limitations of molecular and/or biochemical testing, information about the natural history of a disorder, and resources for patient information and support groups.

## DNP Essential: Clinical Prevention and Population Health for Improving the Nation's Health

Through involvement with my state's newborn screening program, my clinical practice also incorporates the population health aspect of DNP Essential VII: Clinical Prevention and Population Health for Improving the Nation's Health.

Newborn screening began in 1963 with phenylketonuria (PKU) and now may include screening for numerous inborn errors of metabolism, immune disorders, hemoglobinopathies, endocrine disorders, cystic fibrosis, congenital heart defects, lysosomal storage disorders, and hearing screening.[21] As state sponsored public health initiatives, newborn screening programs use low cost, efficient, mass throughput methods to evaluate infants for conditions for which intervention soon after birth may significantly change outcome. All infants undergo newborn screening, regardless of birth setting, unless families specifically opt out. This population health program allows for identification, diagnosis, and management and/or treatment very early, usually prior to clinical presentation of symptoms. Early identification and changes in medical management greatly reduce the morbidity and mortality of these rare disorders. However, it is a screening program and the tests performed are not diagnostic. There is the possibility of a condition that requires further management, but there is also the possibility of false positive results and infants who are screened-positive require further confirmatory testing. My clinical practice is a state-designated genetics referral center for infants who are screen-positive for inborn errors of metabolism. We receive screen-positive referrals from the state laboratory and coordinate confirmatory diagnostic testing for infants identified through newborn screening. We also provide families with the opportunity to ask questions, discuss plan of care, and receive genetic counseling.

The clinical prevention aspect of DNP Essential VII is relevant to my practice through application of evidence-based guidelines after patients/families receive a diagnosis. Individuals and families with genetic diagnoses receive surveillance and management recommendations specific to their diagnosis in order to prevent or reduce morbidity and mortality. For example, it is recommended that patients with Beckwith-Wiedemann syndrome have periodic abdominal ultrasounds and measurement of serum alpha-fetoprotein to monitor for embryonal tumors for which they are at increased risk.[22] Surveillance and management guidelines such as these allow for early detection of sequelae of these rare disorders, which reduces adverse outcomes. Clinical prevention in the form of risk reduction for families also takes place when families have a full understanding of recurrence risks and can then make informed family-planning decisions.

## DNP Essential: Advanced Nursing Practice

A practitioner in the field of clinical genetics must be aware that genetic disorders are often complex, affecting not only physical health, but also impacting familial, psychological, financial, ethical, legal, and social matters. In my practice, I have experienced that the principles of the previously discussed DNP Essentials combine to form the highly developed assessment and practice skills needed to handle these complicated and often sensitive matters, as described

in DNP Essential VIII: Advanced Nursing Practice. As in DNP Essential I, through formal coursework and through serving as a resource for other providers, I seek to increase the understanding of genomics as a foundational science for nurses across roles, specialties, and educational levels. As in DNP Essential II, I apply my understanding of organizations and systems when working with other stakeholders at the institutional, local, and state levels on endeavors such as implementation of new disorders on newborn screening. As in DNP Essential III, I use my clinical scholarship skills to evaluate new evidence and appropriately apply it to patient care and development of practice policies. I similarly critically evaluate and selectively use new technologies and information sources, as in DNP Essential IV. In DNP Essential V, I work with my team to develop practice level policies that address the physical, psychosocial, and financial needs of our patients. In DNP Essential VI, I have the privilege of providing expert guidance to both patients and families and fellow health care professionals for situations that are often unique and complex through interprofessional collaboration. In DNP Essential VII, my practice includes consideration of the individual, familial, financial, and psychosocial issues that affect clinical prevention when caring for patients and families. On a larger scale, my practice also includes consideration of the ethical, financial, social, and cultural implications of population health programs such as newborn screening. The DNP graduate is uniquely prepared to combine the concepts in *The Essentials of Doctoral Education for Advanced Nursing Practice* with the specialized and complex aspects of clinical genetics advanced nursing practice.

# PRACTICE OUTCOMES

My education, experience, and creation of my role have allowed my team to provide improved service delivery in outpatient clinics and inpatient consultation to optimize clinical care, patient satisfaction, and interprofessional collaboration. We have been able to provide more timely response to requests for inpatient consultation, and increased consistency and long-term follow-up for patients seen in inpatient consultation. For example, for infants in the neonatal intensive care unit who have protracted stays, we are able to consistently update both the family and the other members of the care team as results return and potentially change medical management. This provides tailored information and support sooner, increasing satisfaction for both patients/families and other members of the health care team. Also in the inpatient setting, I work with the referrals laboratory to consider the financial interests of the institution and review testing options to recommend timely, cost-effective, and clinically appropriate testing. We have also made improvements to our newborn screening follow-up structure. When an infant is referred to our state-designated regional genetics referral center as screen-positive, we work with primary care providers and families to coordinate confirmatory testing and initial management. Since my role was created, we are now also able to offer the option of an immediate appointment in our metabolic genetics clinic, typically within a few days of the referral from the state newborn screening program. With this option, we can coordinate the diagnostic process internally and provide prompt face-to-face education, support, and resources. Also, when confirmatory labs are ordered and collected internally, we receive results directly which increases efficiency.

The creation of my role has also allowed us to add services for our patients with lysosomal storage disorders receiving enzyme replacement therapy at an affiliated infusion center. Previously, the history and physical prior to each infusion was completed by providers outside of our division. Patients were often seen by a different provider each week. Now, I complete the history and physical for a group of patients prior to each weekly or biweekly infusion. We have received feedback from the staff at the infusion center that they appreciate having a consistent point of contact for any questions or concerns that may arise. Through evaluating the same patients weekly or biweekly, I have also had the privilege of building solid therapeutic relationships. Frequent evaluations from a consistent provider allows the detection of subtle changes that may otherwise go unnoticed. The frequent evaluations are also an opportunity to build rapport and trust. The chance to discuss questions and concerns with a trusted provider is invaluable and can positively impact management. For example, one family recently agreed to influenza vaccination for the first time for a school-aged child, and another family agreed to pursue a recommended procedure that they had been delaying. This added service gives these medically complex patients increased consistency and improved coordination of care without having to schedule a separate visit. In addition, by providing evaluations for these patients at every infusion visit, our division has gained previously uncaptured revenue.

## PROFESSIONALISM

I have served as an ambassador for both nursing and genetics and strive to be a bridge between genetics nurses and genetic counselors. I have promoted the nursing profession through dissemination of my capstone project, collaborations on publications, and presentations at meetings for regional, national, and international professional societies. My capstone project was disseminated through poster presentations at a regional meeting of the National Association of Pediatric Nurse Practitioners and at the annual World Congress of the International Society of Nurses in Genetics. I have also been an invited speaker at an annual national education symposium presented by the Florida Association of Neonatal Nurse Practitioners, as a presenter for both a podium general session and the presenter of the genetics portion of the board review track attended by trainees from all over the nation. As another example of interprofessional collaboration, I have also co-authored an abstract with a physician neonatologist for a respected national annual pediatrics conference. I am also a member of the International Society of Nurses in Genetics professional practice committee.

## CONCLUSION: IMPACT OF THE DNP DEGREE

As a result of obtaining my DNP degree I have the knowledge and skills needed to integrate the foundational science of genomics into clinical practice as a practitioner, educator, consultant, researcher, and leader. I work collaboratively with team members to identify, organize, and summarize pertinent medical and genetics information to assess, diagnose, treat, and communicate with patients, families, and other health care providers. I provide information and education regarding natural history, prognosis, management, recurrence, diagnostic methodologies, possible alternate courses of action, and guidance through potential ethical, legal, and social issues. My capstone project has impacted the education of future nurses by contributing to the growing body of evidence regarding the provision of genetics and genomics content to graduate level nursing students. I have applied my clinical scholarship and interprofessional collaboration skills to quality improvement initiatives and the preparation of abstracts and manuscripts for publication. Through active engagement in professional activities, I have reached nurses on the national and international levels to promote the field of genetics and genomics nursing. I continue to expand my knowledge of complex genetic issues and new technologies and use my clinical scholarship skills to critically appraise new information and apply it to evidence-based practice. My DNP education, experience, and creation of my role have contributed to improved efficiency and enhanced service delivery in both the inpatient and outpatient settings to optimize clinical care, leading to improved patient satisfaction, therapeutic relationships, and interprofessional collaborations. The science of genetics and genomics is rapidly evolving, and its application to clinical practice provides an exciting opportunity for the clinician to engage in life-long learning for the continual improvement of genetics and genomics related health outcomes for individual patients and patient populations.

## ACKNOWLEDGMENTS

To my family, this journey would not have been possible without your limitless patience, love, and support. You are my greatest accomplishment. I would also like to thank my colleagues, whose dedication to our organization and to our patients has transformed a career into a mission. Finally, thank you to my patients and their families. It is an honor to be allowed into your most difficult moments and an inspiration to witness your strength.

# REFERENCES

1. Who are genetic counselors? National Society of Genetic Counselors. Accessed December 29, 2019. https://www.nsgc.org/page/whoaregeneticcounselors-473

2. American Nurses Association. *Essentials of Genetic and Genomic Nursing: Competencies, Curricula Guidelines, and Outcome Indicators.* 2nd ed. American Nurses Association; 2009.

3. The essentials of doctoral education for advanced nursing practice. American Association of Colleges of Nursing. October 2006. Accessed December 29, 2019. https://www.aacnnursing.org/DNP/DNP-Essentials

4. Thompson HJ, Brooks BV. Genetics and genomics in nursing: evaluating essentials implementation. *Nurse Education Today.* 2011;6:623-627. doi:10.1016/j.nedt.2010.10.023

5. Greco KE, Tinley S, Seibert D. *Essential Genetic and Genomic Competencies for Nurses with Graduate Degrees.* American Nurses Association and International Society of Nurses in Genetics; 2012.

6. Talwar D, Tseng TS, Foster M, Xu L, Chen LS. Genetics/genomics education for nongenetic healthcare professionals: a systematic literature review. *Genet Med.* 2017;19(7):725-732. doi:10.1038/gim.2016.156

7. Calzone KA, Jenkins J, Culp S, Bonham VL, Badzek L. National nursing workforce survey of nursing attitudes, knowledge, and practice in genomics. *Per Med.* 2013;10(7):719-728. doi:10.2217/pme.13.64

8. Jenkins JF, Calzone KA. Are nursing faculty ready to integrate genomic content into curricula? *Nurse Educ.* 2012;37(1):25-29. doi:10.1097/NNE.0b013e31823836ec

9. Maradiegue AH, Edwards QT, Seibert D. Five-years later: have faculty integrated medical genetics into nurse practitioner curriculum? *Int J Nurs Educ Scholarsh.* 2013;10:245-254. doi:10.1515/ijnes-2012-0007

10. Genetics education and training. Secretary's Advisory Committee on Genetics, Health, and Society. February 2011. Accessed December 29, 2019. https://osp.od.nih.gov/wp-content/uploads/2013/11/SACGHS_education_report_2011.pdf

11. Bensend TA, Veach PM, Niendorf KB. What's the harm? Genetic counselor perceptions of adverse effects of genetics service provision by non-genetics professionals. *J Genet Counsel.* 2014;23(1):48-63. doi:10.1007/s10897-013-9605-3

12. Bonadies DC, Brierley KL, Barnett RE, et al. Adverse events in cancer genetic testing: the third case series. *Cancer J.* 2014;20(4):246-253. doi:10.1097/PPO.0000000000000057

13. Brierley KL, Blouch E, Cogswell W, et al. Adverse events in cancer genetic testing: medical, ethical, legal, and financial implications. *Cancer J.* 2012;18(4):303-309. doi:10.1097/PPO.0b013e3182609490

14. Vadaparampil ST, Scherr CL, Cragun D, Malo TL, Pal T. Pre-test genetic counseling services for hereditary breast and ovarian cancer delivered by non-genetics professionals in the state of Florida. *Clin Genet.* 2015;87(5):473-477. doi:10.1111/cge.12405

15. Skirton H, O'Connor A, Humphreys A. Nurses' competence in genetics: a mixed method systematic review. *J Adv Nurs.* 2012;68(11):2387-2398. doi:10.1111/j.1365-2648.2012.06034

16. Morgan KM. *Integration of Genetics and Genomics Elements in a Graduate Nurse Practitioner Program: A Curriculum Quality Improvement Project.* Doctoral Capstone. University of South Florida; 2018.

17. Ward LD, French BF, Barbosa-Leiker C, Iverson AE. Application of exploratory factor analysis and item response theory to validate the genomic nursing concept inventory. *J Nurs Educ.* 2016;55(1):9-17. doi:10.3928/01484834-20151214-05

18. Ward L, Haberman M, Barbosa-Leiker C. Development and psychometric evaluation of the genomic nursing concept inventory (GNCI). *J Nurs Educ.* 2014;53(9):511-518. doi:10.3928/01484834-20140806-04

19. Recommended uniform screening panel. United States Health Resources & Services Administration. February 2019. Accessed December 29, 2019. https://www.hrsa.gov/advisory-committees/heritable-disorders/rusp/index.html

20. Loebsack, D. H.R.3235: access to genetic counselor services act of 2019. Congress. June 2019. Accessed December 29, 2019. https://www.congress.gov/bill/116th-congress/house-bill/3235/text

21. About newborn screening. Baby's First Test. Accessed December 29, 2019. https://www.babysfirsttest.org/newborn-screening/about-newborn-screening

22. Shuman C, Beckwith JB, Weksberg R. Beckwith-Wiedemann syndrome. GeneReviews. August 2016. Accessed December 29, 2019. https://www.ncbi.nlm.nih.gov/books/NBK1394/

# CHAPTER 3

# Utilizing the DNP Essentials to Deliver High-End Care in the Home

*Tracie L. Moore, DNP, FNP, ACNP, ACNS-BC*

## Introduction

The Doctor of Nursing Practice (DNP) is a terminal clinical nursing degree that utilizes the American Associates of Colleges of Nurses Essentials of doctoral education for advanced nursing practice. The DNP Essentials were utilized to start a mobile primary care practice in Memphis, Tennessee. With the education that the DNP degree provided, I can deliver high-end primary care services in the home. Entrepreneurship is a viable career choice for the DNP, and any business model can be utilized.

I obtained my DNP from the University of Tennessee Health Science Center and am certified as a family and acute care nurse practitioner by the American Nurses Credentialing Center. I am also certified as an adult health clinical nurse specialist and certified medical examiner. I hold a master's degree in nursing education. When not providing primary care services in the community, I am also an emergency nurse practitioner and adjunct graduate faculty for the Loewenberg College of Nursing at the University of Memphis. Owning a practice was not something I had ever considered within my reach. I started off as a single mom with a dream of becoming a nurse. That was it. I wanted to work in a hospital setting, take care of people, and provide for my son. No one in my family had ever completed college. The thought of having a job that was not considered "labor" was all I wanted to achieve. I wanted to do something different. I wanted to be somebody that beat the odds. I started off with an associate degree in nursing and ended up with a DNP terminal degree from the University of Tennessee Health Science Center in 2010. Fast forward to 2016 and I started a mobile primary care practice. I travel around the city and provide care to people who are unable to make it to an office setting. Moore Healthcare is a mobile-based clinic that is credentialed with most insurance carriers. Clients are assigned to our services by their insurance carriers or are referred by either home health agencies or families that need assistance with their loved ones. It is based out of my home in a specialized space carved out for business purposes only. Obtaining the DNP degree gave me the confidence and tools I needed to provide such a service.

## The DNP Degree in This Practice Setting

The DNP is a terminal nursing degree focused on providing nursing care at its highest level. It is also a translational

Benson LA, ed. *The DNP Professional:*
*Translating Value From Classroom to Practice* (pp 27-35).
© 2021 SLACK Incorporated.

degree aimed at bringing the research to the clinical setting. The degree is an integration of ethics, psychosocial, analytical, biophysical, and organizational science[1] and brings it directly to the patient. No other degree achieves this on an educational level or scale. The DNP skill set provided a way to develop and evaluate new practice approaches using theories from not only nursing but other disciplines. It also allowed us to understand thinking from Newtonian and quantum perspectives.

In my role as a practice owner, I had to first evaluate the market to find the niche that was needed. I needed to discover what was going to set my clinic apart from all the other clinics around the city. My focus was on the community at large. Primary care services are certainly not new and most people who have insurance have a primary care provider (PCP). But, in looking for a way to service the community, I had to find a model that set Moore Healthcare apart from all others. It initially started off like every other clinic; in a building with overhead. I soon discovered a way to provide the service using little overhead and being much more of an asset to the community at large. I was able to develop, evaluate, and carry out delivery of care to a community that needed health care services that were oftentimes out of reach for them.

# INCORPORATION OF DNP ESSENTIALS AND OUTCOMES

There are 8 DNP Essentials that were used when developing this practice and are continuously used as a foundation for what I do every day.

## DNP Essential: Scientific Underpinnings for Practice

In order to bring evidence-based practice to the bedside or client side, it is imperative that the research is understood and implemented. This speaks to the translation of research into practice. There had to be an understanding that I was bringing evidence-based practice to the community at large. There also had to be a commitment on my part to life-long learning by being a part of professional organizations, attending annual continuing education conferences aimed at my specialties, and lending support to the political action committees that stood for what mattered to myself and my clients the most. I had to be prepared to address current and future practice issues. The integration of science into everyday interactions with the client made the difference. In my community, diseases such as hypertension, hyperlipidemia, diabetes, and obesity have wreaked havoc on its citizens. I have been able to get hemoglobin A1cs down to goal for better diabetes management and hypertension controlled with diet, medications, and weight loss maintenance. I use

up-to-date research, treatments, and therapies to assist the client in reaching their health care goals. The outcome of applying this DNP Essential has been an ongoing labor of love. I am continuously reviewing standards of patient care as they relate to the disease processes that I am treating the most.[1]

## DNP Essential: Organizational and Systems Leadership for Quality Improvement and Systems Thinking

This speaks directly to the goals of eliminating health disparities and the promotion of patient safety.[1] In the African American community, health care disparities are still an issue. The social determinants of health including racism, poverty, access to health care services, education, violence, and justice[2] are an issue in 2019 just like it was in 1919. Being able to address health disparities by meeting people where they are is a much-needed service and one realized and elucidated in the DNP education and Essentials. Understanding the principles of practice management along with balancing productivity with quality care is essential for being out in the community and providing this indispensable service. With the understanding of the disparities and the importance of the role I have created in the community, my hope is that I am breaking barriers and closing the gaps. I also use advanced communication and documentation techniques that oversee continuous process improvement and quality initiatives. The electronic medical record (EMR) that I have invested in uses state-of-the-art services that allow patients real time access to their records, secure communication with the provider, and tracking of needed screenings and services. It also allows secure e-prescribing for the safety and security of the practice and the patient. The outcomes have been successful. I can attest annually for Merit-based Incentive Payment System (MIPS) which is a performance-based payment system for Medicare Part B, making sure that I meet quality guidelines and easily keep up with what is needed to meet these guidelines at least >80% of the time in all measures. It also allows the tracking that most insurance companies now require for their performance standards and guidelines.[1]

## DNP Essential: Clinical Scholarship and Analytical Methods for Evidence-Based Practice

As a DNP practitioner, I generate evidence that informs the research. Research and practice have a cyclical relationship. As the practitioner translates the research into practice, the outcomes are communicated back to the researcher in one form or another. I had the pleasure of designing and implementing my own policies and procedures to use in a different practice setting: the patient's home. I had to create a standard of care that mirrored what they would expect at a traditional clinic setting but was intimate and appropriate enough to happen in their living room or at their kitchen table. A home visit from a health care provider is a service that most people think is out of reach. Most people believe these services are out of their reach. With the DNP, the dissemination and integration of new knowledge brings state-of-the-art practitioner care to the client. It also allows a new and fresh perspective when communicating patient needs to other health care stakeholders. This allows high-end participation in collaborative research. I am prepared to use analytical methods to critically appraise the literature and implement evidence-based practice, design and implement processes to evaluate outcomes in my practice, and participate in continuous improvement practices for the practice. This is the patient care model implemented to its fullest potential. Outcomes for this standard are ongoing also. I am now at the point that I am beginning to write and self-report my outcomes for research purposes.[1]

## DNP Essential: Information Systems/Technology and Patient Care Technology for the Improvement and Transformation of Health Care

For Moore Healthcare, an electronic health record (EHR) was purchased to assist with billing. But it is also used to track quality measures such as diabetes and hypertension control, breast and colorectal cancer screening, immunizations, and e-prescribing, for example. Patients can communicate with the provider via the patient portal and via secure text messaging. They also have 24/7 access to their medical records using their email address. The ability to attest for meaningful use is essential when working with Medicare for reimbursement purposes and for process improvements. The EHR is a tool that is the basis for providing quality care. Access to the medical records for tracking, trending, and continuous evaluation can take place on the provider and patient end. This creates the partnership that is needed for healthier outcomes. The outcomes for this measure have been greatly fulfilled. Patients have reported being able to pull up their visit summaries, labs, and educational material that I have sent them via the patient portal to their family members and other specialists that they have been referred to. They have been able to view billing and send secure messages to the provider. Pharmacies, insurance providers, referral correspondence, etc all come through the EMR for secure communication to the practice. I am also able to take credit card payments via the EMR with no need to buy expensive terminals. This is an investment that proved to be well worth it. Prior to switching to an EMR that was intuitive, the process of keeping up with required screenings, testing, and patient needs would be done manually. This would lead to missing out on scheduled testing, needed medications, or timely screenings. With this available now at a glance at all times, I am >80% compliant in all measures that my practice has decided to attest for. For instance, Moore Healthcare does not administer immunizations, therefore this screening is not reported for attestation. However, it still appears in the patients EMR so that I can remind them when it is due, and I can tell them the last time they had it done. At a glance, I can see their last Pap smear, mammogram, colon malignancy screening, etc. This has allowed the practice to capture payments made by insurance companies for timely screenings.[1]

## DNP Essential: Health Care Policy for Advocacy in Health Care

Health care policy creates the framework that can either assist or impede progress in the delivery of health care services to an aggregate.[1] Providers on all fronts are guided by the policies created whether involved in the decision-making process or not. There has always been a professional push to be involved in professional organizations for this reason. Nursing professionals have a duty to be at the table to assist with policy making and influence policy change. Political activism is a hallmark of higher education as the stakes hit closer to home. Advocating for patients who may not have seen the inside of a doctor's office in years due to a disability (eg, mental, physical, and/or emotional) is where health care must lead. In the goal of leaving no one behind, this is a population that has been loosely included. Health care policy that includes the delivery of care, disparities in care, cultural sensitivity, ethics, access to care, quality of care, health care justice, and social trauma, to name a few, are all on the frontline of health care topics that the DNP expert is ready to take on. As a DNP graduate, I am prepared to design, influence, and implement those policies that frame these issues, thereby bringing this expertise to the home of individuals that need it most. Those voices can now be heard on local, state, regional, national, and international levels. I am that critical interface between practice, research, and policy. As an outcome, I have not been able to participate as much as I should during the start-up phase of the practice, but have been able to donate money to the political action committees through the American Association of Nurse Practitioners (AANP). It is a future goal to be fully involved in order to break down the barriers that hold nurse practitioners back from going out into the community and making a difference.[1]

## DNP Essential: Interprofessional Collaboration for Improving Patient and Population Health Outcomes

The Institute of Medicine (IOM) has mandated safe, effective, timely, efficient, equitable, and patient-centered care[3] for a health care system which would include all delivery models. Providing in-home primary care services requires that all community resources are utilized effectively. Generating a network of specialists, home health agencies, therapists, imaging centers, etc requires networking and an understanding that it truly "takes a village." Without a PCP working on their behalf, these patients would have to weather the red tape alone if they are not knowledgeable of the resources. Most have no clue regarding the resources available to them or how to access them. In the state of Tennessee, access is still an issue as nurse practitioners are unable to sign home health orders and physician signatures are still required. Admittingly, physicians do not go into the home to see patients and most patients are unable to get to that provider. Over time, the home health orders and services become abandoned and the patients are on their own with only a few family members who have stayed around to assist. Rural areas are hit the hardest in this scenario due to transportation and help with leaving the home. As an outcome to this DNP Essential, I was able to form a network of community specialists and agencies that I work with closely for the patients that I service. These include home health agencies, mobile imaging centers, free-standing imaging centers, physical therapists, psychiatric providers, and occupational therapists to name a few. For the contacts, I started off cold. I called the agencies and spoke with either their managers or directors and let them know who I was and what I was able to provide. A few of the agencies reached out to me through the word-of-mouth network. Once I started referring my patients to their services, true professional relationships started to form. Peers also refer patients to my service from hospital discharges, inpatient rounds, and emergency room visits.[1]

## DNP Essential: Clinical Prevention and Population Health for Improving the Nation's Health

Clinical prevention includes routine screenings and immunizations which have been proven to reduce disability and death.[4] Utilization of these services prevent and detect illnesses and disease in the disease prevention and health promotion stages, thereby decreasing mortality and morbidity. Even with access to Medicaid and Medicare, these preventive services do not usually reach chronically ill, homebound patients. Clinical preventive services have the tremendous promise of saving millions of lives and to also help people live better.[4] This is an excellent place for community-based nurse practitioners to insert their expertise at the community level. Population health's focus is bringing significant health concerns into focus and serves as an opportunity for health care organizations, communities, and systems to improve outcomes for the communities they serve.[5] The foundation of DNP and nurse practitioner education is health promotion and disease prevention at the implementation stage. We are trained to understand and implement standards of care. Ongoing education and active involvement on the local, state, regional, and national levels make sure that the standards are reaching our marginalized community population. I am prepared to lead in efforts to integrate evidence-based clinical preventions including population health services for individuals, aggregates, and populations[1] in the home. The outcome has been phenomenal. Most homebound patients have not had mammograms, colonoscopy or fecal immunoassay tests (FIT), Pap smears, diabetes screening, etc in years. Although I do not perform Pap smears in the home, I am able to refer patients to appropriate providers and track that these screenings are timely and to follow up effectively when patients miss appointments. I also assist with scheduling transportation to these appointments with local medical travel companies. I receive a report card from most insurance agencies quarterly with a list of their patients that I care for, quality measures met and unmet, and a score. I consistently score > 80% in all measures.[1]

## DNP Essential: Advanced Nursing Practice

Distinct specialization is a hallmark of the DNP graduate. Professionally, I am educated and certified as a family nurse practitioner (FNP-BC), adult health clinical nurse specialist (ACNS-BC), and as an acute care nurse practitioner (ACNP-BC). All roles have served me well in my career. The FNP-BC has been most valuable in the community whereas the ACNP-BC is valuable in the secondary role as an emergency room nurse practitioner and hospitalist. The ACNS-BC has been invaluable as an educator to both nursing students and practicing nurses. Specialization in nursing is essential because it is recognized that an umbrella title does not guarantee a knowledge base in any one area. Because of this admission, mastery is tested in differing areas such as: pediatrics, gerontological, adult, women's health, psychiatry and mental health, anesthesia, administration, neonatal, acute care, primary care, and mid-wifery. The health care system is complex and needs individuals who have completed rigorous training in a single specialty.[1] This does not take away from people who have attained several specialties but does accept that the knowledge is too vast to put in only one program. Individual expertise must be proven. My education and subsequent certification ensure the community that I can conduct a comprehensive and organized assessment of health and illness limitations in complex situations. The DNP ensures the community that I have been educated at the highest level of clinical nursing and can design, implement, and evaluate implemented interventions based on nursing science. I can develop and sustain relationships with community stakeholders that facilitates optimal outcomes and excellent patient care. The outcome of this DNP Essential is a win-win for the community. I can affect patient outcomes from different perspectives based on my individual areas of expertise.[1]

## BUSINESS PLAN: MOVING TO THE COMMUNITY

The decision to become a PCP is a huge one that carries a lot of responsibilities. In the state of Tennessee, nurse practitioners are recognized in state policy as PCPs.[6,7] There must be a collaboration agreement between the nurse practitioner and a physician that has agreed to review and sign 20% of the nurse practitioner's patient's charts.[6] This is not an issue if the practitioner is employed by a physician based group. There are policies and processes as to how the physician on record will co-sign charts. For an independently functioning nurse practitioner, this requirement is a barrier to practice and can be very expensive. Physicians may not be as willing to sign off on charts of a nurse practitioner that they have not worked with, if they are not in a relationship with the patient, or are not available in real time to also see the patient if needed. Deciding to go out and start the business despite these obstacles is what most nurse practitioners in states that do not have full practice authority (FPA) usually do with hopes of finding a partner later. Other barriers include getting fully credentialed on some health insurance panels, getting referrals from hospitals either from emergency room visits or post discharge, getting privileges or being recognized at hospitals, and the lack of legal authority to sign off on home health patients and other state documents.[8] Even with these barriers for some, the advantages outweigh the disadvantages. They include autonomy, efficiency of a single person making decisions, personal time management, titration of income, and adding on or deleting services as needed. Other advantages to practice ownership include the nurse practitioner deciding how the practice is run and the lengths of the patient visits. The nurse practitioner chooses all employees and pay structures, decides on an appropriate workload based on their time, availability and profit desired, and controls quality.[8] Advantages to the patient include the benefit of a combined nursing and medical model of care in which the patient usually gets more time with the provider, better access to the provider, and the patient may also pay less for more service.[8]

Initially, my practice began in an office setting. My first step was to apply for credentialing from every insurance company I could think of including Medicare and state Medicaid. I found an ideal location nestled within the community that I knew could use my services the most. I took out a business loan (that I later regretted), hired an office manager and a nursing assistant, signed a collaboration agreement with a physician, and opened the doors. I held an open house for the community and previous patients that was quite successful and netted a few patients. It took about 3 days for the patients to start coming in. Unfortunately, it took a little longer than that for the reimbursements to start coming in, but when they did, I could not have been happier.

## BUSINESS PLAN: FINANCES AND CREDENTIALING

A business plan is the first step in starting a business. Sitting down and writing out all the specifics related to the plan should be a dose of reality (Table 3-1). Looking at what is essential and what can wait (such as model of care, care delivery, and providing health equity) is an important decision. Likewise, deciding on the business structure such as concierge, cash only, insurance based (eg, Medicare, Medicaid, private insurance, etc) is just as important. Other options include deciding to be theme based: weight loss, intravenous hydration, adult or pediatric primary care, disease specific, mobile or office based, med-spa, high-end clientele, or community care, etc. These are all options that nurse practitioners are free to explore and this is just the tip of the iceberg.

The business plan I used was very thorough and looked at the numbers realistically (see Table 3-1). Making a business plan can be a bit daunting because it makes you really analyze where your monies will be going and what is doable. I saw early on that I was going to have to keep a part-time or as needed position until the clientele picked up and the claims starting coming in. The big question was, "Will reimbursement cover the expenses?" Expenses can include rent, payroll, quarterly state and federal taxes, office supplies, medical waste removal, utilities, recurrent supply expenses, accountant fees, insurance (eg, malpractice, business, compensation, etc), business travel, collaborative physician fees, hospital privileges fees, advertising, etc. The list can go on and on. Physician office start-up can be upwards of $200 000.[8] In a mobile business model gas and vehicle upkeep is also a consideration, but expenses are substantially less.

Credentialing was a task that I took up on my own. I needed to obtain a national provider number (NPI), Drug Enforcement Agency (DEA) number, and a clinical laboratory improvement amendment (CLIA) waiver to perform lab draws. I also had to open a business checking and savings account. I went on to Medicare and Medicaid's website and applied there first, then I contacted each insurance carrier and filled out an application if they were open for new providers in my area. After about 30 days the approval letters started rolling in. There are agencies that will do this for a fee, but I took on the task myself.

As far as a collaborating physician, I was able to secure a very good collaborator, Dr. Grady Saxton, who served in that role until he passed away in October of 2018. Dr. Saxton was a highly decorated cardiologist who was partially retired. I

### Table 3-1

## NURSE PRACTITIONER PRIVATE PRACTICE EXPENSES

| TYPE OF EXPENSE | OFFICE EXPENSES | MOBILE EXPENSES |
|---|---|---|
| Rent | $13 200 per year | n/a |
| Utilities | $1300 per year | n/a |
| Supplies | $5000 to $7000 per year | $1000 per year, no held inventory |
| Professional license | $200 every other year | $200 every other year |
| Certification | $300 for each, every 5 years | $300 for each, every 5 years |
| Malpractice insurance | $2500 per year | $2500 per year |
| Business insurance | $750 per year | n/a |
| Staff salaries | $30 000 to $45 000 per year | n/a |
| Physician salaries | $65 000 per year | $65 000 per year |
| Equipment maintenance | $1000 per year | n/a |
| Cleaning | $1500 per year | n/a |
| Paper and medical waste removal | $840 per year | $240 per year |
| Taxes | $12 000 per year | Variable |
| Security | $500 per year | n/a |
| Phone services (cellular and office) | $3600 per year | $2400 per year |
| Hospital privileges fees | $400 per year | $400 per year |
| Business loan repayment | $1200 per month | $1200 per year |
| Cable and internet | $900 per year | $900 per year |

used his internal medicine designation to run my practice. After he passed away, it took me about 2 months to replace him. During that time, the practice was at a standstill. Dr. Jyothishree Pinnaka soon filled the gap and the practice was back in full swing. Dr. Pinnaka is a community nephrologist. I also used her internal medicine designation to run my practice. In my city, the field for home based primary care was and is still wide open. It was very easy to identify patients that had been all but abandoned by their PCP and family members years ago by the home health agencies and by mouth-to-mouth referrals. My referral base has grown, and I have been busy networking with all types of community resources. It is a field that I highly recommend to any practitioner thinking of starting their own practice. It is also a good start for people who eventually want to open a practice. It allows the provider to start with very little overhead and build the practice into an office setting in the future if desired.

# PEARLS/TAKEAWAYS

Prior to starting a community-based mobile practice make sure that you do your homework. Revisit the goals of the services you want to provide. Be open to using the DNP Essentials[1] and form a conceptual framework for yourself (Figures 3-1, 3-2, and 3-3). Be clear on what you want to do and if you are truly committed to the long-term success of your entrepreneurship in this area. Start forming relationships with physicians in your current workspace. If you are in a state that does not have FPA then you will be at the mercy of finding a collaborator. Set boundaries for the practice, your patients, and family members. Having your own practice will bring family members, drug seekers, and uninsured patients to your door. Make sure you have policies and procedures in place for all of these and know your state laws regarding them. Delivering high-end primary care services in the home is a wonderful career and entrepreneurial goal. It is a career perfect for self-starters, individual practitioners, independent thinkers, and people who wish to live life on their own terms.

The DNP education and degree has been a blessing to the practitioners that obtain it and the community at large. There had never been a degree that promised so much to the community and for the practicing nurse practitioner prior to this. Although the degree has more opportunity to be actualized to its fullest potential in any practice setting, it has the capability to solve problems in all areas that process improvement and where quality care is a goal. This includes academia, hospital settings, corporate board rooms, community forums, public health, local, state, regional, and national leadership forums, and the list goes on. In the words of Dr. Scharmaine Lawson-Baker, DNP, "You won't get wealthy by making house calls, but your spirit will be filled. You won't have a skyline office view, but you will have the cutest 105-year-old lady dressed in her Sunday best with a pot of sweet peppermint tea waiting on you when you arrive for that house call because she knows it's your favorite. It doesn't get any better."[9]

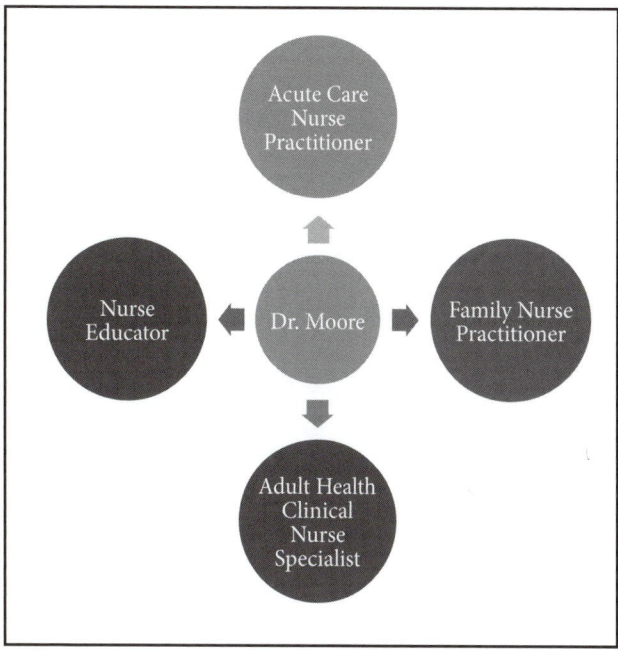

**Figure 3-1.** Personal conceptual framework.

# CONCLUSION: IMPACT OF THE DNP DEGREE

As a result of obtaining the DNP degree, I have been provided with a strong foundation for entrepreneurship. The impact that the DNP Essentials have created provides a strong foundation in which to build a practice. Utilization of the theoretical framework created by the American Association of Colleges of Nursing (AACN) assists in building a lasting relationship with the community and the health care system with the DNP practitioner as a facilitator for both. This foundation suits the needs across disciplines in the health care paradigm. As a DNP practitioner, I am ecstatic about bringing forth the DNP Essentials operationally conceptualized to my patients.

The DNP Essentials outlined demonstrates that AACN was calculating and comprehensive when building a foundation that all clinicians could utilize to bring nursing into the next phase regardless of what path was chosen. In reviewing the Essentials impact of a community-based DNP practice, it is easy to see how this framework suits the need of the community:

1. DNP Essential I: Scientific Underpinning for Practice provides a scientific basis for providing evidence-based care. It explains why care is provided in a particular manner, and its basis is scientific evidence.

2. DNP Essential II: Organizational and Systems Leadership for Quality Improvement and Systems Thinking addresses the quality initiatives that can be completed on patients in the field. Quality of care is essential for optimal patient outcomes. System thinking allows the tying in of patient-side findings back to the health care system. The community provider communicates directly to health care systems about how the patients are faring in the field and what can be done on the health care system side to assist with home care and management. Without clinicians in the field, these systems would be unaware of how their interventions affected outcomes.

3. DNP Essential III: Clinical Scholarship and Analytical Methods for Evidence-Based Practice allow the generation of the evidence that informs the research. As the research scientists create new knowledge, I bring that evidence back to the patient. The generation of evidence creates a cyclical relationship and a continuous need for both clinicians and researchers to improve and optimize outcomes.

4. DNP Essential IV: Information Systems/Technology and Patient Care Technology for the Improvement and Transformation of Health Care includes the integration of a functional comprehensive EHR. Choosing an EHR that allows intuitive documentation, prompts for screenings and testing, communication with vendors (eg, lab, radiology, etc), patient communication, secure messaging, and billing meets all quality indicators. As a part of the Health Insurance Portability and Accountability Act, Affordable Care Act, Centers for Medicare & Medicaid Services, and other regulatory agencies, the inclusion of the EHR in the DNP practice allows for easy integration of the required elements without the worry of how to check off the boxes individually. A good EHR completes all of these items simultaneously. The education in the DNP program did not go in-depth regarding all of the available options, but it did educate on the importance of information systems and technology.

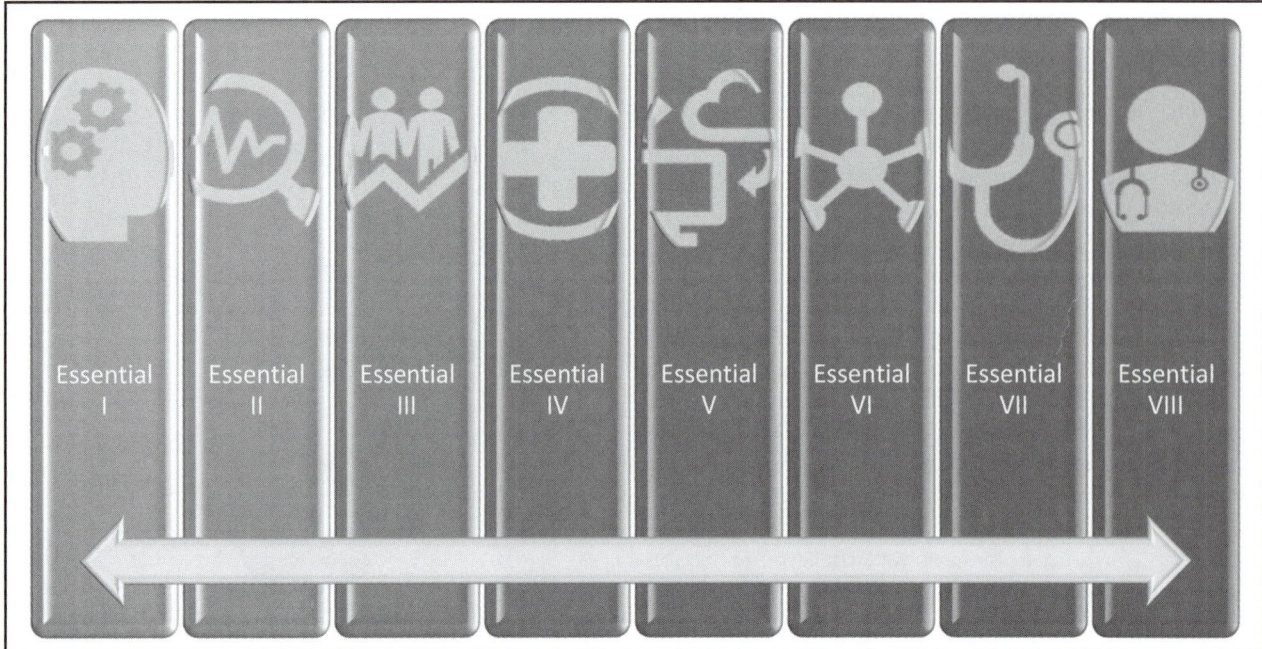

**Figure 3-2.** DNP Essentials.

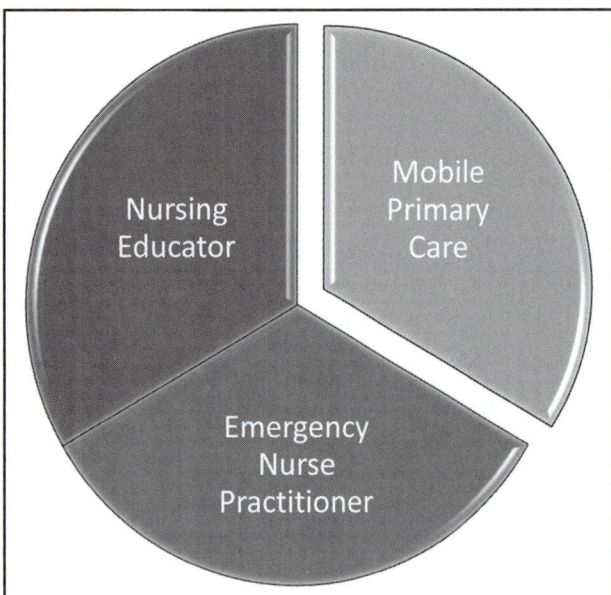

**Figure 3-3.** Personal use of education.

5. DNP Essential V: Health Care Policy for Advocacy in Health Care assisted in understanding why policy and advocacy are essential every day. Advocating for not only the needs of the patient but also the needs of the provider is essential. DNP field practitioners have specific needs that policymakers need to understand. That includes the ability to sign home health orders for the patients they are providing care for, signing for diabetic equipment and supplies, and other limitations that have been placed by regulatory agencies. Supporting the PACS and organizations that take these issues to the policymakers allows them to fight on our behalf more comprehensively. This fight also includes one for FPA, which causes an undue financial burden on DNP field practitioners.

6. DNP Essential VI: Interprofessional Collaboration for Improving Patient and Population Health Outcomes includes generating a network of specialists that includes home health agencies, therapists, imaging centers, and labs to provide the services that will be needed. Knowledge of obtaining public transportation, food pantries and services, and other resources as needed is an essential aspect of providing community health care. The DNP practitioner will not be able to provide all these services alone. They also require a relationship with an in-house physician or service line to admit their patients into the hospital. These relationships require networking. Education in the DNP program emphasized the importance of collaboration, and its importance was quickly realized while putting the practice together.

7. DNP Essential VII: Clinical Prevention and Population Health for Improving the Nation's Health guidelines brought timely screening to community members. This DNP Essential encourages timely screenings, including mammograms, prostate, lipid panels, diabetes, and hypertension, to a community of patients that may not be able to get to a clinic regularly. The act of bringing these screenings to them ensures their timeliness, accurate monitoring, and education in these areas for the population served. The impact of this DNP Essential is tremendous.

8. DNP Essential VIII: Advanced Nursing Practice is a DNP Essential that brought it all together. My expertise as a triple-certified APN is advantageous to the

patients. The courage that the DNP education and scholastic mentoring provided encouraged me to step out on my own with these Essentials as a footstool in which to uphold my practice and how I administer care. I have been trained and tested rigorously according to the standards set by AACN.

Ultimately, earning the DNP degree gave me the confidence, wherewithal, and tools to impact quality patient outcomes for not only Moore Healthcare but my local health care systems. The DNP prepared me to implement evidence, provide care, evaluate the care, network in my community, and inform other providers of care via quality data and outcomes. The DNP degree served as a foundational tool that ultimately prepared me for a role that took my life and career to another level. I would encourage any nurse who wants to move up the career ladder or provide a firm foundation in their entrepreneurship to consider and obtain the DNP degree.

## Acknowledgments

I would like to thank and acknowledge my husband, Martin E. Moore Jr. His role in the development and maintenance of the practice is paramount. His love and ability to push me into my thoughts and dreams is exactly what I needed. He has truly been a partner throughout this process. I would also like to acknowledge my children, Derrick, Alexis, and Ariel. They have always been my inspiration and sources of strength.

## References

1. The essentials of doctoral education for advanced nursing practice. Duquesne University. Accessed June 6, 2019. https://www.duq.edu/assets/Documents/nursing/dnp/_PDF/DNPEssentials.pdf

2. Noonan AS, Velasco-Mondragon HE, Wagner FA. Improving the health of african americans in the USA: an overdue opportunity for social justice. *Public Health Rev.* 2016;37:12. doi:10.1186/s40985-016-0025-4

3. Six domains of health care quality. Agency for Healthcare Research and Quality. Accessed June 6, 2019. https://www.ahrq.gov/talkingquality/measures/six-domains.html

4. Clinical preventive services. HealthyPeople. Accessed June 1, 2019. https://www.healthypeople.gov/2020/leading-health-indicators/2020-lhi-topics/Clinical-Preventive-Services

5. Division of population health. Centers for Disease Control and Prevention. Accessed June 5, 2019. https://www.cdc.gov/nccdphp/dph/index.html

6. Tennessee scope of practice policy: state profile. Scope of Practice Policy. Accessed May 5, 2019. http://scopeofpracticepolicy.org/states/tn/

7. Rules of tennessee department of finance and administration bureau of tenncare. Tennessee State Government. Accessed May 5, 2019. https://www.tn.gov/content/dam/tn/health/documents/1200-13-01.pdf

8. Buppert C. *Nurse Practitioner's Business Practice and Legal Guide.* Jones & Bartlett Learning; 2018.

9. Baker SL. *House Calls 101: The Only Book You Will Ever Need to Start Your Housecall Practice.* A DrNurse Publishing House; 2014.

# SECTION II

## NURSE PRACTITIONER AND CLINICAL NURSE SPECIALIST COLLABORATION EXEMPLAR

# ACUTE CARE DNPs
## IMPROVING INTERPROFESSIONAL PRACTICE ONE PATIENT AT A TIME

*Susanna Sirianni, RN, DNP, ACNP-BC, ANP-BC, CCRN and Maria Teresa Palleschi, RN, DNP, ACNP-BC, CCRN*

## INTRODUCTION

Dr. Sirianni practices with the surgical intensive care unit (SICU) service at a university-affiliated inner-city hospital, where she serves as the lead nurse practitioner (NP) for the hospital. In her clinical role, she manages critically ill and injured patients along with the SICU resident team. She is an integral part of the SICU team serving both as a care provider and mentor to the numerous outside rotating residents on the service and nursing staff.

In addition to her clinical work, Dr. Sirianni has been instrumental in multiple evidence-based practice (EBP) change initiatives. She has an active role in the education of residents, nursing staff, and NP students. Furthermore, she is active on multiple committees both at the hospital and system level. She is the hospital sepsis lead and has helped the hospital achieve a sepsis mortality rate of just more than 10% by ensuring application of EBP.

Dr. Palleschi was the clinical nurse specialist for 22 years over 4 adult medical surgical critical care units in a university-affiliated hospital. She serves as nursing advisor to multiple shared decision-making and performance-improvement councils. Dr. Palleschi has chaired the interprofessional system-level critical care council for more than 5 years and

has developed and revised policies and evidence-based initiatives for the 8-hospital system and 80-hospital enterprise. She has worked in critical care for more than 40 years and has mentored many staff registered nurses, advanced practice registered nurses (APRNs), respiratory therapists, and physicians. A consummate advocate for the bedside clinician patients and families, she has worked diligently to support their engagement and enrichment. Dr. Palleschi has partnered with many intensivists to bring about collaborative evidence-based changes to the critical care environment for the hospital and system enterprise. Because of her experience and education, she has transitioned to a director-level position over sepsis care and Magnet designation for 3 hospitals within the system.

## ROLE CREATION

The Doctor of Nursing Practice (DNP) degree prepares APRNs at the highest level of leadership in practice and scientific inquiry.[1] Upon completion of the DNP degree, APRNs are prepared for a variety of specialized nursing practice roles such as leadership, education, health care policy, and clinical practice. The overarching goal of DNP-prepared nurses is to improve patient care and health care outcomes

Benson LA, ed. *The DNP Professional: Translating Value From Classroom to Practice* (pp 39-49).
© 2021 SLACK Incorporated.

for the population. Utilizing a variety of theoretical models, DNP-prepared nurses evaluate and develop new practice approaches to deal with the ever-changing complex health care arena. The complexity of today's health care issues requires someone with knowledge of system-level change, leadership, and practice expertise to successfully implement the evidence.

Incorporating EBP into daily care is inherent in the practice of the NP and clinical nurse specialist. As advanced practice providers (APPs), both authors were continuously looking for opportunities to improve patient outcomes within their own practices. While in their pre-DNP positions, both APPs were very involved in many initiatives that involved practice changes within the intensive care units (ICUs).

The critical care environment lends itself to many opportunities to incorporate EBP to improve morbidity and mortality. Upon completion of the DNP, the authors took on a broader role in implementing EBP at the hospital, system, and enterprise level. However, the authors quickly realized that other units within the system and enterprise would benefit from the practice changes. The authors evaluated best practices for many hospital initiatives and partnered with the interprofessional team for successful implementation of multiple practice changes. The authors collaborated to address targeted initiatives for improvement including but not limited to sepsis, mobility, nutrition, cost containment through the Choosing Wisely initiative and reduction in hospital-associated infection. The authors became the driving force behind the changes in process and care that extended beyond their own ICUs to the numerous hospital systems within the enterprise. Utilizing the DNP knowledge that the authors gained from coursework and experiential knowledge, the authors were easily able to tailor their roles into that of a DNP-prepared nurse. Although the authors remained in their respective roles, the newly acquired DPN knowledge gave them new insight into the analysis and implementation of changes for multiple initiatives. With this newly acquired knowledge, the authors gained a better understanding of implementing large-scale practice changes and improving health care for patient populations within either the large hospital systems setting or in the community.

# Incorporation of DNP Essentials

The authors have both chaired multiple hospital, system and enterprise-level critical care committees, and initiatives which have resulted in implementation of EBP. Both authors were well seasoned professionals who worked in critical care as APPs for more than 30 years. This experiential knowledge, along with the DNP education, assisted them to integrate science into their practice and facilitated their energy to make evidence-based changes. The highest level of nursing is gained using nursing science that is integrated with

knowledge from many aspects of organizational, biophysical, psychological, and analytical sciences in addition to ethics (DNP Essential I). The DNP authors were leaders in their institutions and brought a balanced perspective using both clinical nurse specialist and NP roles to make changes across the market. Both developed into leaders who assessed the organization needs, identified system concerns, and then led hospital and multiple market level interprofessional committees to drive agendas to meet the needs of current and future patient care populations (DNP Essential II). The enterprise consisted of academic and non-academic affiliated hospitals. An analysis of current critical care practices was conducted by the authors and numerous gaps in standards of care such as sedation practices, mobility, and nutrition were identified. Work groups based on evidence-based literature were developed to initiate change. The authors were strategically selected to lead many of the initiatives given their knowledge, experience in the setting, collaborative approach, influence, and evidence-based nursing backgrounds.

Through analytical and critical analysis of current existing literature, the authors advocated for change and program development (DNP Essential III). They put in place multiple audits and research projects to investigate needs and outcomes of the critical care initiatives. Working collaboratively with many levels of professionals enabled the authors to be successful. Analyzing complex practice and organizational issues was accomplished by engaging and integrating input from multiple types of professionals and facilitated the success of the processes.

The DNP authors decided to team up together and lead 5 separate enterprise-level critical care work groups. Their combined efforts led to critical care evidence-based processes for mobility, sedation, sepsis, targeted temperature management, and nutrition. The authors designed processes to evaluate and monitor outcomes associated with the changes through manual and information technologies (DNP Essential IV). Metrics and policies were associated with each of the work group outcomes and ongoing analyses were initiated at the system-level meeting and at each of the 4 adult hospitals. Each hospital system within the enterprise was also charged with reviewing metrics, outcomes, and developing action plans.

Change and implementation of evidence is always difficult. The status quo is always much easier for individuals and hospitals than making changes, even if the changes will result in better patient outcomes. The authors knew full well that bringing evidence into 80 hospitals would be a challenge, and failure mode analysis revealed many potential barriers. The first barrier or challenge the authors had to overcome was the intensive oversight required by the for-profit enterprise. Making changes to 4 adult hospitals was considerably easier than moving change through 80 hospitals within a for-profit enterprise. The sheer number of diverse hospitals (urban vs community) with very different patient populations seemed insurmountable. Perhaps the most difficult barriers the authors faced was the implementation of EBP in community hospitals that were quite content with the "we have always done it that way" mindset. Patient populations, resources, and engagement of change agents varied across sites. Electronic medical record (EMR) types and versions differed so what worked at one site for electronic charting or alerts did not work at another. Many sites did not have doctorally prepared nurses, and many did not have APRNs. Many of these community hospitals were non-academic and had physicians at the helm of implementation of EBP changes rather than APRNs. While the authors worked collaboratively in their own institutions, collaboration was a bit more challenging in the non-academic setting.

The other huge challenge or barrier that the authors faced was trying to implement EBP while remaining cost neutral. This was extremely difficult when trying to roll out an early mobility (EM) protocol when most of the literature clearly recommended a team for EM. The authors had to develop creative ways to engage staff and looked for inexpensive adjuncts that would help the interprofessional team implement the changes.

# PROFESSIONAL MISSION AND PASSION

Every 2 minutes, someone develops sepsis in the United States, leading to more than 500 deaths per day. The lack of care and causes of death are multifaceted. First and foremost, only 65% (an increase from 22%) of the US population know the word "sepsis." However, while 72% in the United States can recognize the signs and symptoms of stroke, only 12% can recognize the signs or symptoms of sepsis.[2] The lack of recognition of sepsis symptoms leads to a delay in seeking medical assistance which subsequently results in delays in treatment. Early identification and treatment are the mainstay of sepsis survival, yet treatment cannot start if patients do not present to the hospital early in the course of sepsis.

As part of their combined DNP project, the authors researched improving sepsis care in their hospitals and published *An Interprofessional Process to Improve Early Identification and Treatment for Sepsis*. Soon after the publication, both authors experienced sepsis in their own families. Dr. Sirianni's brother died of septic shock at the age 46 and Dr. Palleschi's mother survived septic shock with the onset of acute myeloid leukemia. The pair noted that if their families, who were well aware of sepsis, could be afflicted with the mortality and morbidity of sepsis, what about others who had no concept of the devastating effects of sepsis (DNP Essential V)? In 2015, they partnered with the Sepsis Alliance and started the first-ever sepsis awareness event in Michigan (Stomp Out Sepsis Rochester). This annual event has generated more than $100 000 to date and launched many additional opportunities to spread public awareness regarding sepsis. The authors have partnered with the media to help raise public awareness. They have been featured on the radio and have recorded public service announcements

discussing the signs and symptoms of sepsis and how imperative seeking immediate treatment is to survival. They have also authored articles in community newsletters and have been featured speakers at numerous events and conferences. Recognizing the tremendous need for early identification of symptoms by the public, the authors partnered with the Michigan Hospital Association (MHA) to educate other health care systems on public awareness strategies. In 2017, the authors, together with MHA, were instrumental in having the governor of Michigan declare the month of September as Sepsis Month (DNP Essential V).

Increasing sepsis awareness so more lives can be saved is inherent to what the authors wholeheartedly believe. In 2017, the authors were honored for their ongoing work in sepsis by the Sepsis Alliance in New York City. Sepsis Alliance is a 501(c) nonprofit organization whose mission is to educate the public about sepsis. The nonprofit hosts an annual event to honor Sepsis Heroes, individuals who the charity recognizes as having made a significant contribution to improving sepsis awareness with the public or health care providers.

# BUSINESS PLAN

Upon completion of their DNP work, the authors returned to their roles as APPs. While neither author had a change in title, they embraced their DNP education to expand their roles. Since neither their titles, nor their roles, changed initially, no formal business plan was utilized to delineate the DNP impact. With this new knowledge, the authors were quickly able to demonstrate that the cost of a DNP-prepared nurse was minute when compared to the benefits associated with having nurses practice at that level. The authors facilitated the initiation of multiple projects that reduced ICU discretionary cost per day such as medications, length of stay (LOS), laboratory, and utilization of resources without increasing mortality. The average ICU cost per day varied based on patient populations and ranged from $210 to $360 with observed vs expected mortality of 0.3 to 0.6 compared to other enterprise units of $240 to $315 with observed vs expected mortality of 0.7 to 1.2. Pharmacy costs per day related to pain management and sedation strategies decreased from $350 per day to $275 in each ICU. Utilizing knowledge of science-based theories and concepts (ie, DNP Essentials), the authors were able to drive major EBP changes that improved care, costs, and decreased morbidity and mortality. The value and expertise that the DNP brings to the table far exceeds the cost of their employment.

Critically ill patients in the ICU usually require extensive diagnostic imaging and laboratory studies in the initial hospital days to determine their course of treatment. However, staff members often continue to perform routine diagnostic testing and phlebotomy, whether or not it is indicated. While radiographic imaging is an important diagnostic tool in the management of the critically ill adults, excessive and cumulative imaging leads to unnecessary radiation exposure and increased risk of cancer.[3] In fact, evidence notes that very few routine chest x-rays result in any significant change in patient management.[4] Routine phlebotomy has also been shown to be detrimental to patient outcomes leading to hospital-acquired anemia (HAA). Approximately 98% of ICU patients have anemia by hospital day 3, largely due to phlebotomy. This practice leads to an increase in cost due to infections and blood transfusions.[5] In 2014, the Society of Critical Care Medicine (SCCM) released the Choosing Wisely initiative in an attempt to reduce unnecessary chest x-rays and phlebotomy.[6] The authors assisted an interprofessional group with the development guidelines for ordering of both x-rays and phlebotomy. The group partnered with the information technology department to develop reports to monitor compliance. The use of new guidelines led to a decrease in both unnecessary phlebotomy and lab draws thereby decreasing discretionary cost of care. Laboratory costs reduced from $140 per day to $127 per day and chest x-ray frequency reduced from 0.88 to 0.73 per day.

Implementation of the numerous evidence-based interventions has led to cost avoidance as evidenced by a decrease in LOS from 6 days to 4.5 days and a decrease in ICU morbidity. In 2012, the authors led several practice initiatives based on the American Association of Critical-Care Nurses (AACN) and SCCM's Assess, Prevent, and Manage Pain; Both Spontaneous Awakening Trials (SAT) and Spontaneous Breathing Trials (SBT); Choice of analgesia and sedation; Delirium: Assess, Prevent, and Manage; early mobility and exercise; and Family engagement and empowerment.[7] The implementation of the ABCDEF bundle incorporated major changes in practice that involved nursing, respiratory therapy, physical therapy, and APPs along with intensivists and residents. ICU care prior to the implementation of the ABCDEF bundle resulted in higher costs of care related to cost of sedation medications, ventilator days, number of patients with delirium, and both hospital and ICU LOS. The presence of delirium alone increases LOS and cost of care. Furthermore, patients who have delirium have an increased likelihood of death within 6 months or 1 year.[8] Everyday a patient on the ventilator is delirious, their chance of mortality increases by 10%. Each of the 4 hospital systems demonstrated a marked decrease, especially in the amount of benzodiazepines utilized. The use of continuous benzodiazepine drips are known to cause delirium. Reports were developed to demonstrate the number of patients who tested positive for delirium on a daily and monthly basis (Table 4-1). The number of patients with delirium decreased substantially with the implementation of evidence-based sedation practices. Changes included delirium screening every 12 hours, improvement in mobility, reduction in benzodiazepine use, facilitating sleep practices, and increased focus on timely liberation from mechanical ventilation. The authors utilized these reports as a way of monitoring a change in practice. By decreasing benzodiazepine use, the authors were able to decrease delirium and subsequently allowed patients to be weaned off the ventilator more readily.

Furthermore, patients were more able to participate in EM which resulted in a decrease in deconditioning. The implementation of the ABCDEF bundle led to a decrease in both ICU and hospital LOS, a decrease in hospital cost, and more importantly a decrease in patient deconditioning. By mitigating the risk of deconditioning and the development of post-intensive care syndrome (PICS), physical, psychological, and cognitive morbidities associated with substantial burden for patients, families, and society are reduced.[9] Many patients do not return to work because of persistent functional or cognitive impairments and have ongoing medical conditions that require substantial support that reduces quality of life.

The authors noted that this work is just the tip of the iceberg when learning and identifying ways to decrease the devastating side affects of PICS and ICU acquired weakness. With continued research and implementation of new evidence, practitioners can only improve patient outcomes. After the successful implementation of the ABCDEF bundle at the 4 adult hospitals, it was later incorporated at the enterprise level. The research they led proved that the mobility educational intervention was sustainable over time. While it is difficult to clearly attribute a monetary value on mobility practice changes, patient LOS was reduced after the implementation of the bundle. In addition to the practice changes led in the critical care arena, the authors also demonstrated a reduction in cost in relation to sepsis care. The cost of caring for a patient with sepsis varies greatly depending on the severity of the sepsis and whether or not the sepsis was present on admission. The cost of care can range from $16 324 for a septic patient without organ dysfunction to $24 638 for a patient with severe sepsis to as much as $38 298 for the patient with septic shock.[10] The development of sepsis in the hospital leads to an even bigger cost burden of approximately $51 022 vs $18 023 for the patient with sepsis that is present on admission.[10] The variability in cost of care is impacted by the severity of sepsis but also depends on the hospital and ICU LOS, length of antibiotics, organ failure, and complications associated with sepsis. The average LOS for sepsis is affected by the severity of sepsis ranging from 4.5 to 16 days depending on the degree of sepsis.[11] The LOS for sepsis is approximately 75% higher than other conditions.[12] However, early identification and implementation of the sepsis bundle throughout the hospital demonstrates a decrease mortality and cost of care.[13] Similar outcomes were actualized by the authors through their DNP research project and ongoing EBP implementation. The authors demonstrated a significant decrease in cost of care and a decrease in the sepsis mortality (all cause) from 16% to 10.26% (Table 4-2). National mortality from severe sepsis at the time varied from 14.7% to 29.9% depending on patient population and methodology of analysis.[13]

## Table 4-1

### DAILY DELIRIUM SCORING

| INTENSIVE CARE UNIT | TOTAL PATIENTS | TOTAL PATIENTS WITH A/B RESPONSE | % WITH A/B RESPONSE TOTAL | TOTAL $\geq 4$ | % $\geq 4$ |
|---|---|---|---|---|---|
| 4E | 22 | 3 | 13.64% | 4 | 18.18% |
| 5B | 26 | 2 | 7.69% | 4 | 15.38% |
| 5C | 22 | 4 | 18.18% | 6 | 27.27% |
| 5W | 11 | 1 | 9.09% | 1 | 9.09% |
| 6W | 19 | 2 | 10.53% | 4 | 21.05% |
| 8W | 18 | 1 | 5.56% | 5 | 27.78% |
| 2N | 16 | 2 | 12.50% | 3 | 18.75% |
| 2W | 26 | 6 | 23.08% | 3 | 11.54% |
| 2S | 25 | 4 | 16.00% | 2 | 8.00% |
| Total | 319 | 25 | 7.84% | 30 | 10.60% |

## Table 4-2

### SEPSIS CARE MORTALITY

| FACILITY | ALIVE | EXPIRED | TOTAL PATIENTS | MORTALITY |
|---|---|---|---|---|
| *All Sepsis Diagnosis Codes* | | | | |
| Hospital 1 | 98 | 11 | 109 | 10.09% |
| Hospital 2 | 62 | 8 | 70 | 11.43% |
| Hospital 3 | 45 | 7 | 52 | 13.46% |
| Hospital 4 | 105 | 10 | 115 | 8.70% |
| Detroit Medical Center total | 315 | 36 | 351 | 10.26% |
| *Severe Sepsis Without Septic Shock R65.20* | | | | |
| Hospital 1 | 31 | 2 | 33 | 6.06% |
| Hospital 2 | 8 | 0 | 8 | 0.00% |
| Hospital 3 | 6 | 0 | 6 | 0.00% |
| Hospital 4 | 19 | 1 | 20 | 5.00% |
| Detroit Medical Center total | 65 | 3 | 68 | 4.41% |
| *Severe Sepsis With Septic Shock R65.21* | | | | |
| Hospital 1 | 15 | 8 | 23 | 34.78% |
| Hospital 2 | 12 | 6 | 18 | 33.33% |
| Hospital 3 | 8 | 5 | 13 | 38.46% |
| Hospital 4 | 16 | 6 | 22 | 27.27% |
| Detroit Medical Center total | 51 | 25 | 76 | 32.89% |

# OUTCOMES AND INCORPORATION OF EVIDENCE-BASED PRACTICE

Prior to the DNP work, the hospital system did not have a formal EBP process for identification and management of patients with sepsis. While the hospitals had attempted to implement components of the identification and management process, the success of the implementation was disjointed and less than favorable. An electronic sepsis alert to help identify septic patients early had been developed and incorporated into the existing EMR. The sepsis alert had been developed to automatically page the rapid response team (RRT) nurse with critical sepsis data with a goal of having the RRT evaluate the patient and start evidence-based sepsis care and management.

The EMR sepsis alert process was intended to be used hospital wide, thereby affecting providers including but not limited to: registered nurses, APPs, physicians, and patient care associates. As the EMR alert was rolled out, the authors quickly identified that neither the sepsis alert process nor the implementation of the EB sepsis protocol were successful. In order to bridge this gap, the authors provided intensive interprofessional education to many levels of health care providers. Furthermore, the DNP research initiated by the authors included the innovative introduction of point of care testing for lactate by RRT for patients with suspected infection and systemic inflammatory response syndrome criteria. The interprofessional education and practice change resulted in an increased application of the evidence facilitated by the RRT sepsis protocol process developed by the authors. The RRT sepsis protocol enhanced the completion of the sepsis bundle in a timely manner. Evidence identifies that administering antibiotics early, obtaining blood cultures, and normalization of lactic acid levels along with fluid resuscitation demonstrate an improvement in patient care outcomes. The DNP research project resulted in many of the improvements in implementation of important components of sepsis care including reduction in the time to administration of antibiotics by 91 minutes (from 182.09 minutes pre-intervention to 91.62 minutes post-intervention). Interprofessional education also resulted in more frequent blood cultures (from 35% pre-intervention to 42% post-intervention ) and the completion of more lactic acid tests (from 25% pre-intervention to 48% post-intervention ) being drawn in patients who were deemed septic. Given the challenges associated with practice changes, the authors assisted with the development and application of electronic EBP order sets. The DNP research also resulted in an improvement of use of the sepsis PowerPlan.[3]

While the authors were successful in bridging the knowledge gap at 4 adult hospitals, they soon realized that other hospital systems could benefit from some of the strategies that they utilized to improve outcomes. The authors soon partnered with the MHA and helped other systems improve sepsis care, mobility, and delirium. Dr. Palleschi worked with the MHA and a delirium toolkit was developed for use to prevent, identify, and treat delirium from a non-pharmacological and pharmacological perspective.[14]

Recognizing that sepsis extends beyond the hospital walls, the authors began to work with the Michigan Peer Review Organization (MPRO) to help educate nursing home administrators regarding sepsis. The authors participated in a series of process improvement initiatives with a variety of nursing homes educating them on implementation of EBP for sepsis. They educated the facilities on the research behind the sepsis bundles, discussed practice change strategies, and coached them through some of the struggles associated with practice change.

Immobility is associated with increased ventilator acquired pneumonia (VAP), ICU and hospital LOS, mortality, ICU acquired weakness, as well as an increased risk for deep vein thrombosis, and pressure injury. In addition, as the population continues to age resulting in an increase in older patients, the development and implementation of interventions to prevent or interrupt mobility limitation becomes even more essential. Immobility and frailty are some of the most important hospital-adverse events resulting in a poor prognosis for independent functioning, increased use of health care services, and mortality.[15,16]

Combating barriers to mobility are numerous, including but not limited to the following: staffing, equipment, lack of protocol, lack of leadership support, referrals for physical therapy or occupational therapy, delirium, over sedation, safety, patient hemodynamic tolerance, rotating staff and residents, and skeptical clinicians.[16] Immobility and deconditioning affect multiple organs and systems, yet nurse adoption remains a barrier. Patient safety, staffing, potential complications, patient habitus, and equipment are also frequently cited as barriers to adoption.

The DNP-prepared authors chaired an enterprise-wide interprofessional group to develop and implement protocols for mobility and pain, agitation and delirium (PAD) with input from physicians, nurses, respiratory therapists, pharmacy, and physical and occupational therapists. Delirium scoring was initiated to identify patients at risk. A 5-phased EM protocol was developed to address deleterious effects of immobility. Bariatric, stroke, and deconditioned patients presented a challenge for meeting the mobility goals for nursing and therapy staff, therefore the implementation of novel therapy was required. Verticalization/tilting beds allowed registered nursing staff, in collaboration with physical and occupational therapists, to stand deconditioned and bariatric patients. By progressively increasing the degrees of height and time in the vertical position, staff could evaluate patient tolerance and strength in a safe and controlled environment.

# DATA MINING AND PRACTICE OUTCOMES

The authors partnered with the information technology department to develop reports to help track the progress of the numerous initiatives. Several reports have been developed and adjusted based on review of the data obtained. Some reports that were generated were quite helpful, while others did not provide meaningful data. While the concept of an electronic alert to help identify sepsis is definitely helpful, it is only helpful if one can answer the question of whether sepsis is present. Therefore, the report on sepsis alerts and compliance with the bundled elements of care was redesigned to report data on patients with a discharge diagnosis of sepsis.

Some of the automated reports that were developed include the following:

- A daily sepsis report that includes all patients with a sepsis alert:
  - The report includes some demographic data time of the alert, whether the sepsis PowerPlan was used, if there was compliance with the 3-hour bundle, alert form, and emergency department alert form.
- A daily sepsis report developed to aid in tracking bundle compliance:
  - The report includes a number of important data points: site, patient name, and identifier; age; weight; time of arrival to emergency department or unit; source of infection; sepsis PowerPlan use; if patient was admitted to ICU; onset of sepsis; lactate draw time; lactate value; time of antibiotic administered; time between blood culture, lactate drawn, and antibiotic administration; time between onset and antibiotic administration; time of fluid administration; time of vasopressor administration; and attainment of 3-hour bundle (by indicating a yes or no). The report is submitted daily and reviewed for improvement opportunities related to sepsis bundle compliance and care.
- A sepsis monthly report was developed to capture all patients with a coded discharge diagnosis of sepsis that includes mortality, compliance with the 3-hour bundle elements, use of the PowerPlan, and discharge disposition (Table 4-3).

The authors studied whether an evidence-based educational intervention influenced critical care nurses' decisions to institute early mobilization in the ICU. This study was conducted in the adult ICUs at 3 Midwest academic medical center hospitals. Using a pre- and post-test, non-experimental design, data was collected at 4 intervals: Time 1 baseline (pre-test, n = 102); Time 2 after an educational intervention to the critical care nurses (88); and Time 3 and 4 data collected following 2 quarters post-intervention (a post-test with interrupted time-series design, n = 110 and 110, respectively). Immobility and deconditioning poses a huge threat for both patients and staff. In an effort to decrease the deleterious effects of immobility, the authors developed a 5-phased EM protocol by leading an interprofessional group consisting of an RN, physician respiratory therapist, physical therapist, occupational therapist, and patient care associate or tech. Interprofessional educational modules were developed and reinforcement occurred during bedside rounds as part of the ABCDEF bundle. These methods provided a basis for informing and reinforcing new processes. Preselected orders were added to admission order sets for "initiate mobility protocol" and EMR RN documentation for real time phase of mobility.

The RNs attitude and practice decisions to mobilize ICU patients matched or exceeded the phase of mobility based on readiness criteria and was sustained over time. The results showed a statistically significant difference ($P < .001$) from Time 1 baseline to Time 2. Additionally, each post-test period was found to be similar as there was no statistically significant difference between Time 2, Time 3 and Time 4 ($P = .180$).

Post-intervention critical care RNs increased mobility and ambulated most patients more frequently and in congruence with their ability when compared to baseline data. However, opportunities remained for challenging patients related to patient size and debilitation.

Weakness due to immobility contributes to disability and reduced quality of life for months or years following ICU discharge. Evidence-based education to improve and enhance patient mobility can impact and influence the attitudes and practice of nurses and thereby improve patient outcomes. Attitudes and practice decisions of critical care nurses were influenced by the provision of evidence-based EM education. The results were statistically significant and sustained over time.

Post-implementation findings and a performance improvement pilot identified that recognizing deconditioning and the care of bariatric patients presented the greatest challenges for the staff. The APRNs in this study went back to the drawing board and investigated other options for care including verticalization. A pilot of technology associated with verticalization/tilting of patients using both beds and a chair was performed. Further research in the efficacy of verticalization technology that could safely mobilize and strengthen patients without extraordinary staffing support or equipment is required.

The authors were able to demonstrate that evidence-based education targeted at improving and enhancing patient mobility can impact and influence the attitudes and practice of nurses and thereby improve patient outcomes. Attitudes and practice decisions of critical care nurses were influenced

## Table 4-3

# SEPSIS DATA ANALYSIS AND COMMUNICATION: EXAMPLE OF MONTHLY REPORT DEVELOPED FOR CENTERS FOR MEDICARE & MEDICAID SERVICES SEPSIS 3-HOUR BUNDLE COMPLIANCE

| PATIENT # | MISS REASON | UNIT | SEPSIS PRESENTATION | CASE COMMENTS | OUTCOME |
|---|---|---|---|---|---|
| x66 | Initial lactate level collection | 2S | Sepsis presentation: 2/8 1235<br><br>Source: 1235<br><br>ICU progress note: severe sepsis<br><br>SIRS: n/a<br><br>Organ dysfunction: n/a | • To hospital 1/31 for aneurysm clipping. Admitted to ICU after surgery 1/31 at 2235.<br><br>• No sepsis alert fired. Sepsis PowerPlan was not used.<br><br>• 2/7: patient had elevated theta/beta ratio, WBC; BC and U/A sent (UTI). ABX started. No clear organ dysfunction documented. ICU progress note says "Severe Sepsis." No lactate ordered. | Home |
| xx321 | Initial lactate level collection | 8W | Sepsis presentation: 2/8 0035<br><br>Source: 2/8 0035<br><br>H&P: severe sepsis<br><br>SIRS: n/a<br><br>Organ dysfunction: n/a | • To emergency department 2/7 C/O missed HD, SOB, diarrhea, pain, fever, upper respiratory infection symptoms. Treated for possible influenza. Admitted to 8W 2/7 at 2057.<br><br>• Sepsis alert did not fire. Sepsis PowerPlan was not used.<br><br>• H&P: "Severe Sepsis"; lactate was done in emergency department at 1521 2/7, but no lactate was ordered/ done within 3 hours of time zero ("Severe Sepsis" documentation time). | Expired |
| xx8341 | Broad spectrum or other antibiotic administration | 4W | Sepsis presentation: 2/23 2330<br><br>Source: 2125<br><br>Progress note: Problem list includes infection with drug resistant organism; CXR at 0108: pneumonia<br><br>SIRS: 2330 T 38.8; heart rate: 120<br><br>Organ dysfunction: 2330; SBP 88 | • To emergency department 2/17 C/O leg pain, missed his surgery appointment for RLE amputation. Admitted to 4W 2/17 at 1415. Had surgery 2/19; 2/24 at 0108 CXR showed pneumonia.<br><br>• Sepsis alert fired 2/23 at 2322. Sepsis PowerPlan was not used.<br><br>• The resident ordered blood cultures 2/24 at 0006, antibiotics not ordered until 2/24 at 1000, 9 hours after CXR result showed pneumonia. | Facility |

Abbreviations: ABX = antibiotics; BC = blood cultures, C/O = complains of; CXR = chest x-ray; HD = hemodyalisis; H&P = history and physical; RLE = right lower extremity; SBP = systolic blood pressure; SIRS = systemic inflammatory response syndrome; SOB = shortness of breath; T = temperature; U/A = urinalysis; UTI = urinary tract infection; WBC = white blood cell count.

by the provision of evidence-based EM education. The results were statistically significant and sustained over time.

To support the mobility initiative, daily delirium reports were developed to include delirium scores and those patients that were not able to participate in the scoring process. Active in-house patients responses are from "yesterday" through the current runtime of the report (see Table 4-2). By implementing the ABCDEF bundle, the authors were able to decrease the number of patients who developed delirium. Patients who did develop delirium were identified earlier in their hospital course and the authors were able to develop strategies to mitigate the effects of delirium. Staff nurses were educated to discuss delirium during daily intensivist rounds and seek interventions for risk reduction and treatment for those who screened positive.

# INTERPROFESSIONAL COLLABORATION

As DNP-educated NPs, both authors have opportunities to collaborate with many professionals. Interprofessional collaboration is paramount in order to implement EBP. As APPs, the authors interact daily with many interprofessional team members to ensure that patients receive the best possible care. Daily interactions with nurses, physicians, physical, occupational, and respiratory therapists, and patient care associates allow for opportunities to educate and reinforce best practice as implemented. The authors have both chaired a number of hospital, system, and enterprise-level interprofessional committees as they facilitated the implementation of the following programs, protocols and guidelines:

- Sepsis protocol, order sets, PowerPlan, sepsis alert development and implementation
- Point-of-care testing for sepsis alert
- RRT protocol and process development and management for acute sepsis care
- Early and aggressive mobility program
- PAD guidelines
- Enteral nutrition protocol
- Targeted temperature management
- Choosing Wisely initiative
- Standardization of critical care equipment across market
- Standardization of critical care policies across market
- Alcohol (ethanol) withdrawal guidelines and order set
- Market level shared decision-making council

As sepsis care experts, the authors envisioned a process across the hospital market for analyzing data in relation to bundle compliance. They advocated for reports and personnel to review clinical data and processes to identify ongoing gaps and facilitate communication and education to RN staff members and providers. A role was developed in the hospitals to advocate for protocol-based care. A system-wide interprofessional committee was developed to review site analyses and facilitate market level changes.

In addition, the authors helped develop the ICU standardization and structure policy delineating expectations for interprofessional teams for the system which was later adopted enterprise wide. The policy encompassed SCCM standards for the intensivist role, coverage and rounding, interprofessional team composition, definitions for levels of critical care, collaboration with nursing leadership for management and clinical concerns, and data measurement processes.

# PROFESSIONALISM

Knowledge is power and in order to be powerful, DNPs must share their research and knowledge so that patients can have excellent outcomes. Numerous opportunities to disseminate the knowledge acquired through the DNP coursework and research are available and are utilized. The authors initially presented the results of their research at numerous venues in lecture or poster format. Initially, the authors gave local nursing presentations at their respective hospitals and for the Michigan Council of Nurse Practitioners, Madonna University, and Wayne State University. The presentations quickly expanded to include presentations for their physician and APP colleagues as well. The authors quickly began to disseminate their research and knowledge of sepsis management at prestigious conferences such as the AACN's National Teaching Institute & Critical Care Exposition and the National Doctors of Nursing Practice Conference. They have also developed webinars for various organizations as another method to disseminate knowledge of sepsis.

As their expertise in sepsis continued to grow, they published in the *Journal for Healthcare Quality* and in local journals such as *Healthcare Weekly, Italian American News,* and *Neighborhood News*. Recognizing that sepsis identification extends beyond the hospital, the authors partnered with emergency medical services to educate them on the importance of early identification and treatment. Furthermore, the authors work with MPRO to help educate nursing homes and subacute rehab facilities on the perils of sepsis. Future plans include working with home care agencies to help identify sepsis early and to reduce sepsis readmissions.

Together with the Sepsis Alliance, the authors continue to increase public awareness. They have partnered with local US and Canadian radio hosts to help spread the message about early identification of sepsis as they enter the fifth year of the annual Stomp Out Sepsis event. In addition, the authors serve as advisors on the Sepsis Alliance's Sepsis Coordinator Network, helping to provide best practice resources and guidance to sepsis coordinators and other health care providers across the country. The DNP-prepared authors have been expert panel speakers at sepsis-coordinator sessions at AACN National Teaching Institute and have provided multiple webinars for professionals and the public.

Education of our future DNPs and NPs is imperative. Acting as adjunct faculty and capstone members of several DNP projects, the authors have been able to impact the education of future DNPs. Both authors are active preceptors for numerous universities in both the DNP and NP programs at Madonna University, Wayne State University, Michigan State University, University of Michigan–Flint, Vanderbilt University, and University of South Alabama where they help shape our future DNPs.

The role of the DNP extends far beyond the walls of educational institutions, hospitals, clinics, and nursing homes. Leadership roles offer yet another opportunity to put the DNP at the forefront of health care by influencing large groups of providers. As president of the Michigan Council of Nurse Practitioners, Metro chapter and the regional representative for the Metro and Ann Arbor chapters, Dr. Sirianni was able to discuss the role of the DNP and mentor future NPs and DNPs.

# Conclusion: Impact of the DNP Degree

As a result of obtaining their DNP degrees, the authors were instrumental in the development of critical care and interprofessional strategies for their hospital market and enterprise for mobility, sedation, sepsis, targeted temperature management, and nutrition. Sepsis care research was conducted that resulted in practice change, improvement in bundle compliance related to time to antibiotic administration, and an increase in frequency of blood cultures and lactic acid completion. All-cause sepsis mortality reduced from 16% to 10.1%. Data reporting was developed and designed to identify bundle compliance in patients with the diagnosis of sepsis. Through education, advocacy, and fundraising, the authors continue to foster sepsis care through prevention approaches in the community and the professional setting.

The DNP authors were instrumental in initiatives that resulted in financial cost avoidance and a reduction in LOS from 6 to 4.5 days. Mobility improvements resulted in a decrease in the frequency of benzodiazepine use, an increased focus on liberation from ventilation, and a reduction in delirium. The pair were responsible for innovations in mobility by advocating for new technology in verticalization treatments to promote weaning from ventilation for improved mobility, especially in the morbidly obese.

The DNP is not a job or a role, but rather a degree that provides individuals with the tools to critically analyze the literature and develop processes and structures to improve patient morbidity and mortality. The DNP education allows nursing professionals the opportunity to lead teams to participate in partnerships, nurture role model behavior, mentor staff to influence and impact changes in practice, and improve patient care outcomes. Whether it is in the hospital, in the community as an activist, on nursing advisory boards, presenting work at conferences or the Michigan Council of Nurse Practitioners, acting as faculty, or mentoring students and peers, the span of influence is infinite.

Find your passion. Make a difference…. Research it…. Teach it…. Live it…. Love it….

# Acknowledgments

No one has been more important to us in the pursuit of our DNP than our family members. Most importantly, we wish to thank our loving and supportive husbands, Joe Sirianni and Arduino Palleschi. Without them, our educational pursuits would not have been possible. We are grateful for the love and support of our children who witnessed their mothers in school for most of their lives. We are especially indebted to Dr. Nancy O'Connor and Dr. Regina Malley who were visionary in the development of our DNP and life's work.

We would like to express our gratitude to all our mentors, interprofessional colleagues, and nursing staff members who have facilitated and supported all our initiatives and life's work. We are forever grateful to our chief nursing officers Shawn Levitt, BSN, MBA, MS, RN, FACHE, CPHQ and Christine M. Bowen, MSN, RN, CCRN for their support to allow us the latitude and confidence to implement changes.

# References

1. The essentials of doctoral education for advanced nursing practice. American Association of Colleges of Nursing. October 2006. https://www.aacnnursing.org/Portals/42/Publications/DNPEssentials.pdf

2. Patients & Families. Sepsis Alliance. https://www.sepsis.org/education/patients-family/

3. Initiative to reduce unnecessary radiation exposure from medical imaging. U.S. Food & Drug Administration. June 2019. https://www.fda.gov/Radiation-EmittingProducts/RadiationSafety/RadiationDoseReduction/ucm199994.htm

4. Fasanya A, Sharara R, Leap J, Pelinescu A, Mickus T, Thirumala R. Routine daily chest radiograph in the medical ICU: stop it! the evidence is not there. *Chest.* doi:http://dx.doi.org/10.1016/j.chest.2016.08.308

5. Ahmed AH. Prevention and management of hospital acquired anemia. *Hosp Med Clin.* 2014;3(1):71-84.

6. Critical care societies collaborative: critical care. Choosing Wisely. January 2014. Accessed July 7, 2019. http://www.choosingwisely.org/societies/critical-care-societies-collaborative-critical-care/

7. Morandi A, Brummel NE, Ely EW. Sedation, delirium and mechanical ventilation: the "abcde" approach. *Curr Opin Crit Care.* 2011;17(1):43-49. doi:10.1097/mcc.0b013e3283427243

8. Salluh J, Wang H, Schneider EB, et al. Outcome of delirium in critically ill patients: systematic review and meta-analysis *BMJ.* 2015;350:h2538.

9. Barr J, Fraser GL, Puntillo K, et al. Clinical practice guidelines for the management of pain, agitation, and delirium in adult patients in the intensive care unit. *Crit Care Med.* 2013;41(1):263-306.

10. Hopkins R, Mitchell L, Thomsen G, Schafer M, Link M, Brown S. Implementing a mobility program to minimize post-intensive care syndrome. *AACN Adv Crit Care.* 2016;27(2):187-203. doi:10.4037/aacnacc2016244

11. Paoli CJ, Reynolds MA, Sinha M, Gitlin M, Crouser E. Epidemiology and costs of sepsis in the United States: an analysis based on timing of diagnosis and severity level. *Crit Care Med.* 2018;46(12):1889-1897. doi:10.1097/CCM.000000000000334

12. Overview of the national (nationwide) inpatient sample (NIS). Agency for Healthcare Research and Quality. Accessed August 1, 2019. https://www.hcup-us.ahrq.gov/nisoverview.jsp

13. Hall MJ, Williams SN, DeFrances CJ, Golosinskiy A. Inpatient care for septicemia or sepsis: a challenge for patients and hospitals. National Center for Health Statistics. June 2011. Accessed August 1, 2019. https://www.cdc.gov/nchs/data/databriefs/db62.pdf

14. Dammeyer JA, Mapili CD, Palleschi M, et al. Nurse-led change: a statewide multidisciplinary collaboration targeting intensive care unit delirium. *Crit Care Nurs Q.* 2012;35(1):2-14. doi:10.1097/cnq.0b013e31823b1fec

15. Schweickert W, Pohlman M, Pohlman A, et al. Early physical and occupational therapy in mechanically ventilated, critically ill patients: a randomised controlled trial. *Lancet.* 2009;373(9678):1874-1882. doi:10.1016/s0140-6736(09)60658-9

16. Engel HJ, Needham DM, Morris PE, Gropper MA. ICU early mobilization: from recommendation to implementation at three medical centers. *Crit Care Med.* 2013;41:S69-S80. doi: 10.1097/CCM.0b013e3182a240d5

# SECTION III

## CLINICAL NURSE SPECIALIST EXEMPLARS

# CHAPTER 5

# THE NURSING CLINICAL QUALITY SPECIALIST

## A PERFECT POSITION TO CAPITALIZE ON THE DNP ESSENTIALS

*Linda A. Benson, DNP, ACNP-BC, CPHQ*

## INTRODUCTION

The setting for this practice is a 1009-bed academic teaching hospital along the Western Central–Gulf Coast of Florida. The hospital is the number 1 ranked hospital in the Tampa Bay area according to the US News and World Report. It is also recognized in 5 different specialties. The hospital is both Joint Commission accredited and a 4-time Magnet-designated facility.

The nursing clinical quality specialist (CQS) is a member of the nurse executive team. The CQS reports directly to the chief nursing officer (CNO) who is also a senior vice president of the organization. The CNO has her Doctor of Nursing Practice (DNP) degree as well. This allows for a deeper understanding of how to fully integrate the DNP skill set into practice. Initial job requirements included preference for a DNP degree and Certified Professional in Healthcare Quality (CPHQ) certification. I entered the position with my DNP degree and was able to obtain my CPHQ certification within 9 months of taking the position. Shortly after hire and as part of orientation, I met with all nursing divisional leaders, most in either director or vice president roles as well

as other multidisciplinary leaders within the organization. I was able to learn more about the organizational culture and do an initial evidence-based gap analysis on nursing practice. In retrospect, meeting key organizational stakeholders during orientation proved invaluable. The CQS is employed within nursing administration and is a member of the nurse executive team. I also collaborate closely with the chief quality officer, meeting monthly to ensure that department of nursing goals align with the organizational goals.

In general terms, the CQS role is similar to that of a typical clinical nurse specialist role with the addition of the DNP skill set. The CQS is responsible for coordinating the department of nursing quality improvement initiatives. Annually, the CQS in conjunction with the CNO develops the comprehensive nursing strategic quality plan for the fiscal year. The quality plan needs to be inclusive of both nursing sensitive process and outcome measures. The measures need to be evidence based and data driven. The CQS is responsible to ensure involvement and engagement by all levels of nursing staff toward attainment of the designated quality metrics. This is accomplished through ongoing continual data dissemination including a quality committee structure that supports this communication.

Benson LA, ed. *The DNP Professional:*
*Translating Value From Classroom to Practice* (pp 53-61).
© 2021 SLACK Incorporated.

# CURRENT ROLE: THE NURSING QUALITY STRATEGIC PLAN

The nursing CQS is the linchpin for the department of nursing's quality structure. Annually for each fiscal year, a strategic plan is developed and proposed by the CQS for review and approval first by the CNO and then the entire nurse executive team. A Donabedian framework has been utilized wherein both process and outcome measures are placed onto the plan to be monitored throughout the year.[1]

Based on the Institute of Medicine's initial work in *Crossing the Quality Chiasm*, quality has been defined as having the following domains: safety, timeliness, effectiveness, efficiency, equity, and patient-centeredness.[2] The Agency on Healthcare Research and Quality (AHRQ) proposed to target a decline in hospital-acquired conditions to save 8000 lives and $2.9 billion in costs by the end of calendar year 2019. Various patient safety indicators (PSIs) have been designated by AHRQ for hospitals to monitor.[3] The 4 major categories comprising the nursing quality strategic plan include patient care experience, infection prevention, prevention of harm and injury, and the PSIs 11, 12, and 13 (Table 5-1).

# EXPANSION OF THE ROLE WITHIN THE PRACTICE SETTING: COMMITTEE STRUCTURE AND GEMBA WALKS

The role of the CQS expanded from that of my predecessor as the DNP Essentials were incorporated. A robust quality committee structure was developed so that both data dissemination and specific evidence-based strategies to optimize the data could be put into place. The Nursing Leadership Committee is chaired by the CNO. The CQS primarily presents the data related to the metrics and where the department has been successful and where opportunities still exist. This meeting takes place on a monthly basis. The CQS chairs the Nursing Quality Council which also meets monthly. The intent of this committee is to present strategies for improvement of the strategic plan metrics that have not reached goal. The CQS formulates interventions after gaps between practice and the evidence have been identified. Other nursing committees also report up to the Nursing Quality Council such as the Nursing Peer Review Committee. Case studies

are presented on an as needed basis with either success stories from high performing units or units that have identified opportunities that exist with recommendations for practice that may affect the entire department. The CQS also presents to the different nursing divisional committees with frequencies determined by either the associated nursing vice president or director. The CQS also developed a unit-based nursing Quality Champions program. The Quality Champions are unit-based clinical nurses or nurse clinicians who served as quality experts by attending monthly meetings where new data and interventions to improve the data are discussed. They disseminate data through a variety of methods including posting the data for display on the unit quality boards. They present unit-based data in staff meetings or education blocks and discuss urgent topics in shift huddles. The quality champions also provide surveillance and monitoring of quality processes and identify opportunities for performance improvement of the nursing metrics on a unit level. The CQS has mentored several of the nursing quality champions to present quality improvements or innovations internally during Nurses' Week and National Healthcare Quality Week as well as at regional and national nursing conferences.

The CQS discussed the idea of conducting Gemba walks utilizing the nursing quality boards. The CNO was familiar with the concept and agreed to this implementation. *Gemba* refers to the place where value is created.[4] In manufacturing, the gemba is the factory floor. It can be any site such as a construction site, sales floor, or where the service provider interacts directly with the customer. For nursing, gemba occurs on the nursing unit as an activity that takes management to the frontlines. Gemba walks denote the action of going to see the actual process, understanding the work, asking questions, and learning. It is also known as a fundamental part of Lean management philosophy.[5] While this process began with the Toyota company, it is still widely used today to allow management to interact with, engage, and empower the staff at all levels. Using Strengths, Weaknesses, Opportunities, Threats (SWOT) analysis techniques taught at the doctoral education level, the CQS routinely conducts quality rounds. This SWOT analysis technique has also been taught by the CQS to the nursing leadership across all divisions. Staff are empowered to discuss all quality metrics on the nursing quality boards on each unit. It is paramount that staff are allowed to celebrate their successes and discuss what they do well first. Next, staff are asked to identify weaknesses and opportunities for those metrics that are not meeting goal and what interventions are needed to meet the targeted goal for the fiscal year. Frontline staff are optimally positioned to discuss threats or barriers that they are facing. I often take notepads on rounds so that I can address barriers immediately after rounds. This follow-through is important so that staff feel that they are supported by the nursing administration.

**Table 5-1**

# Nursing Strategic Plan

| DOMAIN | METRIC TYPE | METRIC WITH DESCRIPTION |
|---|---|---|
| Patient Experience | O/P | Manager/bedside shift report, drivers for nursing communication goal<br>Manager ("yes" response)<br>Bedside shift report ("always" response) |
| | | Proactive toileting and response to call lights, key driver for responsiveness goal |
| | | Bundled care and door closure, key drivers for quiet at night goal |
| | | Indications and side effects, key drivers for medication communication goal |
| | | Anticipating discharge needs/providing the after visit summary are drivers for discharge communication goal |
| Safety | P | CAUTI bundle compliance, key driver to preventing CAUTIs |
| | O | CAUTI/1000 catheter days |
| | P | CLABSI bundle compliance, key driver to preventing CLABSI |
| | O | CLABSI/1000 catheter days |
| | P | Multidrug-resistant organism handwashing and decolonization, key drivers preventing multidrug-resistant organisms<br>Handwashing compliance (nursing) |
| | | Chlorhexidine gluconate and mupirocin decolonization |
| | O | *Clostridioides difficile* infections/1000 patient days |
| | | Methicillin-resistant *Staphylococcus aureus* infections/1000 patient days |
| | P | Overall chlorhexidine gluconate operative bath compliance per patient, key driver to reduce surgical site infections |
| | | Mobilization (out of bed) is a key driver to decrease incidence of HAPIs |
| | | Incidence of patients with pressure injuries |
| | | Utilization of fall mats and remaining within arm's reach while toileting patients, key drivers for reducing falls with injury |
| | | Utilization of restraint alternatives is a key driver for restraint reduction |
| | P | Blood administration vital signs at 15 minutes is a key driver in the prevention of an anaphylactic reaction from transfusion |
| Mortality | P | PSI 11 post-operative respiratory failure: provision of incentive spirometry and oral care are key drivers in preventing post-operative respiratory failure<br>Oral care compliance |
| | | Incentive spirometry documentation |
| | | PSI 12: perioperative venous thromboembolism: applying sequential compression devices and reducing missed doses of anticoagulation are key drivers in reducing perioperative venous thromboembolism<br>Sequential compression device documentation |
| | | Missed doses of anticoagulation incremental reduction |
| | | PSI 13: post-operative sepsis rate/sepsis mortality prevention |
| | | Obtaining blood cultures and antibiotics within 3 hours of patient sepsis presentation are key drivers in reducing sepsis mortality. Blood cultures drawn before antibiotics. |
| | | Antibiotics administered within 3 hours of identification of sepsis |

Abbreviation: O/P = outcome and process metrics.

# Incorporation of the DNP Essentials: Evidence-Based Practice, Interprofessional Collaboration, Policy Review and Ethics

It is the responsibility of the CQS as the quality leader for the department of nursing to perform evidence-based reviews periodically to determine where gaps occur in practice. Several methods can be used, including but not limited to traditional literature searches, reviewing best practices identified through databases, webinars or conferences, and reaching out to best practice facilities. All have been useful in developing strategies to optimize the nursing quality metrics. Practice must be evidence based and data driven. The CQS has leveraged data to drive the nursing department and unit-specific performance when needed. Quality town meetings were recently initiated to assist units that may not be meeting specific metrics as strategies, opportunities, and barriers were addressed. These meetings were conducted by the CQS but the CNO attended and was instrumental at getting rapid-fire solutions to barriers identified. Examples of evidence put into practice and data mining with information technology (IT) department collaboration will be elaborated more specifically further into this chapter.

The CQS also collaborated with multiple interprofessional key stakeholders to advance both the department of nursing and organizational goals. Monthly meetings are held with the chief quality officer as together they co-chair both the organizational sepsis committee and the code blue committee.

There has been opportunity to work with physician providers via continuous performance improvement teams (CPIT) that were in place within the organization. These teams are multidisciplinary in nature. The CQS has worked with the medicine CPIT to assist with treatment of sepsis and alcohol withdrawal. In addition, data was provided to the neuroscience CPIT to outline opportunities for the service line.

There is also routine collaboration with pharmacy on many different projects including improvement in medication education, improvement in antibiotic administration times for sepsis, decreasing delays in chemotherapy times, optimizing practice to screen for and treat delirium and review of medication adverse events from a system perspective.

The CQS has reviewed or developed policies, procedures, or protocols as needed in relationship to the nursing strategic metrics. The standards have been presented to the nursing standards committee, and the nurse executive team as needed. Also, as it relates to the DNP Essentials, the CQS is the nursing executive team representative on the hospital-wide ethics committee.

# Cost-Benefit Analysis of Role in Relationship to Nursing Sensitive Indicators

The CQS is able to demonstrate a cost savings since joining the organization due to a significant reduction in hospital acquired conditions. The average cost per incident has been estimated to be $10700 for hospital acquired pressure injuries (HAPIs), $13316 for falls, and $45814 for central line bloodstream infections (CLABSIs).[6-8] The CQS served as an organizational leader for nursing quality by providing unit-specific data on progress toward goals and ensuring that the most current evidence was put into practice. To prevent HAPIs the CQS promoted use of criteria-based prophylactic skin dressings and micro-positioning for the critically ill patient population. These were adopted by the Wound and Skin Project Team and then further implemented. To reduce falls, unit-specific fall strategic programs were put into place. Based on AHRQ recommendations, the CQS developed policy, procedure, and education for obtaining orthostatic blood pressures to prevent falls.[9] Soon after starting, the CQS collaborated with the clinical research nurse to find and implement a new pediatric falls risk assessment tool as opportunities existed within that patient population as staff felt that their existing tool was not providing enough sensitivity. With regards to CLABSI reduction, the CQS developed evidence-based criteria for central venous line removal that was incorporated into the electronic medical record for daily review of device necessity. In the 5 years that the CQS has been at the practice setting and provided multi-level leadership for nursing on quality, there has been a 94.3% reduction in HAPIs, a 28.7% reduction in falls, and a 59.3% reduction in CLABSIs. This would have resulted in an approximate concomitant cost savings of $7682032 for all 3 nurse-sensitive hospital-acquired conditions over a 5-year period.

# Implementing Evidence Into Practice to Improve Nursing Processes for Patient Safety Indicators 11, 12, and 13

In order to increase nursing awareness of the AHRQ and value-based purchasing, the CQS added nursing process measures for PSIs 11, 12, and 13 to the nursing strategic plan.

PSI 11 is post-operative respiratory failure. Initially, ventilator associated pneumonia (VAP) prevention bundle and oral care were placed onto the nursing strategic plan. The compliance with the VAP bundle remained high across those units with bundle compliance for ventilated patients generally greater than 95%. Eventually, incentive spirometry was put in its place to improve lung expansion based on AHRQ recommendations.[10] Oral care improved over time to reach goal at greater than 91% compliance. At the same time, aspiration pneumonia demonstrated a 13% reduction.

Venous thromboembolism (VTE) reduction was the focus for PSI 12 which looks at perioperative VTE. Nursing-sensitive processes added to the strategic plan were reduction in missed doses of anticoagulation and sequential compression device (SCD) wearing. The literature demonstrates that missed doses of prophylaxis increased VTE risk and improving adherence to prophylaxis compliance decreased VTE rates.[11,12] A gap analysis was performed to determine if the facility's current practice differed from best practice evidence-based standards. It was determined that the most significant opportunity was for a reduction in missed doses of anticoagulation. The missed doses could be a result of either patient refusal or those doses held prior to diagnostic testing. Initial emphasis was placed on decreasing refused doses of prophylaxis through a variety of methods. Nurses were encouraged to determine the etiology of the patient and family refusal. Topical pain products were made available to the nursing staff. Use of Lovenox (enoxaparin) when appropriate was encouraged for those patients refusing due to thrice daily injections. Education was ramped up so that pharmacists and providers collaborated with nursing staff to discuss refusals with patients and families. VTE case reviews were led by the CQS. The case reviews were multidisciplinary in nature with providers (many times nurse practitioners or physician assistants) presenting the cases and determining the appropriateness of anticoagulation based on Caprini Risk Assessment Scale.[13] Nursing leadership reviewed the cases for missed doses of anticoagulation, SCD documentation, mobility, and central venous line removal based on criteria. The CQS also worked with Interventional Radiology and the Gastroenterology Center to identify low-risk procedures and add verbiage to the electronic medical record so consideration would be given to not hold anticoagulation. The CQS also participated in a hospital-wide committee to examine ways to reduce VTE which included changes to order sets to better identify risk. Overall, there was a 24% reduction in refused doses of anticoagulation through enhanced patient education and a 67% reduction in overall VTE PSI 12 rate to below the national median.

PSI 13 focuses on post-operative sepsis but a more global approach was taken to reduce sepsis mortality hospital wide. The nursing processes placed onto the strategic plan were to obtain blood cultures before antibiotics and broad-spectrum antibiotics within 3 hours of sepsis presentation. The CQS worked to have blood culture draws prioritized including those obtained by phlebotomy. Collaborating with pharmacy,

Zosyn (piperacillin/tazobactam) was stocked in the medication delivery systems on each unit to expedite antibiotic delivery. The medical director for informatics brought to the organization a predictive analytics tool for sepsis. This tool was built into the electronic medical record and provided a probability score of the likelihood that the patient would develop sepsis. Based on previous work with an anion gap acidosis report, the CQS determined the score that would be used to contact the rapid response team for a septic patient. The CQS over a series of months rolled out the predictive analytics tool to advanced practice providers, medical doctors, a select group of pharmacists, and then the staff registered nurses. Also, once the staff registered nurses were educated on the analytics, the score was then placed onto the charge nurse tool so that patients with a high probability of sepsis would be immediately recognized. In the interim, a sepsis specialist who was a master's-prepared registered nurse had her previous role converted with a shift toward a primary focus on sepsis. She reported to the CQS the majority of the time. System-wide solutions were put into place and interprofessional case reviews that focused on compliance with the sepsis bundle were initiated. The sepsis mortality index declined for 5 consecutive months after the onboarding of the sepsis specialist who partnered with the CQS.

# DATA MINING, PRACTICE OUTCOMES, AND BENCHMARKING

Technology can be leveraged to yield data that in turn is utilized by nursing management and staff to transform and improve practice. Informatics serves as the linchpin providing the information on which to build and change practice. The CQS joined forces with the business intelligence analysts (BIAs) and system analysts in the IT department to develop a series of compliance and safety reports to optimize the nursing scorecard measures. The CQS presented the desired report logic and the IT professionals constructed the report build. The compliance reports covered a series of nursing sensitive indicators including but not limited to pain reassessment, utilization of the Pasero Opioid-Induced Sedation Scale,[14] SCD documentation, chlorhexidine gluconate bath completion, device infection bundle implementation, vaccine administration, and blood administration. Specialty unit compliance reports were also developed. For example, compliance with the American Association of Critical-Care Nurses' ABCDEF bundle was also tracked with separate reports for ventilator days, delirium screening, and mobilization.[15] Compliance with normothermia in the operating room was tracked as well. At present, there are nearly 20 total compliance reports that are disseminated monthly.

With the initial reports, compliance was analyzed to determine if the percentage improvement was statistically significant. Independent *t* tests were conducted to determine

| Table 5-2 |
|---|

### PRE- AND POST-STATISTICAL SIGNIFICANCE FOR ELECTRONIC MEDICAL RECORD COMPLIANCE REPORT DEVELOPMENT

| REPORT | P VALUES USING INDEPENDENT T TEST TO COMPARE COMPLIANCE PRE- AND POST-REPORT |
|---|---|
| Pain reassessment within 1 hour | < .01 |
| Chlorhexidine gluconate pre-operative bath | < .01 |
| SCD documentation every 4 hours | < .01 |
| Vaccinations | < .01 |
| Mobility documentation twice daily | .01 |
| Urinary tract infection bundle | .05 |

the statistical significance of the compliance improvements. All nursing metrics demonstrated statistically significant improvement after 6 months of report build and usage (Table 5-2).

Data was mined or obtained from the electronic medical record. The data was utilized to engage and motivate nursing leadership and staff to achieve the nursing quality metric goals. Data was disseminated electronically and discussed at meetings and on walking quality gemba rounds.

Benchmarking has been stressed by the CQS so that comparisons can be made against similar hospitals. For nursing excellence, the hospital has recently received its fourth Magnet designation. The National Database of Nursing Quality Indicators (NDNQI) was utilized for hospital benchmarking with the following nurse sensitive indicators: HAPIs, falls with injury, catheter associated urinary tract infections (CAUTIs), and CLABSIs.[16] Unit-based benchmarking is available for multiple drug resistant organism data. The CQS served as the database site coordinator for the hospital ensuring that all data were entered for inpatient, ambulatory, operative, and emergency areas. Benchmarked data were displayed as z scores on the unit nursing quality boards. Education was completed by the CQS for the nursing leadership and staff on the definition of this benchmark statistic being equal to the hospital mean minus the population mean divided by the standard deviation. This was then incorporated into quality gemba rounds so that staff could speak to whether their unit was better than benchmark on any of the 4 major metrics. In order to maintain Magnet designation, the hospital had to have the majority of its unit metrics better than benchmark.

The Vizient Clinical Data Base was also utilized for quality benchmarking.[17] The Vizient Clinical Data Base uses the Institute of Medicine definition incorporating safety,

mortality, efficiency, effectiveness, equity, and patient centeredness. Nursing most typically influences safety, patient centeredness, and mortality. The safety domain incorporates more than 90 indicators but includes metrics on HAPIs, falls with injury, CAUTIs, CLABSIs, multiple drug resistant organisms, post-operative respiratory failure, VTE, and sepsis. Nursing had addressed patient centeredness by including the metrics of nursing communication, responsiveness, quietness of hospital environment, medication communication, and discharge communication on the nursing strategic plan. As of this writing, both patient safety and patient care experience were between the top 10th to 20th percentile when compared to other hospitals in the database. Nursing has focused on mortality primarily by attempting to recognize and treat sepsis more appropriately via a bundled approach. Going forward, nursing will add efficiency and effectiveness process measures to the strategic plan in order to address length of stay and readmissions.

## INTERPROFESSIONAL COLLABORATION

As previously mentioned, the CQS engages in interprofessional collaboration by chairing committees with the chief quality officer and attending both service line and CPIT meetings. The CQS was recently asked to coordinate the oncology service line initiatives for the Commission on Cancer (CoC) accreditation. Initiatives being studied include decreasing the admit to chemotherapy start times, improving genetic screening for cancer patients, and decreasing readmissions post-chemotherapy. This responsibility generally includes providing data so that the interventions to be taken are clarified. The CQS worked with the nursing director of the service line, both surgical and medical oncologists, and nursing leadership for the inpatient oncology units and the director for the infusion center. After working with an IT system analyst, several reports were constructed. The admit time to chemotherapy start time report looked at various points in the process map to identify opportunities for discussion with the interprofessional workgroup.

After conducting literature reviews and finding the evidence lacking, the CQS formed multidisciplinary committees to address 2 other quality initiatives: both delirium resolution times for older adults and CAUTI reduction in the emergency room (ER). The interprofessional performance improvement initiative to decrease delirium resolution times for older adults was born from the fact that 11% to 56% of older adults develop delirium during their hospitalization.[18] This leads to concomitant increases in length of stay, cost, post-operative complications, functional decline, new requirements for nursing home placements, and increased mortality. Based on previous literature, the time to delirium resolution ranges from 4.2 to 7.4 days.[19]

The purpose behind this interprofessional performance improvement initiative was to identify older patients on an Acute Care of the Elderly (ACE) unit with delirium more expeditiously by using an evidence-based screening tool and to reduce delirium resolution times. As patients screened positive for delirium with the Intensive Care Delirium Screening Checklist (ICDSC), a list of nursing interventions was made available in the electronic medical records from which the registered nurses could individualize their patient care. The registered nurses could also activate consults to the unit-based pharmacist for medication reviews and to the psychiatric nurse resource team for a review of both delirium etiologies and interventional strategies. A chart review of the first 12 patients who screened positive for delirium revealed that the mean day to develop delirium from admission was 6.0 days. Documented delirium resolution was 1.84 days. Subsequently, an automated report was built and demonstrated a quarterly report for the ACE unit with 87 episodes of delirium and an 18-hour mean resolution time. Through the utilization of a proven screening tool and activation of multidisciplinary consults, older patients on an ACE unit had earlier resolution of the symptoms of delirium as compared to that previously published.

After review, internal data suggested that an opportunity to reduce insertion-related CAUTIs in the ER existed. Because a majority of the catheters are inserted in the ER, a change was piloted involving dual-licensed personnel insertion and implementation of a "safety time-out." As part of our continuing efforts to improve the quality of patient care, a group that included the CQS and nursing research specialist, representatives from the ER, and the infection prevention department collaborated on strategies to reduce CAUTI rates in the ER. The evidence shows that there are 3 steps in the process where opportunities for improvement can be made: insertion, compliance with maintenance and care of the catheter, and timely and appropriate catheter removal.

The practice change involved 2 licensed personnel first reviewing together the essential procedural steps for urinary catheter insertion derived from the policy. The catheter was then inserted by an registered nurse with either a registered nurse or licensed practical nurse being solely responsible to ensure that proper technique was followed for the essential procedural steps during insertion. The procedure was stopped if proper sterile technique was not followed. A data collection checklist developed by the CQS was completed and signed post-procedure indicating that proper technique had been followed. As a result, the hospital reduced its indwelling urinary catheter utilization ratio by 23% among patients in its emergency department (ED). It also decreased the number of insertion-related CAUTI attributed to the ER by 75% ($P = .05$).[20] The CAUTI rate in the ER went from 6.9 infections per 1000 catheters inserted to 1.7 per 1000 in 18 months. Insertion-related CAUTI was considered any CAUTI occurring within 7 days of insertion of an indwelling urinary catheter. The utilization ratio was based on the number of urinary catheters inserted per 1,000 ER visits. Due to the success of the pilot, dual person urinary catheter insertion has now become standard practice in the ER. In addition, it is considered on a hospital-wide basis for specific cases with difficult insertion where technique may be jeopardized during insertion.

# PROFESSIONALISM

After graduating with my DNP degree, I looked to publish my capstone project. At the time, I was practicing as a nurse practitioner on an all–nurse practitioner rapid response team. My capstone project focused on the impact of this team on sepsis outcomes. There is a definite realization that nurse practitioner outcomes are not always measured or disseminated, so I felt it was important to publish our model and the sepsis outcomes. Having published multiple times before, I was not a novice to publication. However, finding the journal to be the right fit for my manuscript proved to be slightly daunting. From out right rejection to publisher agreement to print only a few pages of the manuscript due to page space limitations, I found some initial frustration with this publication journey. Finally, I was able to find the right fit with the journal editor from the *Dimensions of Critical Care Nursing* who agreed to publish my manuscript in its entirety.[21] Persistence paid off.

My DNP education also highlighted for me the importance of legislative involvement. I was fortunate enough to be able to incorporate some legislative policy review for my state senator in Michigan as part of my DNP practicum. My state senator was also the chair of the Senate Committee on Health Policy. I was able to review bills that were pending before the committee and provide my senator with valuable input from the viewpoint of a DNP student. During this same time, the state of Michigan was making legislative determinations on allowing nurse practitioners, certified nurse-midwives, and clinical nurse specialists to prescribe Schedule II to V drugs under delegation and non-scheduled drugs autonomously. I was able to discuss the importance of this with the senator so that advanced practice nurses could practice to the full extent of their education. I would recommend a legislative health policy practicum be incorporated as a small portion of the main DNP practicum.

Due to educational preparation for both the clinical nurse specialist and nurse practitioner roles (master's and post-master's education), I have been fortunate to practice in both roles solely in acute care hospital settings. During my professional career, I have always been active in my professional organizations including both local chapters and at the national level. I have served as a local American Association of Critical-Care Nurses chapter president, as well as a clinical nurse specialist regional consultant for the American Association of Critical-Care Nurses. I have also been fortunate to present at national conferences for the National Association of Clinical Nurse Specialists, the American Association of Nurse Practitioners, and the National Doctors of Nursing Practice Conference. Participation in professional organizations and conference presentations has served to increase my leadership skill set and presentation capabilities.

Since obtaining my DNP, I have had the opportunity to precept multiple Bachelor of Science in nursing students with their leadership projects, master's students with their capstone proposals, and DNP students with their capstone projects. I find that working with the DNP students to help develop and then implement their projects to be a rewarding experience for both student and preceptor. I was honored to receive the 2018 Excellence in Preceptor/Mentor Award from the Florida Organization of Nurse Executives. Giving back by precepting, mentoring, and role modeling is an important part of the profession.

## Pearls/Takeaways

Incorporation of the DNP Essentials into my role as the nursing CQS was made markedly easier by reporting to a CNO who not only was DNP-prepared herself, but understood the value of having a DNP-prepared advanced practice nurse to lead the nursing quality initiatives. Her support to an outside hire proved invaluable as well and allowed for the success of the DNP-led CQS position.

In moving the quality initiatives forward, it was of paramount importance that all levels of nursing were involved. Change within nursing related to quality was made possible by first performing evidence to practice gaps. Adaptation to change will only occur after the rationale and evidence have been shared. Serving as the change agent by using scientific underpinnings is at the crux of all DNP education. Data mining is also emphasized in DNP programs. It is important to drive change toward goals in not only nursing but with all disciplines. Benchmarked data is the strongest indicator of quality performance as hospital data is compared against similar 500-plus bed academic teaching facilities. As emphasized in DNP practicums, involvement of key interprofessional stakeholders in multidisciplinary initiatives is vital to ensure success of the projects.

Project outcomes must be measured as part of DNP-led projects. Outcomes may involve clinical change, functional improvement, patient satisfaction, and/or cost savings. It is important to both measure and disseminate our findings to add to the body of nursing knowledge, particularly as it pertains to the body of knowledge on DNP impact.

## Conclusion: Impact of the DNP Degree

As a result of obtaining my DNP degree, I have been able to implement change on a systems level having substantial organizational impact. An overall nursing strategic plan that identified nursing sensitive indicators fit into the organizational Institute of Medicine model that was emphasized within the DNP curriculum. Gap analyses were performed to determine opportunities between identified evidence-based best practices and actual practice. New DNP data-mining skill sets allowed for report logic development in collaboration with IT in order to optimize both process and outcome measures. My CQS role allowed me to implement the various performance tools and strategies outlined in the DNP curriculum. As part of Lean philosophy, the frontline staff were engaged in quality through gemba walks. As emphasized in DNP education, key stakeholders were involved in system interprofessional quality initiatives.

Over a 5-year time frame, there was a significant decrease in hospital-acquired conditions particularly those that nursing impacted directly. Evaluation of our performance shows that the hospital is performing better than NDNQI benchmarks in the nursing sensitive indicators for HAPIs, falls with injury, CAUTIs, and CLABSIs when compared to other academic teaching facilities with more than 500 beds. There has been a 94.3% reduction in HAPIs, a 28.7% reduction in falls, and a 59.3% reduction in CLABSIs resulting in more than $7.5 million in savings. Post-operative respiratory failure rate decreased 51.1% and VTE rate decreased 20.9%. Sepsis mortality demonstrated 6 data points below the median indicating a significant change. The hospital has a 10th percentile safety ranking in the Vizient Clinical Data Base.

Having earned the DNP degree, I was ultimately poised and positioned to impact quality outcomes both for the discipline of nursing and across the organization. A DNP degree specifically prepares nurses to be able to evaluate and implement evidence, successfully engage in data mining, and employ various quality improvment tools to optimize both quality processes and outcome measures.

# REFERENCES

1. Donabedian A. *An Introduction to Quality Assurance in Health Care.* Oxford University Press; 2003.

2. Institute of Medicine Committee on Quality of Health Care in America. *Crossing the Quality Chasm: A New Health System for the 21st Century.* National Academy Press; 2001.

3. Patient safety indicators benchmark tables. Agency for Healthcare Research and Quality. Accessed June 15, 2019. https://www.qualityindicators.ahrq.gov/Downloads/Modules/PSI/V60-ICD09/Version_60_Benchmark_Tables_PSI.pdf

4. Womack JP, Shook J. *Gemba Walks.* Lean Enterprise Institute; 2011.

5. Cohen RI. Lean methodology in health care. *Chest.* 2018;154(6):1448-1454.

6. Spetz J, Brown D, Aydin C, Donaldson N. The value of reducing hospital-acquired pressure ulcer prevalence: an illustrative analysis. *J Nurs Adm.* 2013;41(4):235-241.

7. Wong CA, Recktenwald AJ, Jones ML, Waterman BM, Bollini ML, Dunagan WC. The cost of serious fall-related injuries at three midwestern hospitals. *Jt Comm J Qual Patient Saf.* 2011;27(2):81-87.

8. Zimlichman E, Henderson D, Tamir O, et al. Health care-associated infections: a meta-analysis of costs and financial impact on the US health care system. *JAMA Intern Med.* 2013:173(22):2039-2046.

9. Preventing falls in hospitals toolkit. Agency for Healthcare Research and Quality. Accessed June 15, 2019. https://www.ahrq.gov/professionals/systems/hospital/fallpxtoolkit/fallpxtk-tool3f.html

10. Toolkit for using the AHRQ quality indicators. Agency for Healthcare Research and Quality. Accessed June 15, 2019. https://www.ahrq.gov/sites/default/files/wysiwyg/professionals/systems/hospital/qitoolkit/combined/d4h_combo_psi11-postoprespfailure-bestpractices.pdf

11. Louis SG, Sato M, Geraci T, et al. Correlation of missed doses of enoxaparin with increased incidence of deep vein thrombosis in trauma and general surgery patients. *JAMA Surg.* 2014;149(4):365-70.

12. Patil S, Ayad M, Kaushal S, Gopal K, Patel B. Reducing the missed doses of VTE pharmacological prophylaxis is associated with reduction in VTE rate. *Chest.* 2017;152(4 suppl):A460. doi:https://doi.org/10.1016/j.chest.2017.08.487

13. Caprini, JA. Risk assessment as a guide for the prevention of the many faces of venous thromboembolism. *Am J Surg.* 2010;199(1 suppl):s3-s10.

14. Pasero C, McCaffery M. Monitoring sedation: it's the key to preventing opioid-induced respiratory depression. *Am J Nurs.* 2002;102(2):67-69.

15. Balas MC, Vasilevskis EE, Burke WJ, et al. Critical care nurses' role in implementing the "abcde bundle" into practice. *Crit Care Nurse.* 2012;32(2):35-47.

16. Montalvo I. The national database of nursing quality indicators. *The Online Journal of Issues in Nursing.* 2007;12(3):manuscript 2. doi:10.3912/OJIN.Vol12No03Man02

17. Clinical data base. Vizient. Accessed June 1, 2019. https://www.vizientinc.com/our-solutions/clinical-solutions/clinical-data-base

18. Siddiq N, House AO, Holes JD. Occurrence and outcome of delirium in medical in-patients: a systematic literature review. *Age Ageing.* 2006;35(4):350-364.

19. Flaherty JH. The evaluation and management of delirium in older persons. *Med Clin N Am.* 2011;95:555-577.

20. Rhone C, Breiter Y, Benson L, et al. The impact of two-person indwelling urinary catheter insertion in the emergency department using technical and socioadaptive interventions. *J Clin Outcomes Manag.* 2017;24(10):451-456.

21. Benson L, Hasenau S, O'Connor N, Burgermeister D. The impact of a nurse practitioner rapid response team on systemic inflammatory response syndrome outcomes. *Dimens Crit Care Nurs.* 2014;33(3):108-115.

# CHAPTER 6

# The Clinical Nurse Specialist as Chronic Disease Expert

## THE SYNTHESIS OF THE CLINICAL NURSE SPECIALIST COMPETENCIES AND DNP ESSENTIALS

*Ileen Craven, DNP, CNS, MSN, RN-BC*

## Introduction

In 2011 I obtained a Doctor of Nursing Practice (DNP) degree from Chatham University in Pittsburgh, Pennsylvania. In January of 2012, I was recruited by Vidant Medical Center (VMC), a 900-bed rural academic medical center in Greenville, North Carolina. I was VMC's first DNP. For the first 14 months of employment I was a diabetes clinical nurse specialist (CNS), focusing on the chronicity of diabetes, working with nurses, patients, families, treatment team members, and the health system to achieve better outcomes related to readmissions, persistent hyperglycemic events, and hypoglycemia. In March of 2013, I became a medicine CNS working on general medicine units helping care for patients with acute illnesses and chronic comorbidities, which included diabetes, end stage renal disease (ESRD), chronic obstructive pulmonary disease (COPD), heart failure, depression, and other chronic conditions that often plague patients in our communities. Vidant Health (VH), the parent company of VMC, serves 29 counties in eastern North Carolina, all of which are rural, with many patients having little to no health insurance, and all having VH as their primary source of care when hospitalized and after discharge. My position as a CNS in medicine is to assist patients and families with better outcomes, reduce length of stay, and readmissions. In addition, I serve as a clinical expert for the patients and families, nurses, treatment team, and health system. The fusion of the *CNS Core Competencies*[1] and the *Essentials of Doctoral Education for Advanced Nursing Practice*[2] directly influences my role of a DNP-prepared CNS, demonstrating how to best serve VMC and the patients of the 29 counties in eastern North Carolina.

## Practice Setting

VMC is a 900-plus bed academic medical center and Level 1 trauma center located in Greenville, North Carolina, which has a population of 92 000 and whose main employers are VMC and East Carolina University. VH, the parent company of VMC, serves 29 counties, encompasses 8 hospitals, and has more than 12 000 employees, and more than 90 physician practices.[3] VMC is VH's largest hospital, which includes a medical facility, children's hospital, heart institute, and cancer center. In fiscal year 2017, VH cared for more than 63 000 hospitalized patients, had 272 000 emergency visits, and more than 332 000 office visits.[3]

VMC also has achieved Magnet status from the American Nurses Credentialing Center. Magnet-status

Benson LA, ed. *The DNP Professional: Translating Value From Classroom to Practice* (pp 63-75).

hospitals exhibit excellence in professional status and nursing care to patients, along with dissemination of best practices.[4] Magnet hospitals are also known for the quality of safety culture, quality of nursing experience, and increased community awareness leading to philanthropic gifts.[4]

Eastern North Carolina is a rural area, with rampant poverty, scattered access to healthy foods, and where chronic diseases such as diabetes and heart disease are passed along from generation to generation of families. VH's mission is to serve all patients of rural eastern North Carolina[5] who enter their doors regardless of economic or social status.

# ROLE IN PRACTICE SETTING

There are 6 CNSs that practice at VMC. The other 5 CNSs practice in oncology, surgery/trauma, vascular access, cardiac intensive care, and neonatal intensive care. I am the only CNS in medicine and the only one with a DNP degree. I am asked to conduct literature reviews, ensuring best practices are evidence based and understood by the nursing staff.

I practice on 5 general medicine units whose capacity is 160 patients. General medicine patients are routinely admitted through the emergency room by attending physicians whose specialties include nephrology, family medicine, and internal medicine. Hospitalists also admit patients in medicine. Nurse practitioners and physician assistants work with all providers except nephrology. Many patients are admitted for acute exacerbations of chronic illnesses related to diabetes, heart disease, COPD, and ESRD, with many of the renal disease patients on dialysis. Many of our patients have multiple comorbidities and are often hospitalized for complications of their chronic illnesses and for other illnesses which can include sepsis, pneumonia, bacteremia, influenza, and other infectious processes.

I am VMC's first CNS with a vast knowledge of chronic diseases and how multiple comorbidities can be affected during a hospitalization when the stress response is paramount. There are many times when a patient may be admitted for pneumonia or sepsis but suffers respiratory distress due to several factors that have to do with the infectious process and its role in exacerbations of chronic disease. Bedside nurses see me as the clinical expert who can assess a patient for a variety of symptoms, deciding if the patient's acuity requires a change from general medicine to a higher level of care. I have a long-standing relationship with the providers and often notify them of this change in patient status and ask them to reassess the patient or provide measures, such as intravenous fluids or changes in medications that will assist the patient. There are times when a patient will be transferred to a higher level of care such as an intermediate or intensive care unit. On general medicine units 6 patients are cared for by a nurse and nursing assistant. On intermediate and intensive care units there are lower nurse-patient staffing levels.

For 6 years I have taught all newly graduated nurses about diabetes management and education through Diabetes Core. Diabetes Core is necessary because up to one-third of our patients have diabetes or hyperglycemia. The newly graduated nurses are hired in nurse residency cohorts 4 times a year. Teaching Diabetes Core demonstrates to nurses my expertise in diabetes management, and these nurses often consult me to see a patient for a variety of reasons: persistent hyperglycemia, persistent hypoglycemia, the patient's poor understanding of diabetes, newly diagnosed diabetes diagnoses, the inability to afford medication, and the lack of follow-up care. I am also consulted by providers and case managers for the same reasons. Though I am assigned the 5 units as my primary focus, medicine patients are often hospitalized throughout the hospital and I will see patients when consulted. Consults are placed by phone, when I see providers or nurses in interdisciplinary rounds, or formally in our electronic health record.

One of the medicine unit's specialties is caring for ESRD patients who are often on dialysis. Every month, new residents and interns work with attending providers to care for these patients. ESRD patients have complex medical needs due to the complexity of the disease and the comorbidities associated with ESRD. These comorbidities can include diabetes, heart failure, autoimmune disorders, cardiac issues, and others. Patients are often admitted for infections at their catheter sites or other infectious disease processes. Many of these patients are readmitted frequently due to these complex issues, but also due to failure to have dialysis when necessary, depression due to their many comorbidities, and the risk of infections being high in this patient population. I know many of these patients well and will participate in interdisciplinary rounds with the nephrology team, when possible, to serve as a voice for these patients and serve as a clinical expert. The ESRD patients are often seen as "difficult" by nurses and residents because they often project their feelings of poor self-worth on the medical personnel. However, the attending physicians and I often remind others that the patients have many factors leading to their demeanor, including psychosocial issues, and our role is to provide competent and safe care during their hospitalization.

VMC has adopted a shared governance model for clinical decision making. Shared governance is composed of 4 groups which influence nursing practice throughout VMC. All committees have a DNP or PhD to conduct literature reviews and serve as an expert regarding evidence-based practice (EBP) or research. I serve as the DNP on the practice council, which is a council who votes on changes in nursing practice, conducts research, examines new products for patient care, and ensures policies and procedure are evidence based and necessary.

# THE CLINICAL NURSE SPECIALIST ROLE

The CNS is 1 of 4 advanced practice nurses (APRNs) recognized in the United States. Other APRNs include nurse practitioners, nurse-midwives, and nurse anesthetists, all possessing at least master's degrees with many APRNs now pursuing terminal degrees such as DNP or PhD. APRNs are trained to assess diagnosis, order tests, manage patient issues, and prescribe medications. Some states, such as my home state of North Carolina, do not allow the CNS to practice to the full scope of their APRN license and do not allow prescriptive authority.

The CNS was the first category of APRNs in 1956, when Hildegard Peplau, considered the founder of the CNS role, established a master's degree for clinical practice.[5] The majority of CNSs are hospital based, more than 1% have a doctoral degree, with the majority focusing on adult, gerontology, or adult/gerontology, with specialties including diabetes, oncology, palliative care, or hospice.[5]

The CNS practice is diversified, which includes direct patient care; acting as a consultant and/or educator for nurses, staff, and others; leaders of EBP projects; and helping with patient care issues.[6] Many CNSs are unit based and may be responsible for multiple units or may work for the entire health system, which can include different hospitals within that system.[6]

The CNS's 3 spheres of influence are the patient/family, nurse/nursing practice, and organization/system. The CNS is the only APRN to function among these spheres, also assimilating Core Competencies that work among these 3 spheres of influence.[2] These Core Competencies are integrated into the care of the patient, working with nurses, and ensuring partnership with the health care system. CNSs have been shown to decrease patient length of stay and lower costs for postpartum and end-of-life patients, reduce hospital acquired infections for surgical intensive care and post cardiac surgery patients, and lead measures to reduce complications among stroke and TIA patients.[6]

The main emphasis of CNS practice is devoted to the patient/family sphere of influence.[6] The CNS can provide direct and indirect nursing care to the patients, also focusing on clinical outcomes that are fiscally responsible, while improving quality of care.[6] Examples of this can include a CNS-led team looking at best practices and evidence-based interventions to decrease ventilated associated pneumonia (VAP) rates or CNS led post-discharge phone calls that reduced readmission rates.[6]

Improving patient outcomes can also be attained through the CNS nurse/nursing practice sphere related to educational activities, EBP interventions and implementations, and policy development.[6] A palliative care CNS implemented the End-of-Life Nursing Education Consortium for nurses who care for adults and children that aimed at improving patient outcomes at end of life, while also addressing the emotional needs of nurses caring for these patients.[6]

The similarities in all 3 CNS spheres of influence are designed to improve outcomes and ensure safe, quality care, while remaining cost-effective. The organization/system sphere of CNS influence is no different, with a focus on distribution of essential resources and health policies for outcomes

improvement and cost-effectiveness.[6] A wound care CNS conducted a SWOT (Strengths, Weaknesses, Opportunities, Threats) analysis regarding hospital-acquired pressure ulcers (HAPU), which are costly to the medical system and detrimental to patients.[6] The wound care CNS and the wound care team implemented evidence-based interventions for pressure ulcer prevention and were able to significantly reduce HAPUs prevalence rate below the national average.[6]

# THE CLINICAL NURSE SPECIALIST CORE COMPETENCIES

The CNS Core Competencies were adopted in 2010 by the National Clinical Nurse Specialist Competency Task Force. The CNS Core Competencies are based on an organizational framework showing the 3 CNS spheres of influence, intertwined with the Hamric/Spross Competencies of Advanced Nursing Practice and the American Association of Critical-Care Nurses' (AACN) Synergy Model nurse characteristics.

The Hamric/Spross Competencies of Advanced Nursing Practice include direct clinical practice, expert coaching and guidance, consultation, research, clinical professional and systems leadership, collaboration, and ethical decision making.[1] The melding of Hamric/Spross competencies and the AACN Synergy Model allows the CNS to practice as an APRN, taking into account all patient and family relevant issues, while assisting the nurse and nursing practice to grow in the EBP arena to best serve patients and families. It also allows the system/organization to function in a highly safe and quality driven environment, while being fiscally responsible. These 3 CNS spheres of influence work together to fuse a system of care that is highly reliable, safe, delivers high-quality care, and functions best to work with all patient populations for enhanced outcomes.

There are 7 items under the CNS Core Competencies and behaviors with associated sphere of influence and nurse characteristics.[1] Each competency has a subsequent behavioral statement, the sphere(s) of influence affected, and nursing characteristics. Each competency has behavioral statements that can affect 1, 2, or 3 of the spheres of influence. The CNS Core Competencies are direct care, consultation, systems leadership, collaboration, coaching, research, and ethical decision making.[1] The CNS research competency is divided into 3 parts, each with their own behavioral statements. The parts of the CNS research competency are interpretation, translation, and use of evidence; evaluation of clinical practice; and conduct of research.[1]

Later in this chapter, I will discuss how I practice as a DNP-prepared CNS by blending the 7 CNS Core Competencies and the 8 DNP Essentials. This merger allows me to best serve my patients, families, nurses, interdisciplinary team, and the communities of eastern North Carolina.

Upholding the mission of VH is at the forefront of every clinical encounter. Vidant Health's mission is to improve the health and well-being of eastern North Carolina.[7]

# THE DNP ESSENTIALS

The 8 DNP Essentials will be assessed in relationship to the CNS role.[2] Each DNP Essential includes all elements of the CNS Core Competencies and highlights the importance of scientific endeavor, EBP, and their inclusions in caring for patients. Nurses, treatment teams, and health care systems are all significant for health care practitioners. Everything in the health care arena relates back to providing safe, high-quality, and evidence-based care as standard practice to serve patients and families. The DNP CNS brings continued excellence to patient care by highlighting the science and art of nursing, best practices, ethics, collaborations, outcomes, fiscal responsibility, and the individuality of each patient.

Following are the 8 DNP Essentials, each with an example of the collaboration between these Essentials and the CNS Core Competencies. CNSs are advanced practice nurses. With this in mind, all the DNP Essentials relate to DNP Essential VIII, Advanced Practice,[2] and I will only mention DNP Essential VIII in my example of this competence. As a DNP-prepared CNS, I am an APRN every day of my career, striving to achieve and mentor excellence in nursing, while improving outcomes for the patients, nurses, and systems through evidence-based measures.

## DNP Essential I: Scientific Underpinnings for Practice—The Serenity Room

Prior to beginning my DNP, I knew that I wanted to have an EBP project based on the work of Jean Watson and her Theory of Human Caring. I believe the essence of the practice of nursing, with its relationship to art and science, is defined through a caring moment between one person and another. Dr. Watson, through endless studies published by her and other international authors, has proven the science and art behind caring. I chose to teach my nursing students about caring theory and how it relates to their practice and selves prior to venturing out in the world of nursing. I wrote to Dr. Watson during my entire project and she was instrumental in assisting me to find a valid tool for my study and was given a copy of my study upon completion. The outcomes of the study were statistically significant, and the nursing students felt this was an important starting point in their nursing career.[2]

Two years later, when I began as a medicine CNS, I would again delve into the literature to see how I could help a nursing staff that often were negative, stressed out, had little time for breaks, and did not exhibit loving kindness toward themselves or others. This was on my first medicine unit as a medicine CNS and the idea of the serenity room was developed and achieved with the assistance of bedside nurses. When looking at current literature, there were many studies from Dr. Watson and others on the importance of self-care and its link to better patient outcomes. During my literature review, I found a direct relationship to CNS Core Competency F (Tables 6-1, 6-2, and 6-3) regarding all aspects of research from interpretation, translation, and use of evidence to evaluation of clinical practice and implementation of research findings.

Dr. Watson has developed the 10 Caritas Processes, which means love and charity, to illustrate the science and importance of caring.[8] Dr. Watson, through the development of her theory and through further research, found that caring for self is the key to caring and loving others. Dr. Watson believes in the necessity of self-compassion and intentionally practicing loving-kindness to oneself.[8] How many nurses are the caregivers who forget the importance of nourishing our own needs, physical and otherwise?

The year prior to beginning as a medicine CNS, I attended Dr. Watson's annual conference on human caring. There were many attendees speaking of how to better one's nursing practice through caring for ourselves and others. One poster was about a serenity room in which the staff could go and relax, practice yoga, and spend just enough time to feel recharged internally, thus allowing them to best care for all patients while living in the moment.

When I spoke to the manager of the medicine unit about my interest in having a serenity room, she was very enthusiastic as was their leadership who provided the funding. A core group of nurses and I decided what should be in this room and it was unanimously decided to make this a comfortable living area, with a couch, lounge chairs, and 2 lamps that could dimly light the room. The staff and I picked out the furnishings, carpets, and wall color. Later, we added a Monet print of lilies, a large poster portrait of violets, a sound machine, a bible, and a prayer shawl. The room was originally just for staff, but families can use the room to visit with physicians for privacy. All interviews for new staff are conducted in there. On the door to the room is a laminated poster with a quote from Thich Nhat Hanh, often thought to be influential in the importance of mindfulness, about staying in the present moment. Later, the serenity room was dedicated to a nurse manager who died but was influential in helping the serenity room become a reality. The serenity room was opened in October of 2013, just 7 months after I became the unit's CNS. It is the only such room in the hospital and one of my proudest moments in nursing because I created the ability to give moments of joy to nurses and other staff. The collaboration among myself, management, staff, and administration of the hospital ties into the CNS Core Competency D (see Table 6-1) by illustrating collaboration and how to optimize clinical outcomes, which is shown by Dr. Watson's work to be enhanced with self-care.

To measure the room's effectiveness, a survey was given to the staff, with the same survey given a year later. Five questions were asked on a 5-point Likert scale. For the first survey,

**Table 6-1**

## THE DNP/CLINICAL NURSE SPECIALIST: COMPARING THE DNP ESSENTIALS AND CLINICAL NURSE SPECIALIST CORE COMPETENCIES

| DNP/CLINCAL NURSE SPECIALIST WORK | DNP ESSENTIALS | CLINICAL NURSE SPECIALIST COMPETENCIES |
|---|---|---|
| Serenity room | I | D, F |
| Failure to rescue | I, II, III, VI | A, B, C, D, F |
| Diabetes core | III | D, E, F |
| Newly diagnosed patients with diabetes: no readmissions | III, IV, VI | A, B, D, E, F |
| Literature reviews | I, II, III, V | C, E, F |
| Progression of care rounds and supply chain management standardization | II, III, VI, VII | A, B, C, D, F |
| Community service: Stand Down | VII | A, B, D, E, G |
| The Great 100 Nurses of North Carolina | ALL | ALL |
| Note: All 8 works reflect DNP Essential VIII: Advanced Nursing Practice. | | |

**Table 6-2**

## THE DNP ESSENTIALS

| |
|---|
| I. Scientific Underpinnings for Practice |
| II. Organizational and Systems Leadership for Quality Improvement and Systems Thinking |
| III. Clinical Scholarship and Analytical Methods for Evidence-Based Practice |
| IV. Information Systems/Technology and Patient Care Technology for the Improvement and Transformation of Health Care |
| V. Health Care Policy for Advocacy in Health Care |
| VI. Interprofessional Collaboration for Improving Patient and Population Health Outcomes |
| VII. Clinical Prevention and Population Health for Improving the Nation's Health |
| VIII. Advanced Nursing Practice |
| Adapted from The essentials of doctoral education for advanced nursing practice. American Association of Colleges of Nursing. October 2006. https://www.aacnnursing.org/Portals/42/Publications/DNPEssentials.pdf |

the majority of the 51 staff who responded (68%) felt stressed before entering the room, with 82% feeling relaxed after leaving the room, 90% saying they would use the room, 86% feeling the room was a necessary part of the unit, and 90% saying they would encourage their peers to use the room. A year later, the results were very similar. Staff comments included "The entire room is relaxing," "I wish all units had this," and "I am so grateful for a place to go to be centered and reconnect so I can continue to help others." In 2015, at Dr. Watson's annual conference, I presented a poster of the serenity room, with photos of the staff who helped make it

possible. Dr. Watson was informed on the room's presence from inception to reality.

DNP Essential I speaks of enhancing the practice of caring for others based on evidence, ethical decision making, and affecting positive change. In comparing this inception to completion, this DNP Essential I complements CNS Core Competencies D and F by speaking of collaboration to achieve better outcomes and all aspects of research and to show how evidence improves clinical practice and nursing practice.

**Table 6-3**

## CLINICAL NURSE SPECIALIST CORE COMPETENCIES

| A. Direct care |
| --- |
| B. Consultation |
| C. System leadership |
| D. Collaboration |
| E. Coaching |
| F. Research |
| G. Ethical decision-making, moral agency, and advocacy |

Adapted from Clinical nurse specialist core competencies. The National CNS Competency Task Force. https://www.nacns.org/wp-content/uploads/2017/01/CNSCoreCompetenciesBroch.pdf

## DNP Essential II: Organizational and Systems Leadership for Quality Improvement and Systems Thinking— Failure to Rescue

When I began working as a medicine CNS, I often evaluated a patient's change of status, whether it related to vital signs, laboratory values, or changes in mental status (CNS Core Competency A, see Table 6-1). Nurses also asked me to see patients because they just "looked" different (CNS Core Competency B, see Table 6-1). It is this gut instinct that is well known in nursing. General medicine units, with its ratio of 5 to 6 patients, needed patients transferred to either intermediate or intensive care units due to changes in patient status. I was the APRN who would either call our emergency response team (ERT) or ask the provider to reevaluate the patient. ERT is composed of critical care nurses who evaluate patients when called by the nurse, when a modified early warning score (MEWS) is more than 5 (indicative of vital sign changes or sepsis), when a lactic acid is more than 2 (indicative of sepsis), or during code blue or stroke situations. In the beginning as a medicine CNS, the providers did not know me and there was some push back about patient transfers. However, over time, and with positive patient outcomes, due to needed transfers to higher levels of care, I became well trusted by providers and nurses on my units (CNS Core Competency C, see Table 6-1).[2]

VMC shows many events that occur to a patient through a safety intelligence (SI) network. The SI report shows events that could range from a 1 (no patient harm) to a 9 (patient death). SI is not a punitive reporting structure. It is built to assist the hospital to better care for our patients and delve into all events to see how to deter these from happening again. I will assess events more than 5 to see if there were missing links leading to these events. Then, the nurse and I will speak about what could have been done differently. This is a non-punitive interaction and is done in confidence. The nurse also speaks with their manager.

The nurse manager (NM) of ERT was asked by the medicine nursing administrator to collaborate with me about failure to rescue (FTR) events that occurred in our hospital and how to best disseminate these events to staff. FTR is a sequence of events that lead to deterioration in a patient's status and can lead to death.[9] FTR are avoidable events that are not recognized by various clinical staff, not just nursing. FTR can be precipitated by what is seen as subtle occurrence, such as a slight change in patient status or vital signs.[9] These minor changes are why I teach bedside nurses to look at the patient's hemodynamics and laboratory values daily, to avoid events such as FTR.

I conducted a literature review on FTR to see its relevance to practice, which highlights CNS Core Competency F (see Table 6-1). I suggested to the NM of ERT that we conduct nursing grand rounds in our large auditorium inviting all clinical staff to 6 sessions, conducted during day and night shifts, with at least 1 on the weekends. Our FTR team invited nurses of all levels, and other disciplines including advanced practice providers, residents, and respiratory (CNS Core Competency E, see Table 6-1). Other members of our FTR nursing grand rounds team were an ERT nurse (who narrated the grand rounds) and a quality nurse from medicine (CNS Core Competency D, see Table 6-1). We asked risk management what de-identified cases we could use, and we chose 3, all resulting in a patient's death. Prior to the start of grand rounds, all participants received a survey asking about their knowledge of FTR, followed by a post grand rounds survey assessing knowledge gained and if they felt the content was relevant and would help their practice.

We began with a definition of FTR, followed by an interactive patient story. All details were not provided to the audience. We asked what was missed, how this could have been prevented, how we could have prevented missing this, and what discipline(s) contributed to FTR. We did not want nurses to feel they were the sole discipline contributing to FTR events. During our FTR sessions, we also educated our attendees about the importance of listening to family members regarding changes in patient status. One of our FTR cases involved not listening to a spouse and the patient having a poor outcome.

Our post-surveys were the most telling about our FTR nursing grand rounds. All attendees (about 100 through all sessions) ranked our sessions as excellent, necessary to their practice, and something that should be repeated often to staff. We presented a poster on FTR to a Sigma Theta Tau biennial conference in 2017. The plans are to recreate FTR nursing grand rounds throughout the hospital involving different areas of clinical expertise and cases of deterioration not only those resulting in patient death. Three months prior to our inception of FTR nursing grand rounds there were 6 recorded FTR events and 3 months after there were only 3, a significant decline.

I placed FTR under DNP Essential II (see Table 6-1), Organizational and Systems Leadership for Quality Improvement and Systems Thinking. However, FTR also relates to DNP Essentials I, III, VI, and VIII (see Table 6-1). These Essentials cover the essence of the DNP from understanding and interpreting the importance of literature reviews, disseminating the evidence through collaboration aimed to improve patient outcomes by preventing FTR events in the future. FTR blends the DNP Essentials highlighted with 5 CNS Core Competencies (A, B, C, D, and F), which include literature reviews that would have evidence FTR education improves patient outcomes, assists disciplines in safer, directs patient care by stressing collaboration between nurses and other disciplines, and provides active coaching of all disciplines. The combination of DNP Essentials and CNS Core Competencies also reveals how CNS leadership allows us to empower and influence others, implement evidence that results in accountability leading to positive change for ourselves and others to practice, and provide safe, quality, and ethical care.

## DNP Essential III: Clinical Scholarship and Analytic Methods for Evidence-Based Practice—Diabetes Core

I have taught diabetes to nurses and patients since I began working at VMC. Six years ago, I was asked to be the facilitator of diabetes core. Diabetes core is offered to all new nurses at VMC 6 times annually and experienced nurses 2 times annually. This class educates nurses that patients diagnosed with diabetes are a national epidemic numbering 415 million people worldwide.[10] The first 4 years that I facilitated diabetes core it was taught by an interdisciplinary team (CNS Core Competency D, see Table 6-1) composed

of an endocrinologist, pharmacist, dietician, and nurse. Nurses were taught about nutrition for patients with diabetes, current insulins (and their costs), oral medications, using the electronic health record to chart care for patients with diabetes, and diabetes survival skills for successful patient management of diabetes. This class was taught for more than 15 years in this format. I felt this design of diabetes core was better suited for nursing students and not new nurses. I conferred with the education department to change the structure of diabetes core and they agreed we should make it timelier for our bedside nurses. To better understand best practices related to current education of new nurses I began to search the literature. After this literature review (CNS Core Competency F, see Table 6-1), and for the last 2 years, I began teaching in an interactive case study format which covered all aspects of diabetes self-management including hospitalization for diabetes emergencies, insulin pump management, patient education needs, and transitioning patient from hospital to home while setting up necessary after care with a provider and certified diabetes educator (CDE) as necessary (CNS Core Competency E, see Table 6-1). This is a holistic view of our patient population and how we care for them while hospitalized, barriers faced including no insurance or high copays for medicines, and the necessity of ensuring patients are cared for post discharge. The nurses are divided into small groups working on the case studies and presenting them to the group in whatever way they would like. Some nurses act out scenarios of nurse to patient and others just speak to the group, often having the group provide questions and their own opinions. Though I act as facilitator of this group, I work with the nurses on all these case studies and present one to the group, where they will interact with me during this presentation. The nurses often tell me this is a unique way to learn how to care for patients with diabetes and they will remember most of what they learned in this class. The nurses also enjoy the fact that when they are given the case studies, the answers can be found using personal cell phones or tablets. Diabetes core provides new nurses with the tools needed to successfully educate many patients, recognize how to advocate for proper glycemic control, when to consult me for assistance, and review transitions in care to assist in better patient outcomes and fewer hospital readmissions.[2]

Diabetes core is an example of DNP Essential III (see Table 6-1), which shows how evidence is implemented into practice and how scholarship is disseminated to improve care for patients through the use of the case studies corresponding to elements located in the electronic health record necessary for safe patient care. The combination of DNP Essential III (see Table 6-1) also connects with the CNS Core Competencies D, E, and F (see Table 6-1) by highlighting the importance of research, dissemination, and implementation through collaboration, while successfully coaching and educating others based on evidence and best practices.

## DNP Essential IV: Information Systems/Technology and Patient Care Technology for the Improvement and Transformation of Health Care— Newly Diagnosed Patients With Diabetes in Eastern North Carolina With No Readmissions

North Carolina has one of the highest diabetes rates in the country, with eastern North Carolina having significantly higher rates at 11.1%, compared to the national average of 9.6%.[11] Among Black persons in eastern North Carolina, the rate for diabetes is 15.3% compared to 9.9% of White persons in that region.[11] Of the 44 counties in eastern North Carolina, 86% have lower life expectancies than the national average.[11] Compared to the national average, residents of North Carolina with diabetes are more likely to be obese/overweight, have less physical activity, eat less fruits and vegetables, and are also likely to have hypertension and high cholesterol.[2,11]

From January to September 2018, I consulted with 50 patients newly diagnosed with diabetes, assisting with the patient's plan of care. I worked with the interdisciplinary treatment team comprised of bedside nurses, attending physicians, advanced practice providers, pharmacists, nutritionists, and case managers. The center and most important element of this interdisciplinary team were patients and/or family members.

The first thing I look at in the patient's chart is whether they have insurance. If the patient has no insurance or were underinsured, the pharmacist or provider would place the patient on lower-cost insulin, which they can purchase at a specific large chain retailer. In North Carolina, neutral protamine hagedorn (NPH) and regular insulin can be purchased over-the-counter using the brand name ReliOn, which has the lowest cost of these insulins. Insulins such as Lantus (insulin glargine) and Humalog (insulin lispro), basal and bolus insulin can cost up to $500 for 5 pens or a vial, whereas NPH insulin purchased at the specific large chain retailer can costs $20 to $25 a vial. This retailer also sells glucometer, glucometer supplies, and glucose tables at a reduced cost under the ReliOn brand. These items are often costly to the uninsured or underinsured patient. The team members learn to understand that EBP suggests the newer insulins, such as Lantus and Humalog, are better for glycemic control. I educate the providers that EBP is negated if the patient cannot afford these insulins.

Case managers assisted in getting patients forms to fill out for medication assistance in North Carolina. I would locate a free or reduced fee clinic near their home and make the patient a follow-up appointment. Since the patients were newly diagnosed with diabetes, I made appoints for within 7 days of discharge.

The patient and/or family understood the necessity of learning more about diabetes management. They were informed of where to get free diabetes education from a CDE. All the principles of diabetes self-care management can take months to learn and the hospital is not able to provide this education during a patient's admission.

The patient's education was initiated by the bedside nurse and me. Education included were insulin(s) prescribed, when to administer or hold insulins, blood glucose targets, how often to check blood glucose, keeping a log of blood glucose numbers, management and notification for hypoglycemia/hyperglycemia, and follow-up appointments with a provider and CDE. All these items were provided on a 1-page handout located in the electronic health record. This handout, "The Basics of Diabetes," was used to educate the patient and/or family while a written copy was provided when education was provided and at discharge. The bedside nurse or I would review this information, utilizing teach-back to ensure understanding and a safe transition from hospital to home. The bedside nurse or I see the patient as often as necessary to validate understanding and demonstrate necessary tasks such as drawing up insulin or using an insulin syringe. Utilizing this 1-page document makes education easier to understand, enforcing the primary goal of safe discharge. The patients also receive my business card to call me with questions.

None of these newly diagnosed patients were readmitted to the hospital within 6 months of discharge, leading to improved outcomes for the patient, and decreased costs for patients and the health system. I have seen some of these patients since discharge and they reported lower hemoglobin A1c. They also report feeling better physically and mentally when following up with providers and the CDE. The follow-up has enabled them to better understand and implement diabetes management. This model was truly based on safe transitions of care by understanding the patient's needs, providing affordable medication solutions, and timely appointments with a provider and CDE.

This initiative is placed under DNP Essential IV (see Table 6-1). The other DNP Essentials utilized are Essentials III, V, VI, and VII (see Table 6-1). DNP Essential IV (see Table 6-1) speaks of the analysis of data, utilizing EBP, and assisting with the prediction and analysis of outcomes. In DNP Essential III (see Table 6-1) I collected data and evidence through many sources to see how to best serve my patients and disseminate the data. DNP Essentials VI and VII (see Table 6-1) illustrated the importance of interprofessional collaboration to achieve goals, educate others, and plan for enhanced outcomes, while considering the patient past hospitalization and how to be cared for in the community post discharge. The CNS Core Competencies A, B, D, E, and F (see Table 6-1) highlight both the CNS as a direct care APRN who also serves in consultant and collaborator roles for the patient and interdisciplinary treatment team, and the importance of coaching principles while educating the patient and/or family while using EBP methods resulting in better patient outcomes. The blending of the DNP Essentials and CNS Core Competencies stress the necessity of implementing EBP, interdisciplinary communication and education, and safe transitions in care for the patient.

This topic was presented at a plenary session at the Sigma Theta Tau international biennial convention in November of 2019.

## DNP Essential V: Health Care Policy for Advocacy in Health Care—Literature Reviews

When attempting to validate EBP, the first step is conducting a literature review using sources of literature that are not more than 5 years old. I use many different search engines such as the Cumulative Index to Nursing and Allied Health Literature (CINAHL) and MEDLINE, but I also search for articles in nursing journals such as the *American Journal of Nursing* (AJN) or *Clinical Nurse Specialist*. I do not ignore the evidence from medical journals such as the *Journal of the American Medical Association* (JAMA) or the *British Medical Journal* (BJM). All articles should be from peer-reviewed sources that demonstrate validity. I also rely on the Criteria of DiCenso for Evaluation of Health Intervention Studies,[12] which examines criteria for the usefulness and effectiveness of interventions, ensuring the studies were free of bias, and the validity of measured outcomes. I will search for literature reviews that compare interventions and their effectiveness, while also studying systematic reviews. Systematic reviews measure the effectiveness of studies in a systematic method, evaluating and integrating qualitative and quantitative studies.[13] The necessity of conducting a comprehensive literature review is to expand available knowledge, to specify a theoretical structure using an outline of up-to-date evidence to assist one in gaining different viewpoints, to understand the gaps in literature, and to gain further implications of the problem including if an EBP or quality improvement project is necessary after the literature review is conducted.[2,13]

VMC uses a shared decision-making model (also called *shared governance*) to guide their nursing practice. When nurses participate in shared decision making, they gain greater control of nursing practice at their organization, therefore empowering them to take responsibility in their practice. This benefits nurses in the use of EBP to change how they practice based on quality improvement projects and current research.[14] The shared decision-making model at VMC is composed of councils meeting monthly. These councils are the practice council, the EBP and quality improvement council, nurse congress, retention and recognition, night shift council, nurse executive council (nursing leaders throughout VMC), and unit-based councils (for individual units). Each council, other than nurse executive council or unit-based council, has a doctoral level nurse who serves as

the person who searches and synthesizes the literature. I also conduct literature reviews for individual nurses and myself to be further educated on or for new initiatives. What I have learned about EBP is if the patient or family cannot afford or refuse proposed recommendations, then nurses and other health care providers need to reconsider options.

Examples of literature reviews conducted, implemented, and not implemented (due to lack of reliable evidence) at VMC include patient mobility, delirium on medical surgical units, the serenity room, FTR, diabetes education for nurses and staff, interdisciplinary rounding, "What Matters to Me" (an Institute for Healthcare Improvement initiative), the medical-surgical nurse caring for behavioral health patients, nursing validation of the insulin administration, and the modified early warning score (MEWS).

Though I have placed literature reviews under DNP Essential V (see Table 6-1), it is also necessary to include DNP Essentials I, II, and III, (see Table 6-1), since all of these implicate the importance of EBP. Essentials I, II, III, and V allow the DNP to examine and execute EBP that betters the nursing profession while looking at the whole patient through the life cycle and implementing positive interventions to best serve patients. The DNP-prepared nurse is shown how to retrieve and analyze current literature and given tools for evaluating and implementing EBP. The DNP is also equipped with the knowledge to change health policies to assist patient care whether the person is hospitalized or in the community, and to educate others to comprehend the EBP initiatives necessary for these changes, all the while serving as an advocate for nursing and patients.

I have compared DNP Essentials I, II, III, and V (see Table 6-1) to CNS Core Competencies C, E, and F (see Table 6-1). These CNS Essentials are guided by a sense of inquiry to improve and implement evidence while demonstrating the importance of changing, permitting others to influence clinical practice, and allowing for advancement of nursing practice through the translation and dissemination of evidence. The DNP Essentials and CNS Core Competencies noted would not be possible without the literature, where EBP commences.

## DNP Essential VI: Interprofessional Collaboration for Improving Patient and Population Health— Progression of Care Rounds and Supply Chain Management Standardization

In 2017 VH partnered with a group purchasing organization (GPO). There are numerous reasons why a health system would have a need for a GPO. Due to an evolving world of health care costs and uncertainty about payer sources, it is imperative to find methods that were once considered untraditional. The GPO states they can help health systems in various ways: group purchasing, technology, consulting, and advocacy.[15] The GPO globally looks at VH and recognizes ways to improve costs and works on continuous improvement in other areas, such as operations and introducing new initiatives to streamline costs while still delivering excellent patient care.[15] Assistance is provided to VH in order to continue functioning as a fluid health care system by suggesting new or improved methods that can affect safety, quality, and population health.[15] The GPO uses data to make choices, repeatedly analyzing data by suggesting changes and improvements when necessary.[2,15]

The CNS group is seen as clinical experts and has been working with the GPO since 2017. All CNSs are part of supply chain led groups which look at costs, best practices, EBP, and standardization of products. In addition to CNS and the GPO, a large group of representatives from all VH hospitals attend clinical quality value analysis (CQVA), and CQVA-equipment. In addition to the representatives from the GPO and VH supply chain, employee attendees are from multiple disciplines: the entire CNS group, registered nurses, respiratory therapists, information systems, legal services, and more. Costs saving initiatives are emphasized and possible product replacement weighing cost-effectiveness, safety, and the quality of the newer product. Products analyzed have included defibrillators, glucometers, surgical gloves standardization, and linen appropriation, among others. The GPO and VH's partnership have saved the organization millions of dollars in just 2 years.

The GPO also assists VH by collaborating to achieve excellence throughout the health system. A new initiative is progression of care rounds (POCR), a multidisciplinary approach to ensuring a safe and timely discharge for patients. POCR is led by a facilitator (usually a unit's charge nurse), who rounds on each patient with the multidisciplinary team composed of bedside nurses and nursing assistants, providers, case managers, unit management, pharmacy, and other teams (such as respiratory or physical therapy) who work with the patient. Discussed in rounds is the patient's current disposition, expected date of discharge, barriers to discharge, mobility status, and patient's destination after discharge. The facilitator speaks to each member of the team for input and barriers to discharge can be addressed by the case manager and provider or both. Examples include: If the patient is waiting for a test, can the test be done outpatient, or can an antibiotic be changed from intravenously to orally? If mobility is an issue, than physical therapy should be consulted. Mobility is an imperative and expectation of the bedside nurse and nursing assistant because one day in bed can delay discharge by an extra day.

I was asked to be the champion for POCR for VMC. I work with systems and procedures, GPO employees, and the interdisciplinary team to ensure the rounds work as designed. When barriers are encountered, the team assesses interventions that can assist in POCR's success.

Length of stay is a measurement which fiscally impacts health systems. POCR's interdisciplinary approach is one that current literature supports, stating all team members can lead to decreased length of stay.[16] In 4 months, 10 units have implemented POCR with a 0.50% decrease in patient hospital length of stay for those units. The plan is to systematically implement POCR throughout all VH's entities.

Though I have placed VH's and the GPO's work under DNP Essential VI (see Table 6-1), you will notice a theme emerging where there is more than 1 DNP Essential under each category, as well as more than 1 CNS Core Competency. Reasons for this include the melding of work the DNP and CNS accomplish, the combining of many layers for a successful practice, and the necessity to look at all aspect of work for the health system, its employees, and the DNP/CNS.

Other DNP Essentials this work covers are DNP Essentials II, III, and VII (see Table 6-1). Essential II (see Table 6-1) writes about systems leadership and systems thinking. The emergence of VH and the GPO's work highlights this DNP Essential and how the DNP/CNS can contribute. DNP Essential III writes of analytical methods for EBP and the DNP/CNS is asked to conduct literature reviews when the initiative arrives for POCR or working with supply chain management. The literature is then analyzed for efficacy and its relationship to the current initiative. DNP Essential VII (see Table 6-1) writes of "Clinical Prevention and Population Health" and all initiatives are patient-centered to best care for those we serve.

For the CNS Core Competencies, I have included A, B, C, D, and F (see Table 6-1). Core Competency A (see Table 6-1) speaks of caring for the patient, which is primary in POCR. Core Competencies B, D, and F (see Table 6-1) speak of interdisciplinary interaction, leadership in improvement initiatives, and optimizing outcomes which is necessary in all VH and GPO work, and Core Competency C (see Table 6-1) is the influence of clinical practice within and across systems, which is done in working with supply chain management.

## DNP Essential VII: Clinical Prevention and Population Health for Improving the Nation's Health—Community Service/Stand Down

The service of nursing at any level is not confined to the walls of employment. I feel it necessary, especially in my rural communities, to care for patients outside of the hospital. When nurses are visibly working in communities, a healthier community with patients making healthier choices are possible, yielding positive outcomes.[17] I have mentored bedside nurses on the importance of giving back to the community to see the patients we care for in the hospital. These nurses then understand health is not dependent on disease processes.

Nurses then appreciate the patient as an individual with wants and needs similar to their own.[2]

Though I will work at health screenings and attend community events in which I am a speaker, I would like to highlight an event, Stand Down, which has had an emotional impact on me and the other nurses who work beside me. In 1988, Stand Down was created by a grassroots group of veterans who wanted to assist homeless veterans.[18] The original event was held in San Diego, California, and this led to the growth of a national, annual event. Included in this 1- to 3-day event is a list of services offered to homeless veterans. These services can include health screenings for physical and mental health, clothing (including shoes, socks, pants, shirts, and underwear), toiletry items, tents, blankets, free veterinary care, eye exams, dental exams, and haircuts.

The first time I attended Stand Down was December of 2016 and I knew nothing about it. Stand Down was held at a large gymnasium in Greenville, North Carolina. My partner and I were to check vital signs and blood glucose levels. When I entered the gymnasium, I was amazed to see the enormity of services and goods being offered. I was sadly unaware of how many homeless veterans lived in my community. Stand Down humbled me and made me realize the social impact of what it means to be homeless and how many of these veterans were still proud they served the United States, despite disadvantages when they returned.

The first year of serving at Stand Down, I had a 30-something-year-old gentleman in line that smelled of alcohol and seemed depressed. His blood pressure was extremely high, which concerned me. I spoke to him privately and recommended he go to the emergency room. He refused, but we spoke for almost an hour about his failure to stop drinking and his chronic depression. He did not realize alcohol would make someone more depressed. He also said he had been prescribed blood pressure medications but did not take them because of his drinking. In the room were mental health services offered by the Veterans Administration, which he said he may reach out to later. I wondered what happened to this gentleman and if he got some deserved help. The next time I was at Stand Down, I looked for him but did not see him.

During Stand Down, another realization I learned was that the situations others face in life are devastating to their mental and physical well-being. When I see these homeless veterans I can offer assistance, listen, and advocate. I respect that all human beings should be autonomous and have the right to say no. Often, health care professionals label patients as non-compliant without understanding how life can get in the way. A few months ago, I had a homeless veteran admitted for an infection. I saw him for his entire admission. At first, he would barely speak to me, but by listening and being present, I gained his trust. Physicians wanted him to start taking insulin. I advocated for oral medications because the patient stayed in a shelter and had no place to store his insulin or pen needles. When he was discharged, he was placed on oral medications and he thanked me. I still think of him, just as I do the other gentleman I saw at Stand Down. This

patient is homeless, but proud, and I was reminded of his pride during each encounter.

A long time ago, when I was a new nurse, a nurse told me "There but by the Grace of God go I." It is a motto I still live by more than 20 years later in nursing and in my life. It is also what I teach nurses when personal judgment comes into play and gets in the way of care.

DNP Essential VII refers to improving the patient's health through health promotion and clinical prevention. Working in the community, highlighted in Stand Down, is an example of how to work with the people we share space within the community. The event, in the broadest sense, is one of health promotion and health maintenance.

In community events, the nurse works directly with the patient as a consultant, collaborating with those in and out of health care to work with the patient. They can be one's coach and educator, assisting the patient by promoting health despite untoward circumstances, acting ethically when working with all patients inside or outside of the hospital. Community events are reflected in CNS Core Competencies A, B, D, E, and G (see Table 6-1).

## DNP Essential VIII: Advanced Nursing Practice—The Great 100 Nurses in North Carolina

In 1988, a group of North Carolina registered nurses gathered to determine how best to recognize registered nurses in North Carolina. Registered nurses chosen for this recognition would be excellent in the field of nursing by their contributions to this profession, their excellence in nursing, and their service to health care systems and/or their communities.[8,19] Heather Thorne, the organizer of this group, found a program in Louisiana called the Great 100 Nurses Foundation, which encompassed the vision of these North Carolina nurses. In 1989, the foundation named their first cohort of great 100 nurses and provided nursing scholarships to nursing schools.[19]

The Great 100 Nurses Foundation sends out calls for nominations annually. Nurses nominated and chosen are employed from the bedside to the boardroom. Nominees work in hospitals, schools, outpatient facilities, and academia. Any nurse can nominate someone to be a great 100 nurse. Thousands of nominations are received annually.[19] To avoid bias, a nominee's name and affiliation are not included. The only identification comes in a separate form.

Those who nominate a nurse answer questions related to how this nominee is advancing nursing in a positive way in a practice setting and/or community; how this nurse functions in one's scope of practice; demonstrates integrity, honesty, and accountability; commits to patients, families, and colleagues; displays energy, and enthusiasm; helps improve outcome; shows caring; and helps others develop and grow. The last item on the nomination form is giving an example of why this nominee should be a great 100 nurse. All categories are limited to 300 words except for the last item with a maximum of 30 words to be displayed at a gala honoring the great 100 nurses of that year.

A team of nurses reads the nominations. Recipients are named in early summer, and a formal banquet is held in their honor at different locations in North Carolina. I was honored to be named a great 100 nurse in 2017. I was nominated by a CNS in my place of employment. It is an honor to be chosen by a group of nursing peers. There are 117 439 nurses in North Carolina as of July 2019.[20] I am humbled, professionally and personally, to be one of such a small group of nurses to be named in this group.

I chose winning this award because I see it as an embodiment of the work I have done from my associate degree to my DNP. I feel I have made a positive impact on nursing, but the impact I have made on my patients and families, fellow nurses, and the health systems in which I have been employed has been more important. For 23 years, I have worked on a medical psychiatric unit, on a substance abuse unit, in home care, in an assisted living, and for 5 years as a nursing instructor for the last diploma school in Pennsylvania whose students scored a 100% pass rate on the NCLEX exams. After I received my DNP, I was recruited by VMC to be a CNS in both diabetes and medicine. I feel the Great 100 Nurses in North Carolina award is a culmination of my service in nursing and a great professional honor.

I have chosen DNP Essential VIII to place this award. However, I feel that the journey to become DNP-prepared has led me to the current road I am on and choosing all 8 Essentials as lead me on this path. I have also chosen all 7 CNS Core Competencies for the same reason. Being named as a great 100 nurse in North Carolina is an accolade highlighting my nursing career.

# CONCLUSION: IMPACT OF THE DNP DEGREE

In 2011, I received my DNP and I can now reflect on how diverse this degree has served my career trajectory. In 2012, 9 months after receiving the DNP, I was recruited to work for a large academic medical center as a DNP-prepared CNS. I was the first DNP at this institution. To my place of employment, the DNP was a new terminal degree and little was known about its strength for nursing. As a result of obtaining my DNP degree, I serve my patients and families, nurses, and the system. EBP and its power to transform nursing has been the strength of my 8 years at my current position.

My DNP EBP project was on educating nursing students on the art and science of caring as exhibited by Dr. Watson's Theory of Human Caring. Dr. Watson's work serves as a strong foundation for why I am a nurse. In an attempt to put theory into practice, I approached the management and administration of one of my units to build a serenity room for the staff. It was with the evidence I supplied on Dr. Watson's

Theory of Human Caring and how caring for self is primary when caring for others. Conduction of pre- and post-surveys of the serenity room proved how important this space was for a staff that served very acute patients and how staff often needed time to destress, debrief, and relax. This room is for the staff, but also serves patients and families since the staff can recharge when seeing them, allowing for enhanced patient outcomes.

FTR was another EBP project that began with a literature review delving into the topic and solutions to decreasing harm to patients. A small team of us reviewed incident reports which resulted in patient harm by missing clinical signs that should have had earlier interventions. Analyzing the literature with the incident reports allowed this team to delve into nursing grand rounds presenting deidentified patients and having the audience tell us the why and how we could have improved as practitioners. FTR was presented as blameless and helped the audience decide factors in a patient's demise. This undertaking resulted in a 50% reduction in FTR.

The hospital in which I am employed has a capacity of 900 patients, one-third of which have or are diagnosed with diabetes. The nurses must be knowledgeable on clinically managing the patients and provide education for patients and families. There are 3000 nurses at my place of employment, with 300 or more new nurses hired each year. Every new nurse is taught diabetes management and education, with refresher courses for nurses who were previously employed. New literature has showed that lectures are not a prime way to educate our nurses and that interactive lessons, such as case studies, are better methods. Nurses are placed in small teams with different scenarios regarding diabetes. In their evaluations, the nurses found this method better for learning and retention.

Although I have highlighted 3 ways I have helped nurses, patients/families, and the system, my DNP degree has allowed me to serve as an APRN who is seen as a clinical expert. While serving on the practice council, I conducted literature reviews on items such as a Foley catheter nursing protocol, a "What Matters to Me" initiative for nurses and staff to increase satisfaction, and cosigning of insulin medication administration, among others. I am also asked by other teams, such as hospital administration and the clinical value analysis team, to look at literature on various EBP projects such as pulse oximetry use and POCRs. I have collaborated with other disciplines to ensure that patients with diabetes receive affordable medications and timely follow-up care and education.

The role of the DNP-prepared CNS is intermingled to best serve my patients, their families, the nurses, and health care system. By practicing as a DNP-prepared CNS, I affect efforts to lead to the safest, highest quality, and fiscally responsible care. As a DNP, I add EBP as a multifaceted foundation to nursing care, highlighting the achievement of best outcomes through the efficacy of current studies, and reaching the highest level of care for all patients and their families.

Being a CNS with a DNP degree has allowed me to practice at the highest level of my nursing scope of practice, as a clinical expert, a nurse and patient advocate, and one who feels excellence in nursing is achieved with the melding of both DNP Essentials and CNS Core Competencies.

## Acknowledgment

To Paul, my wonderful husband, true love, and life-long partner. Thank you for always being my biggest supporter.

## References

1. Clinical nurse specialist core competencies. The National CNS Competency Task Force. https://www.nacns.org/wp-content/uploads/2017/01/CNSCoreCompetenciesBroch.pdf

2. The essentials of doctoral education for advanced nursing practice. American Association of Colleges of Nursing. October 2006. https://www.aacnnursing.org/Portals/42/Publications/DNP Essentials.pdf

3. Media kits. Vidant Health. https://www.vidanthealth.com/Media/Media-kit

4. Drenkard K. Going for the gold: the value of attaining magnet recognition. *Magnet.* 2010;5(3).

5. Mayo AM, Ray MM, Chambleee TB, et al. The advanced practice clinical nurse specialist. *Nurs Adm Q.* 2017;41(1):70-76.

6. Delp S, Ward CW, Altice N, et al. Spheres of influence…clinical nurse specialists sparking economic impact, innovative practice. *Nurs Manage.* 2016;47(6):30-37. doi:10.1097/01.NUMA.0000483132.20566.cd

7. Our mission. Vidant Health. https://www.vidanthealth.com/About-Vidant-Health/Our-mission-vision-values

8. Giavonnoni J. Perspectives: compassion for others begin with loving-kindness toward self. *J Res Nurs.* 2017;22(1-2):173-178. doi:10.1177/1744987116685635

9. Ghaferi AA, Dimick JB. Understanding failure to rescue and improving safety culture. *Ann Surg.* 2015;261(5):839-840. doi:10.1017/SLA.00000000001135

10. Alotaibi A. Gholizadeh L, Al-Ganmi A. Perry L. Examining perceived and actual diabetes knowledge among nurses working in a tertiary hospital. *Appl Nurs Res.* 2017;6(1):24-29.

11. Morgan M, Downer S, Lopinsky T. The diabetes epidemic in north carolina: policies for moving forward. https://www.chlpi.org/wp-content/uploads/2014/05/2014-New-Carolina-State-Report-Providing-Access-to-Healthy-Solutions-PATHS.pdf

12. Baker JD. The purpose, process, and methods of writing a literature review. *AORN J.* 2016;103(3):265-268. doi:10.1016/j.aorn.2016.01.016

13. Taylor S. How to search the literature. *Am J Nurs.* 1974;74(8):145-1459.

14. Murray K, Yasso S, Schomburg R, et al. Journal of excellence: implementing a shared decision-making model. *Am J Nurs.* 2016;116(4):50-56. doi:10.1097/01.NAJ.0000482137.12424.51

15. What we do. Premier. https://www.premierinc.com/what-we-do

16. Bhamidpati VS, Elliott DJ, Justice EM, Belleh E, Sonnad SS, Robinson EJ. Structure and outcomes of interdisciplinary rounds in hospitalized medicine patients: a systematic review and suggested taxonomy. *J Hosp Med.* 2016;(7):513-523. doi:10.1002/jhm.2575

17. McCollum M, Kovner CT, Ojemeni M, Brewer C, Cohen S. Nurses improve their communities' health where they live, learn, work, and play. *Policy Polit Nurs Pract.* 2017;18(1):7-16. doi:10.1177/1527154417698142

18. Stand down guide. National Coalition of Homeless Veterans. http://www.nchv.org/images/uploads/Stand%20Down%20Guide.pdf

19. The great 100 nurses in north carolina. The Great 100. https://great100.org/

20. Licensure statistics. North Carolina Board of Nursing. August 2019. https://portal.ncbon.com/licensurestatistics.aspx

# CHAPTER 7

# Lead, Follow, or Get Out of Your Own Way

## AN EXPERIENCED REGISTERED NURSE TO DNP JOURNEY

*Carol Essenmacher, DNP, PMHCNS-BC, NCTTP*

## INTRODUCTION

Starting my nursing journey as a single mother with 2 pre-school children has made for an interesting but not ideal start. Having been on welfare for 2.5 years, I felt pulled into nursing in order to gain a marketable skill to support myself and my children. For the longest time, I felt guilty about that but then realized that it had a positive effect on my nursing career. As you read about the path that I traveled to a Doctor of Nursing Practice (DNP) degree, keep in mind the concepts of self-confidence, relationships, and serendipity as these have been critical to the level of my achievements to date.

I had always hoped to earn a bachelor's degree in nursing (BSN), but circumstances led me to explore other options. Once I completed an associate's degree in nursing (ADN) and started working as a new nurse, I got used to following someone else's lead. Stepping into the role of charge nurse and leadership took time, and it was not a smooth journey largely due to my limited belief in my own self-confidence. I did become proficient in my leadership skills usually when the role of charge nurse was thrust onto me. Examples of this involve when the charge nurse called in sick or when I was pulled to another unit to assume the charge duties. It took

me 17 years to return to college, but I was able to finish a BSN in nursing. I found that a lot had changed, including but not limited to technology, health care reimbursement, and documentation requirements since I finished an ADN, so my limited self-confidence nearly prevented me from completing this degree.

Serendipity or fortuitous good chance played a critical first step in my eventual path to earning my next degree. While I was still in the BSN program, a very tough US military veteran registered nurse encouraged me to "stop writing like a housewife." Rather than be devastated, I insisted she explain herself and teach me to write better.

Looking back, this experience was the beginning of my belief in myself. Now that I have the benefit of hindsight, I realize that my fledgling attempts with bold decisions were likely grounded in a sense of "I've got nothing to lose," which led to some conflict and turmoil of my own making. I learned how to take more calculated and informed risks with my career. During a discussion with the aforementioned tough instructor, I told her that I wanted to earn a BSN because I wanted to learn how to stand up for myself. This has served me well.

The experience with this instructor also taught me the value of writing. Something well written serves many

Benson LA, ed. *The DNP Professional: Translating Value From Classroom to Practice* (pp 77-83).

purposes, such as learning how to write concisely and targeting the text to a specific audience. This allows for translation of evidence into new practice as a means of providing research and new clinical practice outcomes. It is also used as a means of documenting a self-discovered innovation and linking it to validated research or practice-based evidence. Writing was one of the first critical skills I learned on my path to a DNP. I continue to hone this skill and I have discovered the old adage is very true, that if you don't use it, you lose it. One cannot translate evidence into practice if one cannot effectively articulate in writing what the evidence is, what it means to the patient, what it means for future nursing practice, and how that evidence gets translated into practice in the clinical settings. As I learned to write better, my confidence level improved, and as my confidence level improved, I was more willing to take calculated risks to learn and practice in academic and clinical settings. This is important, as DNPs should be pushing the boundaries of generating innovations in practice that stand up to the rigors of research and vice versa.

Along the way, serendipity again guided me into a role for which I have become very passionate about. Treating tobacco use and dependency, especially among people with serious mental illnesses, has become my passion. During my master's coursework, a professor who was a dual appointee to a respected university and a clinical researcher with a veterans affairs (VA) hospital in her city, took me under her wing. It has been a worthwhile endeavor, and my ability to think critically and write effectively continues to flourish because of that critical relationship. I learned to accept failure as a necessary part of the learning curve and not a personal failing.

I started my role as the tobacco treatment coordinator (TTC) for my VA facility in 2008, shortly after I passed the American Nurses Credentialing Center (ANCC) clinical nurse specialist board certification (CNS-BC) exam. This role has allowed me to flourish and be creative with my nursing practice. Using graduate-level interventions was daunting in the beginning. Going from passing meds to prescribing meds requires a very different type and level of confidence. Practicing at an advanced level is rewarding and exhausting at the same time. It has also been an enormous creative outlet for me. Mastering skills that were conceptualized by me alone and delivering innovative evidence-based psychiatric nursing care has improved my confidence level. As I gained expertise in delivering care, mentoring others to do the same has become increasingly important and has become a large part of my role.

No matter my confidence level, it was a leap of faith to initiate the pursuit of a DNP in my mid-50s. By that time, I had a clearer picture of what I wanted to accomplish and how that would benefit the patients under my care. I had a much better idea of how to guide others to evidence-based care. I still felt I lacked knowledge and confidence in translating DNP-level practice into my graduate-level role at the VA. Questioning my abilities involved a lot of self-reflection and asking myself how I can move beyond providing excellent care to individuals or groups into creating, evaluating, and implementing interventions for large cohorts or populations of patients.

There are different types of DNP programs. As I had already completed advanced pathophysiology and pharmacology, my CNS-BC credential allowed me to prescribe, so I did not feel the need to pursue a clinically oriented DNP. The program I chose focused more on leadership and education.

Knowing there is often confusion and little acknowledgment or understanding of what a DNP could or would do to improve care at a VA hospital made for an interesting conundrum. There was little guidance at my facility and likely within other health care systems as to what, if anything, a DNP would do differently than what was already being done by advanced practice nurses (APRNs). This was, and still is, due in part to DNPs being a relatively new nursing path that many in leadership are unaware of and lack knowledge of what a DNP can contribute to health care. In hindsight, I recognize that even I did not have a totally clear picture of what I could or would do to improve health care. My line of supervisors had even less of an idea as to what I would do to improve care. Therefore, no advancement or more complex assignment awaited me upon graduation. There was also not any associated increase in compensation. Thus, the responsibility to create my own DNP practice was up to me. While this was a daunting task, it was also extremely rewarding and ultimately beneficial on many levels, with opportunities to improve patient access to quality tobacco treatment care.

Another early experience I was fortunate to have (again, serendipity plays a role) was directly due to the relationships that I have developed along the way. Finishing a master's in nursing degree allowed me to take and pass the ANCC exam for a CNS-BC. About the same time, my VA was searching for a professional to help people stop using tobacco. My credentials and good rapport with psychiatry leadership made possible stepping into the role of the facility's TTC for my main assignment with the VA. Anyone who works for a VA will likely tell you that there are many collateral assignments given to you, but my main job was as the TTC from 2008 to 2018. After 2018, my role as TTC was diminished to 20% of my job, with 80% assigned as a disability examiner for a variety of reasons.

## SWOT ANALYSIS

A tool I learned of in graduate school helped shape my initial steps in understanding what I could do as a result of completing a DNP education. SWOT stands for Strengths, Weaknesses, Opportunities, Threats analysis.[1] A sample of a SWOT analysis that can be used by nurses is found in the link provided in the list of references. This tool can be modified to fit a variety of nursing practices, as the intention is to generate an objective assessment of yourself and your practice.

Table 7-1

# SWOT Analysis of DNP Tobacco Treatment Coordinator Practice

| STRENGTHS | WEAKNESSES |
|---|---|
| • My unique, current, and in-demand skills/professional development: Extensive academic and continued professional education (Mayo Clinic Tobacco Treatment Specialist certification; ongoing motivational interviewing and provision of trainings).<br><br>• My network connections: participant, leader, and provider of tobacco treatment services and education through employment and as a member of American Psychiatric Nurses Association (resulting in several serendipitous professional relationships with leaders in the field of tobacco treatment). | • Neglected opportunities/learning to overcome technological challenges/approach and philosophy toward change:<br><br>• Resources are often not provided to teach nurses evidence-based knowledge and clinical skills to treat tobacco dependence. Bias toward and lack of understanding about effective tobacco treatment weakens effective nursing care. |
| OPPORTUNITIES | THREATS |
| • Are there shortages of skilled information workers in this field? Is the field growing?<br><br>• Tobacco treatment specialists are often not in the discipline of nursing. This creates a wonderful opportunity for nurses to innovate in health behavior change, specifically with tobacco treatment in mind. | • Are there regulatory or other constraints affecting employment?<br><br>• Treating tobacco use is often viewed as a secondary health care problem, creating a lack of sense of urgency. This is particularly true for mental health care patients who suffer increased morbidity and mortality, largely due to higher rates of tobacco use. This bias is demonstrated in clinical practice with the lack of support for a nursing role in tobacco treatment, lack of evidence-based nursing education on the topic of treating tobacco use, and lack of dedicated time to educate nurses in clinical settings. There are challenges at individual, clinic, facility, health care organizational, and large-scale system levels to effective care due to poor distribution of resources, poorly documented care, and inaccurate myths about treating tobacco use. |

SWOT analysis was a very useful tool for analyzing and improving my practice. Table 7-1 provides an example of how I was able to critically and objectively use SWOT analysis for my own practice. It helped me identify the skills I could improve upon, and the VA organizational barriers and facilitators so I could maximize my efforts. I was able to objectively state that I was keeping up in strengths, taking advantage of opportunities, and identifying any potential threats to my new role. I was meeting what I needed to do to overcome my weaknesses. It helped me identify a new skill that I should learn, known as data mining. Data mining is very helpful for the practicing DNP in order to facilitate system change for population health.

# DNP Essentials

In the following pages, I describe the journey I took and the experiences I had in developing my own, unique DNP practice that is solidly grounded in my DNP education. My thoughts about these activities and experiences are framed within the context of the DNP Essentials.[2] As many newly educated DNPs find themselves in charge of creating their DNP practice and defining the contributions they will make to nursing practice, I hope to convey the enormous potential for creativity and nearly endless opportunities that exist to improve the health care of the nation.

Throughout my academic career, I have had instructors or dual-appointed faculty (clinical providers and professors) tell me that they practice where they do because of the quality of the nursing staff at the facility where they provide care. These instructors reported that these up-to-date nurses kept them on their toes by always being current with emerging treatments and interventions. This is a prime example of the first Essential, DNP Essential I: Scientific Underpinnings for Practice, in action. It is truly essential that nurses use the latest evidence in their nursing practice.

Science is specifically useful to me in my role as the TTC, as the evidence I discovered in my quest to remain up-to-date in my practice. Nurses and other clinicians are providing care as if tobacco products are the same as they were more than 25 years ago, which they are definitely not. They contain a wide variety of chemicals, steadily added over the years to make the product more addicting. Additionally, nicotine replacement therapy (NRT; eg, patches, lozenges, gum, inhaler, nasal spray) is grossly underutilized and used incorrectly due to inaccurate instructions perpetuated by clinicians including nurses. Accurate information about the effective use of NRT products is readily available in the literature, but if one does not make it a habit to stay up-to-date with current evidence, myths and mistakes abound.

I have translated current tobacco treatment evidence into practice and have developed and conducted ongoing group, individual, and telehealth treatment for veterans and employees in a wide variety of clinical settings. I prescribe according to the latest 2008 clinical practice guidelines (CPG).[3] As these CPGs are now 13 years old, I am also using more recent evidence-based literature to update my prescribing patterns so that I am in concurrence with published research and what I learned in my specialty training for certification with the Mayo Clinic Nicotine Dependence Center. This has helped me to provide care that is efficacious, cost-effective, and supports my patients' quit rate levels as consistently above those seen at other facilities.

Current literature is also a key component to the continuing education sessions that I provide, not only with the VA, but for members of my various professional organizations at local, state, and national conferences. Because I have provided many educational offerings, my confidence level in providing these in a variety of settings and for a variety of clinicians has improved. This has made for educational offerings that I am told are extremely pragmatic and enjoyable to attend. Consequently, I am often sought out to speak on my areas of expertise which include tobacco dependence treatment, motivational interviewing, VA nursing and military culture, and charge nurse and nursing leadership. All of this has a snowballing effect. The more confident I am in providing evidence-based education, the better the training and educational sessions, the more professional relationships I build when my expertise is sought, and the more opportunities become open to me.

The VA health care system is the largest health care system in the United States.[4] It is by both history and nature, very hierarchical in organizational structure. Additionally, despite the system's expressed desire for innovation, there is some resistance to change. Understanding the organizational structure is critical to interpreting and fulfilling a DNP practice in the VA and is consistent with DNP Essential II: Organizational and Systems Leadership for Quality Improvement and Systems Thinking. As part of my DNP preparation, I monitor national performance measures, adjust the verbiage of the clinical reminders, and provide education to correctly complete attainment of the national standards.

The decision was made by providers so that each regional level VA facility would have at least 1 TTC whose majority assignment was to help people quit using tobacco. As there is a plethora of literature about the health care cost savings realized when people quit using tobacco, this was widely supported. There was no local business plan developed for the use of a person dedicated to tobacco treatment issues. However, the TTC role is supported by local data collected and examined about tobacco treatment interventions (behavioral and pharmacotherapy) through the use of what is called "clinical reminders." These reminders in the electronic health records, known as the clinical patient record system (CPRS) of VA patients, are embedded in each patient's CPRS record and come due at scheduled intervals (eg, annual, monthly). The data gathered from the completion of these reminders is stored in the VA's corporate data warehouse (CDW) and is searchable. Trends discovered continue to support the financial rational for the position of the TTC.

About 10 years ago, I joined the American Psychiatric Nurses Association (APNA). This organization of professionals has provided me with a plethora of personal and professional relationships and opportunities. My DNP leadership skills served me well as the president of the APNA Michigan chapter from 2016 to 2019. Not only did I benefit from developing useful relationships within the organization, I was able to facilitate and link other professionals with each other to provide continuing education, mentorship, and networking opportunities for psychiatric nurses in Michigan.

An emerging threat to population health, especially among youth, is the rapidly expanding use of novel electronic nicotine delivery systems (ENDS). For the purposes of this chapter, ENDS is the term widely used in literature for non-combustible devices such as e-cigarettes, vape pens, JUULs, electronic hookah and pipe, and many other devices designed to facilitate the inhalation of nicotine aerosols. As part of another APNA role I have had as the leader of the Tobacco Dependence Branch of the APNA Addictions Council, I facilitated a summary of current information and evidence about the use of ENDS. The group of professionals I led published an article on the subject, with identified nursing implications and recommended talking points.[5]

These activities with APNA are an embodiment of DNP Essential III: Clinical Scholarship and Analytical Methods for Evidence-Based Practice. Information that I have gained via the analysis of clinically oriented literature has supported ongoing teaching for my peers in clinical settings and for colleagues via conferences and multiple electronic media opportunities. Having a DNP degree has broadened my subsequent reach in the pursuit to provide evidence-based information. While these actions are activities that I could have done while possessing a master's in nursing, earning a DNP degree helped me understand how to formulate and deliver evidence and analysis through an expanded perspective. Linking back to graduate school, networking and the professional relationships that I had cultivated has enhanced my DNP practice. I was well-prepared to engage in the opportunity to examine large data collections.

The activities I engaged in are consistent with DNP Essential IV: Information Systems/Technology and Patient Care Technology for the Improvement and Transformation of Health Care. This opportunity consisted of clarifying the trends and meaning of data collected through clinical reminders embedded in CPRS in the VA health care system. The VA has facilities and community-based outpatient clinics (CBOCs) located in all 50 states and many US territories.[4] Clinical reminders track a variety of preventative and standard care for the purpose of measuring results against national performance measures set by VA leadership and other accrediting organizations such as the Joint Commission. The clinical reminders show what percentage of veterans are asked about possible tobacco use and are offered medications and counseling if they use tobacco. Follow-up supportive care is also tracked. Local clinical reminder results are affected by my efforts and the efforts of all primary care providers. There has been wide variability of results largely related to defining what qualifies as care, difficulties relating to documentation of care, and regular technological glitches. At present, the local VA is currently meeting these performance measures.

To date, I have had the opportunity to collaborate with a very experienced team of VA researchers. As a result, we have discovered and published on findings about trends in treatment such as a higher rate of offered care than the private sector, and that the care is both clinically effective and cost-effective.[6-8] Another manuscript is underway that describes what type of providers, clinics, and facilities tend to complete the clinical reminders as well as identifying areas for improvement. Knowledge discovered through this data-mining endeavor will help to shape and improve VA health care for decades to come. This contributes to DNP Essential V: Health Care Policy for Advocacy in Health Care and DNP Essential VII: Clinical Prevention and Population Health for Improving the Nation's Health. As a DNP, I was sought out and completed a chapter in a nursing text that addresses health behavior change.[9] The chapter focused on nursing use of motivational interviewing (MI). Findings included significant interest in using MI but also found inconsistent documentation of MI training of nurses prior to implementation, poor follow-up of mentoring and monitoring, and inconsistent fidelity to the MI model.

Additionally, my DNP education and networking has led to a recommendation in having me review and provide feedback for an implemented Centers for Disease Control and Prevention (CDC) prevention program, A Million Hearts.[10] This program will provide guidance to clinicians as they create supportive systems in their health care systems to help patients quit using tobacco. While most of my review contributions were used, not all recommendations on recovery language were accepted for this version but they will be incorporated into future iterations of the program.

The networking relationships I have created have also led to other work that contributes to national policy and advocacy. As part of my participation with the Smoking Cessation Leadership Center, I volunteered for and was accepted as a co-leader of a systems change committee through the National Partnership on Behavioral Health and Tobacco Use. This committee focuses on large-scale policy changes that can improve tobacco treatment care. Fellow collaborators on the committee include leaders at top national organizations such as the CDC, the Office of the Surgeon General, and gold standard researchers and educators.

My work with APNA nursing competencies for tobacco treatment will help establish minimum standards of knowledge and practice for all nurses and will shape licensing and certifications examinations. As nurses, we are ideally suited to use our frequent and regular contact with patients to assist them in quitting. This system change stands to have a large-scale effect on the rate and adverse effects of tobacco use and emerging nicotine delivery systems.

There is an African proverb that I love, "To go fast, go alone. To go far, go together." This summarizes what DNP Essential VI: Interprofessional Collaboration for Improving Patient and Population Health Outcomes means to me. Many of the aforementioned activities also demonstrate the interdisciplinary nature of my contributions meeting this essential competency.

In 2015, I was a member of the VA central nursing office (CNO) mental health field advisory committee (MH-FAC). As part of my membership in this committee, I was recommended to serve as an affiliate of a joint department of defense (all military branches represented) and VA task force for the purpose of updating and rewriting the 2009 Substance Use Disorders Clinical Practice Guidelines (SUD CPG). As a member of this task force, I met bi-weekly via phone conference calls and 1 face-to-face meeting in Washington, DC to review current SUD treatment literature and complete a comprehensive update of the document. This document, the *VA/DoD Clinical Practice Guideline for the Management of Substance Use Disorders*, is available online.[11]

The final DNP Essential VIII: Advanced Nursing Practice, has been a journey of discovering what does and does not work in clinical settings. There has been a long-standing expectation that evidence-based tobacco treatment care should include individual, group, and telehealth counseling services and the most updated pharmacotherapy. While I agree that these services are the minimum of what can and should be available to patients, there is room for innovation in the clinical setting. Over the course of 12 years of clinical practice, I have discovered and subsequently implemented other services, mostly geared toward making tobacco treatment unbiased, convenient, and highly individualized. Because the addiction to nicotine is often a relapsing condition, creating an atmosphere of acceptance and having an "open-door" policy has lent itself well to this health care challenge. I find that services that include a high degree of flexibility via very brief telephone follow-up and a variety of other services delivered via secure messaging and video chat options are very much appreciated by busy people struggling with a vexing addiction to nicotine. A review of my most recent patient quit rates reveals a range from 60% to 65% successful quitting for 30 or more days. Those who have not quit tobacco engage in frequent quit attempts and usually decrease their tobacco use by two-thirds or more (leading to increased quit attempts). In comparison, the CDC reports that almost 70% of people want to quit smoking and more than 50% make a quit attempt each year.[12] However, only about 10% of people are actually successful in quitting smoking.[12] Focusing on making cessation attempts convenient with easy and supportive follow-up and treating clients as adults with a difficult addiction has led to my successful quit rates. Should this trend continue to be stable, it may reflect practice-based evidence that validates nursing innovation.

My success in clinical practice as a DNP is directly linked to my most recent employment endeavors. I now have a well-rounded curriculum vitae reflecting the cultivation of meaningful collaboration in professional relationships that support individual, group, and population health. I am exploring the exciting challenges of self-employed, independent practice, and consulting with a goal of teaching and mentoring nursing colleagues and students to promote healthy behavior change. My DNP preparation allowed me to critically evaluate the pros and cons of making this substantial change in employment status.

## Pearls/Takeaways

- Cultivate self-confidence. Of all the challenges nurses face, make sure your own lack of vision and lack of confidence in your abilities is not standing in your way. Consider creating opportunities for small but regular successes (eg, take, pass, and exceed at 1 class toward your next degree, not 3 or 4 classes all at once).
- Create your own opportunities. Luck happens when you are in the right place at the right time. Show up to challenging situations, even when (and especially when) you do not want to be there or cannot think of how this challenge will benefit you or your patients.
- Avoid the tendency to go it alone when working on projects (remember the African proverb), as it may seem harder to include others. The outcomes will be consistently better.

- Always give credit where credit is due, even if it is a small accomplishment by a colleague. People live up to and/or down to what is expected of them, so a little bit of "sugar" can help set up future successful efforts.
- Learn how to listen really well. Since it is unlikely you are already doing this, listen with the main purpose of understanding the meaning behind the words. This is a critical building block to effective relationships with professional colleagues as well as patients.
- Make it a point to collaborate with someone who challenges your thinking and who you do not necessarily agree with. This helps you gain a wider perspective of each clinical challenge.
- Relationships are critical for professional development and knowledge sharing. It does not matter one iota what the "alphabet soup" is behind your name. I learned a great deal from my patients and medical assistants at all levels of nursing staff.
- Keep your knowledge and skills up or prepare to get run over (professionally). Always remember to be the nurse you would want to receive care from if you were ill.
- The possibilities for nursing innovation are limitless. Ask yourself how you can contribute to nursing innovation.

## Conclusion: Impact of the DNP Degree

As a result of obtaining a DNP degree, I have contributed to the profession of nursing and improved patient care in both specific and wide-ranging ways. All of the contributions can be replicated. Specific contributions I have made to the practice of nursing include:

- Conceptualization, development, and implementation of a tobacco treatment program for veterans struggling with addictions and severe mental health issues that achieved consistently good quit rates (17% to 20% vs the widely noted quit rates of 5% to 10% for these patients).
- Conceptualization, development, and implementation of an employee tobacco treatment program for employees that has been highly successful (60% to 65% vs approximately 20% in the general public).
- Conceptualization, development, and implementation of a telehealth tobacco treatment program that consistently realized quit rates in the 80% range.
- Development of nursing continuing education that is firmly grounded in current tobacco treatment evidence and was regularly delivered to local, state, and national levels.
- Initiation and ongoing collaboration to develop a comprehensive list of tobacco treatment competencies for

nurses that can be used to develop curriculum in academic and clinical settings and can also be used as content for certification and licensing examinations.

- As the nursing role in treating tobacco use and dependency is sometimes overlooked, the invitation extended to me to participate in national level multidisciplinary program and policy development was significant and directly linked to my DNP preparation. The value of including nursing contributions is visibly raised. The opportunity for nurses to collaborate with tobacco treatment subject matter experts from highly regarded health care organizations (eg, Mayo Clinic, CDC, Office of the Surgeon General) has the potential to serve as a systems change effort aimed at increasing patient access to improved quality tobacco treatment care.

Finally, my DNP degree has resulted in me identifying important wide-ranging research questions to be explored about psychiatric nursing. It is a conundrum to many that the role of psychiatric nursing has historically been so poorly articulated. Psychiatric nursing can and should be more than simply doing intake assessment paperwork, mundane daily charting of vitals, passing or prescribing medications, and being the treatment team scribe. Research questions that I propose to work on include:

- How do we best measure nursing practice adherence to applicable scope and standards of care?
- What would be the best way(s) to create space for nursing innovation regarding treating tobacco use and dependence and/or health behavior change?
- What is it that is *uniquely nursing* that can be contributed to multidisciplinary treatment about the vexing problems associated with tobacco use and behavior change?

These and other questions would not likely have occurred to me prior to earning a DNP degree. I now have the confidence to address these and many other questions. I will use these queries to guide my DNP practice for the remainder of my career.

# Acknowledgments

It is with gratitude that I dedicate this chapter to my children, Dana Mathes and Abraham Essenmacher. They are my heroes and it was and still is with significant sacrifice on their part that I have completed and practice as a DNP. I also want to acknowledge the life-long love and support I have received from my siblings. It really did take a village to raise me. I give credit to my late parents for the many, many sacrifices they made and the grace, tolerance, and humor they extended to me as I insisted on navigating my own course early in life. I have been fortunate to always have good teachers throughout my life, and these individuals were not always in an academic setting. They have included my patients, my coworkers and colleagues, and included 2 key academic instructors—Dr. Diane Hamilton (who suffers no fools and taught me the basics of writing) and Dr. Sonia Duffy (who finished the job of teaching me to write and introduced scientific inquiry to me). To all I owe a debt of gratitude and probably a dinner or 2.

# References

1. Use a SWOT analysis to build you nursing or healthcare career. The Sentinel Watch. https://www.americansentinel.edu/blog/2017/08/18/use-a-swot-analysis-to-build-your-nursing-or-healthcare-career/

2. The essentials of DNP practice. Springer Publishing Company. http://www.dnpnursingsolutions.com/dnp-nursing-program-overview/dnp-program-essentials/

3. Fiore MC, Jaen CR, Baker TB, et al. *Treating Tobacco Use and Dependence: 2008 Update*. Department of Health and Human Service; 2008.

4. Gordon S. *Wounds of War: How the VA Delivers Health, Healing, and Hope to the Nation's Veterans*. Cornell University Press; 2018.

5. Essenmacher C, Naegle M, Baird C, et al. Electronic nicotine delivery systems (ENDS): what nurses need to know. *J Am Psychiatr Nurses Assoc*. 2012;24(2):145-152.

6. Ignacio RV, Barnett PG, Kim HM, et al. Trends and patient characteristics associated with tobacco pharmacotherapy dispensed in the veterans health administration. *Nicotine Tob Res*. 2018;20(10):1173-1181. doi:10.1093/ntr/ntx229

7. Duffy SA, Ignacio RV, Kim HM, et al. Effectiveness of tobacco cessation pharmacotherapy in the veterans health administration. *Tob Control*. 2019;28(5):540-547. doi:10.1136/tobaccocontrol-2018-054473

8. Barnett PG, Ignacio RV, Kim HM, et al. Cost-effectiveness of real-world administration of tobacco pharmacotherapy in the United States Veterans Health Administration. *Addiction*. 2019;114(8):1436-1445. doi:10.1111/add.14621

9. Essenmacher C. Motivational interviewing and patient activation. In: Frenn M. *Health Promotion: Translating Evidence to Practice*. FA Davis Company; 2021.

10. Home. Million Hearts. https://millionhearts.hhs.gov/

11. VA/DoD clinical practice guideline for the management of substance use disorders. US Department of Veterans Affairs. https://www.healthquality.va.gov/guidelines/MH/sud/VADoDSUDCPGRevised22216.pdf

12. Smoking and tobacco use. Centers for Disease Control and Prevention. Accessed December 17, 2019. https://www.cdc.gov/tobacco/data_statistics/mmwrs/byyear/2017/mm6552a1/index.html

# SECTION IV

## CERTIFIED REGISTERED NURSE ANESTHETIST EXEMPLARS

# CHAPTER 8

# IMPLEMENTING THE DNP ESSENTIALS AS A CHIEF NURSE ANESTHETIST AND PRESIDENT OF THE AMERICAN ASSOCIATION OF NURSE ANESTHETISTS

*Garry Brydges, PhD, DNP, MBA, APRN, CRNA, ACNP-BC, FAAN*

## INTRODUCTION

A Doctor of Nursing Practice (DNP) education prepares the certified registered nurse anesthetist (CRNA) for many roles ranging from evidence-based strategies in clinical prevention, population health, and health care policy development through an array of interdisciplinary collaborations. In my professional career trajectory, a DNP education prepared me in 2 key areas: (1) in my workplace as the chief nurse anesthetist including organizational and systems leadership, programmatic development, and clinical scholarship, and (2) as president of both the Texas Association of Nurse Anesthetists (TxANA) from 2012 to 2013 and American Association of Nurse Anesthetists (AANA) from 2018 to 2019 that included focused areas such as organizational and systems leadership, advanced practice registered nursing (APRN) advocacy through health care policy development, quality and safety outcomes, and transformative patient care strategies.[1] These experiences were the most notable areas in which a DNP education enhanced my professional career trajectory. The following chapter outlines 1 example of how CRNAs and APRNs can apply a DNP education in their workplace.

## ROLE TENURE AND EXPANSION

Early in my tenure, as the chief nurse anesthetist for a large academic center, I was responsible for 36 CRNAs and for overseeing a clinical practice involving 39 anesthetizing locations. Today, the practice has grown to more than 110 CRNAs and 6 nurse anesthesia managers reporting to myself (chief nurse anesthetist). To date, the clinical practice has grown to 65 anesthetizing locations serving more than 200 patients per day. Like many other individuals in leadership roles, I was not promoted into this leadership position based on leadership skills, but rather clinical expertise as both a CRNA and an acute care nurse practitioner (ACNP).[2] In many cases, individuals that exhibit high performance and skill mastery in their clinical role are the individuals typically promoted into leadership positions, which may not necessarily be based on leadership competency.[2,3] This is true throughout most professions but remains prevalent across all health care professions. Leadership and clinical excellence are not synonymous.[2] Early in my leadership career, I acquired a number of clinical degrees and clinical experience augmenting my clinical skill set in the cardiovascular

Benson LA, ed. *The DNP Professional:*
*Translating Value From Classroom to Practice* (pp 87-97).
© 2021 SLACK Incorporated.

intensive care units (ICU), but no education that directly related to leadership experience or formal education in leadership development. For example, many clinical nurses are promoted into charge nurse roles due to their excellent clinical skills, troubleshooting acumen, and complex decision-making skills. While these are important elements for developing into a leader, these are not leadership competencies. One of my strengths was an aptitude for self-awareness and identifying personal growth opportunities. While observing and learning, I utilized experiences to develop competencies in servant leadership. I spent an enormous amount of time with the bedside ICU nurses on rounds discussing their patients in-depth, listening to their concerns, collaborating in planning their care for the patients, and offering resources to ensure the care they rendered was optimal for the patients. I also assumed at least 1 patient assignment when functioning in the charge nurse role. In servant leadership, leading from the frontline is an important leadership competency.[4] After completing 2 undergraduate degrees and 2 graduate master's degrees early in my chief CRNA leadership role, I realized a need to develop a range of leadership acumen and decided to pursue formal leadership preparation specific to the APRN role. While examples such as the ones mentioned previously are not directly related to DNP education, they merely serve as validation to the gaps across the nursing continuum and pathways to expanding the professional role of the nurse through a DNP education.

# Evidence-Based Clinical Scholarship, Applying Analytical Methodologies, Systems Thinking, and Interprofessional Collaboration to Implement Opioid-Sparing Strategies

As the chief nurse anesthetist, I was required to complete classes in organizational management and executive leadership. I recognized the need to pursue a DNP education to better represent the clinicians that reported to me within our organization. One of the most important elements of the DNP Essentials outlined by the American Association of Colleges of Nursing was Organizational and Systems Leadership for Quality Improvement and Systems Thinking.[1] In anesthesia, every intervention rendered to a patient must be measured for an immediate response and translated into an overall outcome for that patient. In an era of opioid-sparing strategies in anesthesia, one of the greatest barriers in advancing clinical practice is executing systems thinking. Opioid-sparing techniques in anesthesia are one element of an overall program known as enhanced recovery after surgery (ERAS).[5] Implementing opioid-sparing strategies in clinical practice requires a paradigm shift toward newer innovations in clinical care. Clinicians tend to avoid adopting these newer strategies due to traditional mindsets and behaviors and overall increased workload with newer techniques.[6] Another barrier challenging practice innovation, such as opioid-sparing techniques, is the range of interdisciplinary collaboration required including surgeons, operating room nurses, recovery room nurses, pharmacists, hospital administrators, and executive leadership.[7] Opioid-sparing strategies require the implementation of newer pharmacological agents, which may directly cost more than traditional pharmacological approaches to clinical care. A DNP education helps address these barriers through evidence-based clinical scholarship, applying analytical methodologies, systems thinking, and interprofessional collaboration focusing on improving patient outcomes.[1]

# DNP Essential: Scientific Underpinnings for Practice

As stated previously, opioid-sparing strategies in anesthesia is a paradigm shift in clinical care. A DNP education enabled me to evaluate the scientific underpinnings guiding a transition in anesthesia care delivery into newer innovative practices. Utilizing science-based theories and concepts to describe a range of approaches to opioid-sparing strategies was imperative to developing and evaluating newer emerging anesthesia practices. The theoretical premise for opioid-sparing strategies involves minimizing inflammation and optimizing immune function of the patients when confronting surgical stress.[8] Ironically, opioids have been found to increase inflammation and blunt immune function, which is contradictory to patient optimization during the perioperative continuum. DNP Essential I: Scientific Underpinnings for Practice was a guiding principle in the evaluation of current practice and adopting opioid-sparing strategies based on emerging health care delivery phenomena. Many anesthesia clinicians challenged opioid-sparing strategies due to unfamiliarity with newer emerging philosophies and an overall resistance to change. A resistance to change in health care delivery has existed for decades and is well-documented by the Institute of Medicine's book *Crossing the Quality Chasm: A New Health System for the 21st Century*, written almost 20 years ago.[9]

# DNP Essential: Clinical Scholarship and Analytical Methods for Evidence-Based Practice

In an effort to transform anesthesia care delivery, comparing and contrasting traditional anesthesia methodologies to opioid-sparing strategies requires a critical appraisal of the existing literature for gaps in patient care delivery, patient outcomes, opportunities in new reimbursement strategies, and overall cost-effectiveness.[10] DNP Essential III: Clinical Scholarship and Analytical Methods for Evidence-Based Practice is one of the pivotal Essentials in fostering practice innovation and implementation.[1] Since opioid-sparing strategies in anesthesia is a significant divergence from traditional practices, a preponderance of evidence focusing on clinical outcomes remains vital in nurturing anesthesia clinicians to adopting these novel strategies. Specific to opioid-sparing strategies, a review of the literature was performed focusing on the scientific underpinnings and theories, pharmacological and physiological foundations, change management, cost-effectiveness, quality outcomes, health care policy, reimbursement strategies, and clinical benchmarks.[10] The reason this DNP Essential is critical is because it connects all other DNP Essentials. Opioid-sparing strategies possess a significant range of variability on how clinicians implement these techniques highlighting the importance of critically evaluating the literature available and tailoring anesthesia care to each patient as a unique individual. After collaborating on a framework for opioid-sparing strategies and applying the strategies, evaluating patient outcomes was instrumental for setting benchmarks. Clinical outcome benchmarks validate the paradigm shift toward opioid-sparing strategies redefining practice patterns and mitigating practice variability.[11,12]

# DNP Essential: Interprofessional Collaboration for Improving Patient and Population Health Outcomes

Through my DNP education, I learned how to critically evaluate clinical scholarship. Core decisions in anesthesia practice are based on scientific underpinnings in order to transform practice innovations, such as opioid-sparing strategies. As the chief nurse anesthetist, a major milestone in adopting change required interprofessional collaboration. One strategy was the implementation of annual professional development goals for CRNAs, which included CRNAs generating evidence-based clinical guidelines in their subspecialty of perioperative oncologic care. These annual professional development goals required a review of the literature, interprofessional collaboration with surgeons, anesthesiologists, nurses, and pharmacists to construct clinical care guidelines. For example, a team of CRNAs in collaboration with physicians described the clinical anesthesia approach to performing awake craniotomies and tumor resections in vital areas of the brain.[13] The awake craniotomy practice approach was later published in the AANA journal.[13] These professional development strategies helped anesthesia clinicians to evaluate clinical scholarship and participate in interprofessional collaboration in defining their current practice. In subsequent years, the CRNAs were encouraged to further reevaluate and enhance their practice guidelines with new or emerging evidence and disseminate the information through scholastic initiatives such as additional publications, abstract presentations, and interdisciplinary lectureship. The strategy evolved over a 5-year time frame fostering 2 key elements: clinical scholarship and embracing change because the CRNAs now owned the change being implemented clinically. The next strategy involved formal comprehensive interprofessional collaboration through textbook publications. Mentoring these CRNAs in maturing their expertise through clinical scholarship and interprofessional collaboration was a unique opportunity for CRNAs to define a clinical subspecialty in oncologic anesthesia care delivery. Over the 5 years, the CRNAs were able to bridge many gaps in anesthesia care specific to the oncologic patient. They were now introduced into formal interdisciplinary teams to construct textbook chapters specific to their subspecialty incorporating the surgical approaches to oncology care, the anesthesia approaches to oncologic care, and critical care approaches to the oncologic patient.[14] Content for each textbook chapter included interprofessional collaboration between nurse anesthetists, anesthesiologists, proceduralists, and surgeons. After 2 years, a textbook entitled *Oncologic Critical Care* was published in 2019 describing subspecialty oncology care across the perioperative and acute care phases of the cancer patient.[14]

# DNP Essential: Organizational and Systems Leadership for Quality Improvement and Systems Thinking

DNP Essential II outlines the importance of business acumen and literacy in health care delivery operations.[1] While the DNP Essentials outline the importance of business, finance, economics, and health policy, an opportunity exists for many DNP programs across the country specific to this DNP Essential. In a study performed by Brydges et al[3], a number of study participants identified DNP programs as lacking in this area of the DNP Essentials, most notably business acumen and financial literacy. In hospital operations, APRNs must be able to translate clinical services into business strategies, which is an area many APRNs tend to struggle with even after completing a DNP education. In my role, I decided to pursue an MBA and PhD focusing on financial literacy in executive nursing leadership. As described previously, one of my responsibilities was to expand anesthesia practices across our organization. In an effort to augment and parallel organizational initiatives, my responsibilities included the development of business plans incorporating economics, finance, and business analytics in order to make sound operational decisions. Early on in my career trajectory, I admittedly struggled with many of these facets of leadership competency. However, self-awareness led me to transform a weakness into a strength through additional formal education, application, and mentors. For example, a few years ago a hospital service line approached me about expanding anesthesia services into a specialty department to help manage various types of lung pathologies. The request required an expansion of clinical anesthesia providers and additional anesthesia supplies and equipment. In collaboration with the requesting department, I generated a business plan that incorporated operational analytics and financial ratios, which provided a robust picture to augment the decision making in determining service volume targets and operational metrics. The specific service line set up a series of meetings, which I attended with enormous interest so I could expand and provide additional anesthesia support. However, to my surprise, when I requested the departments pro forma or business plan to identify the projected case volumes, breakeven analysis, overall expenditures, and market competition/recruitment strategies for new patients, the requesting department did not possess any of the information. In contrast, I was able to provide several market forces influencing the entrainment of new patient volumes and the minimum volume thresholds to break even financially for the service line. In operations required a minimum of 2.5 cases per day to break even in the service line expansion.

# SWOT Analysis, Business Planning, and Financial Literacy

While DNP education assisted somewhat in decision-making analysis, I recognized the gap I possessed in financial analytics and sought to develop that leadership competency. In a rapidly changing health care environment, DNP programs need to introduce the translation of clinical services into business analytics and the value nursing offers a health care entity. Currently, I am responsible for a budget exceeding $50 million per year. One of the most important leadership skills is translating clinical interventions into

quality outcomes and weighing health care delivery interventions based on cost-effectiveness or cost-benefit analyses. Operational decision making must be evidence-based using financial ratio analysis, business plans, pro forma, periodic quality metric reporting, and overall fiscal impact to the organization (Table 8-1).

One of the greatest challenges in health care delivery is translating health care and quality outcomes in terms of business analytics. Although DNP Essentials require business elements and financial literacy as part of a DNP curriculum, many DNP programs lack in this area of education.[3] In a study conducted by Brydges et al,[3] DNP graduates describe their programs as focusing on quality and outcomes, but absent in teaching business essentials or critical elements of financial literacy. Furthermore, Brydges et al,[3] describes financial literacy as one of the most important competencies in executive leadership, but executive nurses identify financial literacy as one of their lowest levels of competency. Since business and financial literacy skills are outlined in the DNP Essentials, the gap in DNP education served as a stimulus for myself to develop a competency in financial literacy. After completing an MBA, incorporating business plans into most of my clinical decision making offered an expanded approach to addressing clinical challenges by translating solutions across the entire health care continuum. For example, opioid-sparing strategies require the use of newer agents that increase the direct cost of care. When intravenous acetaminophen emerged onto the marketplace across the United States, the direct acquisition cost started at $10 to $14 per vial. After the pharmaceutical company Cadence Pharmaceuticals sold the rights of intravenous acetaminophen to Mallinckrodt, the price of intravenous acetaminophen increased to $38 to $42 per vial. As a result, many hospital administrators and pharmacists removed intravenous acetaminophen from hospital formularies due to the increase in direct cost, which was not a sound business decision. After a thorough review of literature, the benefits of intravenous acetaminophen resulted in clinically significant associated reductions in pain scores, post-operative nausea and vomiting, early ambulation, and reduced hospital length of stay, demonstrating a clear benefit to patients and quality outcomes.[15] When hospital administrators and pharmacies focus on direct acquisition costs without understanding or translating the consumable inputs into beneficial outputs, such decisions result in lowering the overall quality of care and reducing beneficial patient outcomes. These types of examples reinforce the value in business plans helping to provide rational decision making such as incorporating a modality of care despite a higher direct cost due to the return on investment. Many pharmacists and hospital administrators seem to overlook this concept. In any business plan, the direct cost must be weighed against the variable cost of patient care outcomes, hospital analytics, and overall revenue generation. In the previous example, using traditional pharmacological approaches to anesthesia, the direct acquisition cost for pharmaceuticals during the perioperative phase of care ranges between $290 to $325 per

**Table 8-1**

## SWOT PROGRAMMATIC DEVELOPMENT

| STRENGTHS | WEAKNESSES |
|---|---|
| • Identify scientific underpinnings for programmatic development | • Business skills development and application<br>• Financial literacy development<br>• Reimbursement strategies |
| OPPORTUNITIES | THREATS |
| • Develop skills in change management | • DNP graduates unable to translate care into financial outcomes |

case. However, these strategies incorporate the use of opioids, which increase physiologic inflammation, decrease immune response, increase post-operative nausea and vomiting, contribute to metastatic translocation long-term in cancer patients, increase the incidence of post-operative ileus, decrease early ambulation, decrease early oral intake and nutrition, and may contribute to 30-day readmission rates.[8] When translating the variable costs of each of these iatrogenic comorbidities specifically related to opioid administration, the cost of care is increased nearly 600% compared to opioid-sparing strategies (direct cost = $1400 to $1500 per case), and a return on investment of $5.60 for every $1.00 spent in favor of opioid-sparing strategies. In contrast, intravenous acetaminophen has profound anti-inflammatory properties, immune preservation, reduced post-operative nausea and vomiting, long-term metastatic translocation reductions in cancer patients, reduced incidence post-operative ileus, early ambulation, early oral intake, and reduced hospital length of stay.[15] As part of any business plan, a critical element for health care delivery is a ratio analysis weighing the direct acquisition costs against variable outcome cost and patient satisfaction. When generating business plans, a market analysis comparing traditional approaches to health care delivery is essential in evaluating against any new idea or paradigm shift. Furthermore, as intravenous acetaminophen direct acquisition costs gained scrutiny across many health care organizations, a focus toward oral forms of acetaminophen were explored as a cost-effective alternative in practice and in the literature.[15] However, another critical skill imparted by DNP education was developing into an informed consumer of clinical research. Unfortunately, all research studies are not created equal and consumers must be astute in identifying the difference between quality and poor research.[16] After Mallinckrodt increased the acquisition costs of intravenous acetaminophen, many studies emerged comparing intravenous to oral acetaminophen and correlating clinical outcomes. Unfortunately, much of the research comparing and contrasting intravenous to oral acetaminophen was extremely poor with sample sizes reaching 32 and lacking any statistical significance.[17] Unfortunately, some health care practitioners based clinical decisions on poor research and limited access to intravenous acetaminophen based on these types of studies. While this gets into unfortunate ethical issues related to poor published research, many hospital systems transitioned to the use of oral acetaminophen.[17] While not published in literature due to patient privacy, many personal examples of patients receiving oral acetaminophen in the pre-operative phase of care still had an intact oral acetaminophen tablet residing in the stomach or small intestines after 3 hours into surgery validating a poor bioavailability of drug due to a highly variable route of administration. In many of these episodes the surgeon was still able to read the labeling on the oral acetaminophen tablets. The typical approach to intravenous acetaminophen is to administer the agent 1 to 2 hours before surgery in an attempt to maximize bioavailability of the acetaminophen compound. In contrast, despite administering oral acetaminophen 1 to 2 hours preoperatively the compound remains intact well into surgical procedure providing no benefit or reaching any appreciable therapeutic index. The goal of pharmacological administration during the perioperative period is to optimize pharmacological bioavailability, which cannot optimally be achieved with oral medications. The rationale is that surgical stress contributes to the fight or flight response and the digestive system activity decreases contributing to the delayed uptake of oral acetaminophen.[18] When opioid-sparing strategies are compared against traditional perioperative pain management strategies, the direct cost is increased comparatively (Table 8-2).

A sole focus on the direct cost of care has plagued health care delivery for decades and lasting effects validated through the increasing costs of health care delivery without appreciable quality of health services. The goal of health care delivery demands an intimate understanding of value. Today, we hear a lot of people in health care define value as the quotient of quality over cost. The tricky part remains a thorough understanding of the numerator (quality) and denominator (cost). DNP education is the methodology nursing explores how APRNs, nursing leaders, and the profession of nursing

**Table 8-2**

## COST OF CARE FOR AN AVERAGE 4-HOUR ABDOMINAL CASE

| TRADITIONAL METHODOLOGY: DIRECT COST | | | |
|---|---|---|---|
| *Drug* | *Cost per Unit* | *Units* | *Total Cost* |
| Midazolam | $2.40 | 1 | $2.40 |
| Famotidine | $2.53 | 1 | $2.53 |
| Sufentanil | $8.00 | 3 | $24.00 |
| Propofol | $2.30 | 1 | $2.30 |
| Cisatracurium | $24.40 | 3 | $73.20 |
| Glycopyrrolate | $46.75 | 1 | $46.75 |
| Neostigmine | $52.85 | 1 | $52.85 |
| Desflurane | $6.99 | 6 | $41.94 |
| Crystalloid | $1.95 | 3 | $5.85 |
| Ondansetron | $0.70 | 2 | $1.40 |
| Bupivacaine | $36.64 | 1 | $36.64 |
| Hydromorphone | $8.08 | 1 | $8.08 |
| Total Direct Cost | | | $297.94 |

| OPIOID-SPARING METHODOLOGY: DIRECT COST | | | |
|---|---|---|---|
| *Drug* | *Cost per Unit* | *Units* | *Total Cost* |
| Gabapentin | $12.00 | 1 | $12.00 |
| Celebrex | $4.15 | 1 | $4.15 |
| Tramadol | $7.35 | 1 | $7.35 |
| Acetaminophen | $35.40 | 3 | $106.20 |
| Alvimopan | $700.00 | 1 | $700.00 |
| Dexmedetomidine | $31.92 | 1 | $31.92 |
| Propofol | $2.30 | 9 | $20.70 |
| Ketamine | $21.24 | 1 | $21.24 |
| Lidocaine 0.4% | $2.53 | 1 | $2.53 |
| Albumin 5% | $83.72 | 3 | $251.16 |
| Sugammadex | $92.00 | 1 | $92.00 |
| Crystalloid | $1.95 | 1 | $1.95 |
| Ondansetron | $0.70 | 2 | $1.40 |
| Bupivacaine | $36.64 | 1 | $36.64 |
| Liposomal Bupivacaine | $285.00 | 1 | $285.00 |
| Hydromorphone | $8.08 | 1 | $8.08 |
| Total Direct Cost | | | $1582.32 |

**Table 8-3**

## OPIOID-SPARING ECONOMIC IMPACT ON PATIENT OUTCOMES

| PATIENT OUTCOME | COST PER EPISODE | TRADITIONAL | OPIOID-SPARING |
|---|---|---|---|
| Post-operative nausea and vomiting | $87.12 | 15.0% to 33.0% | < 7.0% |
| Respiratory depression | $568.00 | 3.3% | < 1.1% |
| Urinary tract infection | $1357.00 | 2.0% | < 0.5% |
| Post-operative ileus | $10 247.00 | 15.6% | < 7.8% |
| Surgical site infection | $34 407.00 | 5.6% | < 3.0% |
| Hospital length of stay | $2 064.00 per day | 6 to 10 days | 3 to 4 days |
| 30-day readmission rate | $11 200.00 | 5.4% | 2.1% |

defines themselves as quality providers and actions that exhibit quality. In anesthesia, I always take the opportunity to teach a simple example of quality when starting an intravenous access prior to going to the operating room. In anesthesia school, CRNAs are taught the physics behind intravenous access and how to achieve optimal flow of fluids. For example, shorter large-bore catheters such as 16 or 14 gauge are optimal for rapidly administering blood products under emergency conditions. Ironically, nurse anesthesia residents in training will opt to place large-bore, short-length intravenous catheters even on routine non-emergent surgical cases prior to going to the operating room. Unfortunately, the patient presenting as a difficult intravenous access tends to have unsuccessful attempts on the first, second, and sometimes third try. A non-emergent "what if" scenario does not define quality. The opportunity to mentor the nurse anesthesia resident in training should focus on elements of quality. For example, inserting a short, large-bore intravenous catheter on an awake patient is not quality, but rather a personal challenge. With respect to quality and patient experience, I teach the resident to prepare the skin with chloro-preparation, deliver a small subcutaneous aliquot of local anesthetic, and massage the infiltrated skin for 60 seconds while speaking to the patient and family member. Then, additional chloro-preparation of the skin is performed and the vein is allowed to fill optimally with blood. While still speaking with the patient and family, the insertion of a short 20-gauge intravenous catheter that inserts unimpeded nearly 100% of the time is completed. This process is followed by a meticulous bloodless removal of the needle and attachment of the intravenous tubing and securement of the catheter to the skin. The sharps are disposed of into the appropriate receptacle, and my dirty gloves are doffed while holding all the trash in hand in order to engulf the trash into the dirty gloves and discard them as a single unit. Typically, the patients comment that they did not even feel the intravenous catheter insertion.

The patient experience is the objective when rendering basic functions, such as nursing care. Quality nursing care defines a positive patient experience and patient outcome. One of the key elements of quality is the patient experience. The process was efficient, with low anxiety, and most importantly, the information gained during the conversation with the patient and family is always targeted toward the plan of care transitioning into the next phase of care. The most underappreciated element is the confidence gained by the patient and family members. In anesthesia, there is no rush to place a short large-bore intravenous catheter for non-emergent surgical cases prior to going to the operating room. Once the patient is in the operating room and anesthetized, if using inhalation anesthesia gases, the vasculature vasodilates, which is when the resident nurse anesthetist can place a short large-bore intravenous catheter leveraging physics and physiology to ensure optimal conditions for a 1-attempt, bloodless, intravenous insertion. At this point, the resident nurse anesthetist demonstrates another element of quality being efficiency. Cost of health care delivery is the other part of value that is grossly misunderstood. A focus of direct cost results in premature decision making in many aspects of health care delivery. Indirect and variable costs are important factors that possess major impact on overall cost and contributions to value. ERAS is the best example to demonstrate the importance of variable costs impact on value. Opioid-sparing strategies result in increased direct costs but substantially reduce indirect and variable costs compared to traditional pain management strategies (Table 8-3).[18-27] For CRNAs and other APRNs, understanding the quality of health care delivery they impart and how overall cost of health care integrates into value-based health care delivery is essential for appreciating the overall impact APRNs make in reimbursement.

A facet of health care delivery each DNP graduate must possess fluently is the evolving reimbursement strategies by the Centers for Medicare & Medicaid Services (CMS).[28] In 2019, CMS imposed new reimbursement strategies, which eliminated the flawed sustainable growth rate (SGR) formula for reimbursement. Under the Medicare Access and CHIP

Reauthorization Act (MACRA), CMS will increasingly reimburse health care providers and health care organizations based on shared risk strategies.[28] A health care provider or hospital system will participate in 1 of 2 programs, the merit incentive payment system (MIPS) or alternative payment models (APM) but not both. There was a marking of a new era in 2019 toward reimbursement for quality health care services and a shift away from quantity of health care services. A business plan must incorporate these short-term and long-term reimbursement strategies as shared risk will continue to increase over the next 5 years. Under the MIPS program, health care providers exceeding national benchmark composite scores can receive up to 4% incentive, standard reimbursement for average composite scores, and up to a 4% penalty for substandard composite scores.[28] These incentives for penalties continue to increase to a maximum 9% in 2022 and onward. More importantly, hospital systems under the MIPS program have a 3 times multiplier, which can result in a 12% incentive or penalty in 2019 and up to a 27% incentive or penalty in 2022.[28] In the APM programs, the most popular strategy is a bundle payment system for an episode of care. For example, the average CMS reimbursement for a joint replacement episode of care is approximately $26 000.[29] A health care system achieving high-quality outcomes will preserve a significant portion of the bundle payment, rather than spend the bundle on iatrogenic causes as outlined in Table 8-3. Despite a modestly higher direct cost in moving to opioid-sparing strategies, the quality of services achieved exceeds traditional strategies due to mitigating much of the variable costs. More importantly, the impact anesthesia services impart outside of the perioperative phase is significant due to a reduced utilization of staff time (indirect costs) dedicated to managing issues (variable), such as pain control, post-operative ileus, respiratory depression, and surgical site infections. Therefore, a business plan is essential in evaluating short-term and long-term revenue generation strategies.

In my role as the president of the AANA, I routinely lectured on these topics across the country. One of the most common questions from the audience is how a department can start an ERAS program or opioid-sparing program. In an effort to render change management in anesthesia, opioid-sparing strategies remain a significant paradigm shift for many nurse anesthetists and perioperative teams. Therefore, a critical appraisal of the literature is essential in developing opioid-sparing strategies in parallel to ERAS programs. First, a comprehensive review of the literature evaluating opioid agents' role in the perioperative phase is needed. ERAS programs focus on mitigating inflammatory stimuli and optimizing immune function.[18] Although opioid-free anesthesia is the objective during the perioperative phases of care, various forms of symptom burden and rescue may require opioid administration (albeit lower doses) despite multimodal approaches to pain management. After establishing the untoward effects of opioids, a review of the literature seeking alternative pharmacological agents and anesthetic approaches to opioid agents must be completed. There are numerous ERAS protocols throughout the literature that offer a myriad of strategies in managing pain with opioid-sparing techniques. In our practice setting, our opioid-sparing framework was tailored to each patient specifically. Practice innovations, such as multimodal opioid-sparing techniques and regional nerve blocks, require a number of stakeholders to ensure the success of the program. In our gap analysis, traditional anesthesia techniques compared to opiates sparing techniques possessed many deviations in practice. The framework must be evidence-based with clear objectives and a strategy outlined in a business plan. Once a framework for the program has been established, stakeholders from across the health care delivery spectrum must be engaged and contribute to the overall plan. Interprofessional collaboration was imperative to warrant reduced practice variability such as initiating opioid-sparing techniques in the perioperative phase and ensuring nursing or surgical colleagues do not routinely order opiates in the recovery phase, essentially eliminating the benefits of opioid-sparing techniques. In the perioperative phase of care, I routinely collaborate with surgeons, physician anesthesiologists, pharmacists, operating room nurses, recovery room nurses, and administrators on a daily basis. I have collaborated with many of these individuals on performance improvement projects, such as opioid waste programs, cost reduction programs, opioid-sparing, enhanced recovery after surgery programs, and workflow efficiency programs. Each of these interprofessional team members understand and recognize the DNP degree because they participated in many of my projects during my DNP education. Additionally, I have mentored and overseen a number of DNP projects within our department focusing on time-driven, activity-based costing (TDABC).[30,31] The overall cost-savings for the DNP projects exceeded $1 million. In many instances, our departmental quality improvement teams frequently request a DNP student to collaborate on process improvement projects, such as opioid-sparing projects. Helping students identify projects benefits the students in their academic pursuits, and the benefits are reciprocated to the hospital department. The DNP student is a starting point to help bridge interdisciplinary collaboration, ensuring non-nursing stakeholders recognize the value nurses contribute to the team. Interdisciplinary collaboration is fundamental to achieving the overall goal of value-based care through high-quality outcomes and reduced costing. In an effort to ensure buy-in from all stakeholders, current costs, outcomes, revenue generation, and financial ratios must be calculated ensuring a baseline for comparisons. National benchmarks provide a comparison for programmatic adaptation. Utilizing health care systems and technology to track outcomes and cost is fundamental to automating trends and demonstrating value of the program.

# DNP Essential: Information Systems/Technology and Patient Care Technology for the Improvement and Transformation of Health Care

In our anesthesia practice, we utilize electronic health records. One of the DNP Essentials is the utilization of information systems such as the electronic health record.[1] As the director of anesthesia, I must monitor every provider practice based on a catalog of outcome metrics. One of the conditions for participation and reimbursement under CMS includes monitoring anesthesia providers' clinical performance and outcome metrics which is achieved through the program known as ongoing provider performance evaluation (OPPE) and focused provider performance evaluation (FPPE).[28] I developed 8 dashboards of metrics for the nurse anesthetist to track and benchmark against national averages. We automated a number of data points captured by the electronic health record to benchmark each CRNA's metric against the overall group and national thresholds. These metrics are reviewed with each CRNA on a quarterly basis. Some examples include on-time antibiotics, post-operative nausea and vomiting prophylaxis, post-operative pain scores, intra-operative normothermia, provider handoff report, medication reconciliation, and electronic health record correction within 72 hours. Each of these metrics are plotted on a run chart over the entire fiscal year. One of the best examples since the implementation of outcome metrics is on-time antibiotics. Prior to tracking on-time antibiotics, our overall surgical infection rate ranked below the 80th percentile on National Surgical Quality Improvement Program (NSQIP) reporting data. After implementing on-time antibiotics tracking through the electronic health record and transparent reporting systems, our surgical site infection rates dropped precipitously, and our team ranks among the lowest in the country despite caring for the immune compromised oncologic patient population. As described earlier, surgical site infections introduce a wide range of complicating factors including patient dissatisfaction, failed surgical interventions, prolonged hospitalization, increased cost of health care delivery, and significant morbidity and mortality. The intent of OPPE was to ensure high-quality anesthesia provision and exceedingly high outcomes for each nurse anesthesia practitioner. The overarching goal was to ensure anesthesia providers assessed their own practice against national benchmarks. Also, the real-time metrics attempts to ensure a self-reflection on the care rendered by each practitioner to our patient population.

Consistent with the DNP Essentials, ensuring accountability for a high-quality health care delivery and patient safety provided the foundation for developing these initiatives. Today, many of these strategies implemented more than a decade ago have become instrumental in several CMS mandates, Joint Commission standards, and reimbursement strategies under MACRA.

# DNP Essential: Health Care Policy for Advocacy in Health Care

Since completing my DNP, I was elected to the TxANA board of directors and ascended to the president of the association in 2012 to 2013. As a DNP graduate, leadership within professional organizations is imperative to share expertise acquired by a DNP-prepared nurse and develop the leaders of the future. One of the DNP Essentials includes health care policy and advocacy in health care. As president of the TxANA, I led a number of advocacy initiatives during the 2013 Texas legislative session. One of the most important advocacy efforts in 2013 was establishing a state association political action campaign (PAC) fund. Today, the TxANA PAC is one of the strongest nursing PACs in Texas. During 2013, the Texas legislative session was robust in APRN legislative bills focusing on the removal of practice barriers to enhance patient access to high-quality, cost-effective health care services. In conjunction with Senator Nelson, the Texas Medical Board, Senate Health and Human Services committee, APRN stakeholders, Rural Hospital Association, and our advocacy teams, we were able to amend some of the language for APRNs in the nursing practice act to include expanding the required mileage for collaborating physicians with APRNs and expanding the ratio of collaborating physicians with APRNs. Since nurse anesthetists practice in different care models (eg, independent practice, collaborative practice, medical direction models) compared to other APRNs, our (TxANA) role was instrumental to ensure nurse anesthetist practices were unencumbered with new legislative language ensuring the citizens of Texas have increased access to health care delivery that is safe and cost-effective, especially in rural communities. More recently, nurse anesthetist practice barriers were proposed by the Texas Medical Board attempting to create restraint of trade through a rule proposal imposing additional supervisory requirements for Texas certified nurse anesthetists.[32] According to the Federal Trade Commission, the Texas Medical Board's proposal was anticompetitive, impairing access to care in 170 of 254 rural Texas counties, in 64 of 85 Texas critical access hospitals where no anesthesiologist exists, and in 33 of 85 critical access hospitals where nurse anesthetists are the only anesthesia providers of anesthesia services.[32]

Shortly after completing my term as the president of TxANA, I was elected to the AANA board of directors and ascended to be president of the AANA in 2018 to 2019. Health care policy on a federal level was very different compared to states legislative efforts, especially in states like Texas. One of the milestones early in my tenure as the president of the AANA was President Trump signing into law the ability for APRNs, including CRNAs, to prescribe medication-assisted treatment (MAT) to help combat the opioid addiction.[33]

Another health care policy advocacy effort was surprise billing.[34] In some instances, third party payers and some Medicare administrative contractors (MAC) denied CRNAs reimbursement for procedures such as pain management or denied access to health service networks. For CRNAs to be reimbursed for their services, a separate bill for anesthesia was sent to patients in addition to the hospital bill. Approximately 17% of the population accessing health care delivery are confronted with a surprise bill for anesthesia services because insurers deny CRNAs access to participate in some health care networks and refuse to reimburse CRNAs for their crucial services in rural communities.[34] Unfortunately, if a CRNA does not render these services in many of these communities, then access to many health care services would be eliminated including pain management, labor and delivery, emergency services, and a range of surgical services. As president of the AANA, we spent many hours working with legislators in Washington, DC to ensure CRNAs are included in health care networks and reimbursed for their services in order to continue to increase access to cost-effective health care delivery specific to anesthesia and pain management services. As an organization (AANA) exceeding 55 000 nurse anesthetists we are in favor of addressing and removing surprise billing in order to preserve or increase access to care for patients.[34]

## PROFESSIONALISM

As students embark on DNP preparation, their involvement in professional associations is critical. There are a number of organizational leadership mentorship programs to help operationalize advocacy and health care policy for the emerging DNP leader. AANA and board of directors mentor DNP students at every national meeting available to teach leadership, health care policy, and advocacy. As the AANA president, I would take DNP students with me everywhere to learn the decorum of leadership, organizational operations, collaboration, health policy development, and advocacy for the nursing profession. In many instances, DNP students should ask their professional association if there are sponsorships and mentorship programs to help them transition into these critical roles. A DNP student benefits from the co-op opportunities to apply learned DNP skills in professional organization participation. These opportunities in many instances are at minimal to limited cost to the DNP student, but the application of learned knowledge remains essential

in solidifying the impact a DNP education imparts onto the student, nursing profession, and overall health care delivery.

## CONCLUSION: IMPACT OF THE DNP DEGREE

As a result of obtaining their doctoral degrees, DNP students and graduates are change agents. These unique professionals must embrace and propagate change throughout organizations. The only way health care professionals recognize the value of the contributions that nurses make to quality programs is engagement and collaboration. DNP students and mentors must seek out the optimal experiences, much like a co-op program. Hospitals need help identifying mutual experiences benefiting the organization and optimizing the DNP student experience. DNP students will embrace the opportunity to help when offered by the organization and can lead to value-added cost savings for the organization as demonstrated.

A robust framework has been defined by the AACN through the DNP Essentials. Using scientific underpinnings and implementing evidence-based practice has led to CRNA performance-improvement projects such as opioid waste programs, cost-reduction programs, opioid-sparing culture change, ERAS programs, and workflow efficiency programs. For ERAS, interprofessional collaboration with key stakeholders was paramount to plan patient specific treatment plans by reducing practice variability such as initiating opioid-sparing techniques in the perioperative phase and standardizing ordering practices in the recovery phase. Business planning is essential in evaluating short-term and long-term revenue-generation strategies. While the direct costs for opioid-sparing strategies are higher, they are offset by reductions in indirect costs such as staffing and variable costs for pain control, post-operative ileus, respiratory depression, and surgical site infections. For nurse anesthetists, and other APRNs, understanding the quality of health care delivery they impart and how overall cost of health care integrates into value-based health care delivery is essential for appreciating the overall impact APRNs make in reimbursement. A strict adherence to the DNP Essentials will build a strong career trajectory across the entire health care delivery spectrum and provide the nurse anesthetist with the tools to define their value and act as a change agent in rendering high-quality, economically sustainable health care services across the United States.

## ACKNOWLEDGMENTS

I want to acknowledge my devoted wife, Dr. Ninotchka Brydges, for giving me the strength and guidance to pursue my many academic endeavors, such as this publication. Also, I want to acknowledge the AANA members, AANA staff,

AANA foundation, the National Board of Certification and Recertification for Nurse Anesthetists staff, and my many mentors over the past decade who provided me the opportunities to excel in many avenues of health care delivery and the chance to impart that learned knowledge to our student body.

# REFERENCES

1. The essentials of doctoral education for advanced practice nursing. American Association of Colleges of Nursing. https://www.aacnnursing.org/Portals/42/Publications/DNPEssentials.pdf

2. Ahmed R, Azmi Bin Mohamad N. Differentiating between leadership competencies and styles: a critical review in project management perspective. *Int J Inf Technol Proj Manag.* 2016;7(1):58-71. doi:10.4018/IJITPM.2016010105

3. Brydges G, Krepper R, Nibert A, Young A, Luquire R. Assessing executive nurse leaders' financial literacy level: a mixed-methods study. *J Nurs Adm.* 2019;49(12);596-603. doi:10.1097/NNA.0000000000000822

4. Choudhary AI, Akhtar SA, Zaheer A. Impact of transformational and servant leadership on organizational performance: a comparative analysis. *J Bus Ethics.* 2013;116(2):433-440. doi:https://doi.org/10.1007/s10551-012-1470-8

5. Parks L, Routt M, De Villiers A. Enhanced recovery after surgery. *J Adv Pract Oncol.* 2018;9(5):511-519.

6. Lowe G, Plummer V, Boyd L. Nurse practitioner integration: Qualitative experiences of the change management process. *J Nurs Manag.* 2018;26(8):992-1001. doi:10.1111/jonm.12624.

7. Ma C, Park S, Shang J. Inter and intra-disciplinary collaboration and patient safety outcomes in US acute care hospitals units: a cross-sectional study. *Int J Nurs Stud.* 2018;8(5):1-6. doi:10.1016/j.ijnurstu.2018.05.001

8. Boland JW, Pockley AG. Influence of opioids on immune function in patients with cancer pain: from bench to bedside. *Br J Pharmacol.* 2018;175(14):2726-2736. doi:10.1111/bph.13903

9. Institute of Medicine Committee on Quality of Health Care in America. *Crossing the Quality Chasm: A New Health System for the 21st Century.* National Academy Press; 2001.

10. Murphy J, Pritchard MG, Cheng LY, Janarthanan R, Leal J. Cost-effectiveness of enhanced recovery in hip and knee replacement: a systematic review protocol. *BMJ.* 2018;8(3):e019740. doi:10.1136/bmjopen-2017-019740

11. Balfour A, Burch J, Fecher-Jones I, Carter F. Understanding the benefits and implications of enhanced recovery after surgery. *Nurs Stand.* 2019;34(7):70-75. doi:10.7748/ns.2019.e11437

12. Memtsoudis SG, Poeran J, Kehlet H. Enhanced recovery after surgery in the united states: from evidence-based practice to uncertain science? *JAMA.* 2019;321(11):1049-1050. doi: 10.1001/jama.2019.1070

13. Brydges G, Atkinson R, Perry M, Hurst D, Laqua T, Wiemers J. Awake craniotomy: a practice overview. *AANA J.* 2012;80(1):61-68.

14. Nate JL, Price KJ. *Oncologic Critical Care.* Springer; 2020.

15. Sun L, Zhu X, Zou J, Li Y, Han W. Comparison of intravenous and oral acetaminophen for pain control after total knee and hip arthroplasty: a systematic review and meta-analysis. *Medicine.* 2018;97(6):e9751. doi:10.1097/MD.0000000000009751

16. Matsuda T, Watanabe Y. IR for educational planning, learning analytics, and educational engineering. *Jpn J Educ Technol.* 2017;41(3):199-208.

17. Plunkett A, Haley C, McCoart A, et al. A preliminary examination of the comparative efficacy of intravenous vs oral acetaminophen in the treatment of perioperative pain. *Pain Med.* 2017;18(12):2466-2473. doi: 10.1093/pm/pnw273

18. Oderda GM, Gan TJ, Johnson BH, Robinson SB. Effect of opioid-related adverse events on outcomes in selected surgical patients. *J Pain Palliat Care Pharmacother.* 2013;27(1):62-70.

19. Bartels K, Mayes LM, Dingmann C, Bullard KJ, Hopfer CJ, Binswanger IA. Opioid use and storage patterns by patients after hospital discharge following surgery. *PLoS One.* 2016;11(1):e0147972.

20. Helviz Y, Einav S. A systematic review of the high-flow nasal cannula for adult patients. *Crit Care.* 2018;22(1):71.

21. Jenks PJ, Laurent M, McQuarry S, Watkins R. Clinical and economic burden of surgical site infection (SSI) and predicted financial consequences of elimination of SSI from an English hospital. *J Hosp Infect.* 2013/2014;86(1):24-33.

22. Legesse Laloto T, Hiko Gemeda D, Abdella SH. Incidence and predictors of surgical site infection in Ethiopia: prospective cohort. *BMC Infect Dis.* 2017;17(1):119.

23. Parra-Sanchez I, Abdallah R, You J, et al. A time-motion economic analysis of postoperative nausea and vomiting in ambulatory surgery. *J Can Anesth.* 2012;59(4):366-375.

24. Shepard J, Ward W, Milstone A, et al. Financial impact of surgical site infections on hospitals: the hospital management perspective. *JAMA Surg.* 2013;148(10):907-914.

25. Touchette DR, Yang Y, Tiryaki F, Galanter WL. Economic analysis of alvimopan for prevention and management of postoperative ileus. *Pharmacotherapy.* 2012;32(2):120-128.

26. Vendler MMI, Haidari TA, Waage JE, et al. Incidence of venous thromboembolic events in enhanced recovery after surgery for colon cancer: a retrospective, population-based cohort study. *Colorectal Dis.* 2017;19(11):O393-401.

27. Wu AK, Auerbach AD, Aaronson DS. National incidence and outcomes of postoperative urinary retention in the surgical care improvement project. *Am J Surg.* 2012;204(2):167-171.

28. 2019 program requirements Medicare. Centers for Medicare & Medicaid Services. https://www.cms.gov/Regulations-and-Guidance/Legislation/EHRIncentivePrograms/2019ProgramRequirementsMedicare

29. Finkelstein A, Ji Y, Mahoney N, Skinner J. Mandatory medicare bundled payment program for lower extremity joint replacement and discharge to institutional postacute care: interim analysis of the first year of a 5-year randomized trial. *JAMA.* 2018;(9):892-900. doi:https://doi.org/10.1001/jama.2018.12346

30. Kaplan R. Improving value with TDABC. *Healthc Financ Manage.* 2014;68(6):76-83.

31. Popat K, Gracia K, Guzman A, Feeley T. Using time-driven activity-based costing to model the costs of various process-improvement strategies in acute pain management. *J Healthc Manag.* 2018;63(4):E76-E85. doi:https://doi.org/10.1097/JHM-D-16-00040

32. FTC comment to texas medical board raises competitive concerns about proposed rule imposing additional supervisory requirements on texas-certified nurse anesthetists. Federal Trade Commission. https://www.ftc.gov/news-events/press-releases/2019/12/ftc-comment-texas-medical-board-raises-competitive-concerns-about

33. Policy brief: legislation addressing opioid epidemic becomes law. National Council of State Boards of Nursing. https://www.ncsbn.org/13104.htm

34. Kellett H, Spratt A, Miller M. Surprise billing: choose patients over profits. Health Affairs. August 2019. https://www.healthaffairs.org/do/10.1377/hblog20190808.585050/full/

# CHAPTER 9

# The DNP Certified Registered Nurse Anesthetist
## Practice and Advocacy

*Debbie Barber, DNP, CRNA*

## Introduction

The complexity of today's health care environment requires the advanced practice nurse (APRN) to be highly skilled in many arenas. In addition to sound scientific knowledge, the APRN must be adept in assessing organizations and systems thinking, have political skills, and possess business and financial skills for practice and cost analysis.[1]

The Doctor of Nursing Practice (DNP) Essentials for Advanced Nursing Practice define the curricular elements that must be present in DNP programs.[1] The DNP Essentials outline the foundational competencies that are necessary for all APRNs, including certified registered nurse anesthetists (CRNAs). DNP nurses possess a blend of clinical skills, leadership, economic, and organizational adeptness that allow them to meet the challenges of the complex health care environment along with the rapid expansion of knowledge.[2]

DNP Essential II is identified as Organizational and Systems Leadership for Quality Improvement and Systems Thinking. This DNP Essential allows for DNP graduates to improve patient care, as well as promote patient safety and excellence in practice.[3] In 2010, the Institute of Medicine (IOM) "The Future of Nursing" report called for nurses to lead change and advance health. These objectives could be achieved by removing barriers to practice and allowing nurses to practice to their full extent of education and training. The report also called for nurses to be involved in the redesigning of health care in the United States.[4]

Prior to entering a DNP program, I worked as the co-owner of an anesthesia practice, Triple Crown Anesthesia, which operates at an ambulatory surgery center in Louisville, Kentucky. I was both a practice and business partner with a collaborating anesthesiologist. The anesthesiologist and I performed our cases independently.

CRNAs are APRNs who are licensed as independent practitioners. The presence of an anesthesiologist is not required in any state, however, the Centers for Medicare & Medicaid Services (CMS) do require supervision of CRNAs. CMS has allowed for an "opt-out" of this supervision clause, in which individual states can seek an exemption from the federal supervision requirement.[5] In 2012, Kentucky became the 17th state to opt-out of the federal supervision requirement.

Prior to 2012, I worked at the surgery center independent of an anesthesiologist, but to meet the CMS requirement, I worked under the supervision of the operating surgeon. After 2012, this was no longer necessary due to the opt-out.

Benson LA, ed. *The DNP Professional:*
*Translating Value From Classroom to Practice* (pp 99-109).

Currently, I am the sole owner of Triple Crown Anesthesia, having bought out my partner who is semi-retired.

I started this anesthesia practice with minimal knowledge about how to run a business. Most of my learning had come from audio books on starting and running a business. We launched the practice with an informal business plan, basically an outline of the steps needed to begin billing for anesthesia services in consultation with the ambulatory surgery center.

As I learned more about the DNP degree, I realized the knowledge I would obtain would be useful in maintaining a business and anesthesia practice. When I read the IOM report, I felt as if I were already involved in redesigning anesthesia care, as only about 1% of all anesthesia practices function as CRNA-anesthesiologist partnerships.[5]

At this time, I was also heavily involved in lobbying with my state association, the Kentucky Association of Nurse Anesthetists (KyANA) and believed a DNP degree would strengthen my abilities in this arena. DNP Essential V addresses Health Care Policy for Advocacy in Health Care.[6] If I was going to continue to fight to remove barriers and protect CRNA practice, I believed I needed a DNP to increase my knowledge related to lobbying and advocacy.

I had the opportunity to hear Dr. Mary Wakefield, DNP, speak at a national CRNA meeting. At that time, she was serving in the Obama administration as the head of Health Resources and Services Administration. As she was speaking, I noticed her credentials, and at that moment I realized I did have goals that were political in nature. The DNP credential behind her name convinced me I needed to seek a terminal degree in nursing to add credibility to my name in the political arena. Dr. Wakefield is credited with the statement, "If nurses want to be sought out as health care resources and to have their views reflected in health policy, nurses have to get off the porch to run with the big dogs."[6]

# Implementing Evidence Into Certified Registered Nurse Anesthetists Practice: Handoffs

In 2010, I returned to my graduate school alma mater, Baylor College of Medicine, to pursue the goal of a terminal degree in nursing and graduated in 2012 with a DNP in nurse anesthesia. During school and upon graduation, I continued my role as co-owner of my anesthesia practice at the ambulatory surgery center. I did not see immediate changes when I first obtained this degree. I did discover my critical thinking and problem-solving skills had improved, and I began to put those to use in the surgery center.

One example is the case of handoffs from the operating room (OR) to the post-anesthesia care unit (PACU). I believed we were deficient in this arena, as this is often where safety fails first.[7] I organized meetings to discuss safety and the need for change. During these meetings, I presented current evidence-based research supporting the need for the change. We were able to create a handoff checklist, which led to greater efficiency (Table 9-1).

# Incorporation of the DNP Essentials

I was able to utilize DNP Essential III: Clinical Scholarship and Analytical Methods for Evidence-Based Practice to present methods and reasons for implementing the changes.[8] Information presented by Potestio et al suggested that anesthesia handoffs are associated with increased adverse events.[9] Presentation of this material to nursing staff, anesthesia providers, and surgeons led to the development of a PACU Handoff Checklist for the center.

The development of a handoff checklist also addressed DNP Essential VI: Interprofessional Collaboration for Improving Patient and Population Health Outcomes. The creation of the checklist allowed for less possibility that an adverse event would occur, and as a result, we were able to improve patient care through collaborative efforts.

DNP Essential VI was also useful in addressing conflict in the workplace. While obtaining my DNP, I gained valuable knowledge on how to address conflict and improve collaboration. The majority of errors in health care occur from communication problems.[10] These issues often arise from conflict. Management of such situations is critical for those working in a high-stress environment such as the OR.

Effective resolution of a conflict requires clear communication and a level of understanding of the perceived areas of disagreement. Conflict resolution is an essential element of a healthy work environment due to the potential for an increase in patient errors.

Often those in management positions have not received any training in how to handle conflict. Handling conflict in an efficient and effective manner results in improved quality, patient safety, and staff morale, along with a reduction of stress for all involved.[11]

The process of conflict management is a learned skill and must be practiced with regularity. According to the standards for Accreditation of Nurse Anesthesia Educational Programs, the graduate of a nurse anesthesia program must demonstrate the ability to utilize interpersonal and communication skills that result in the effective exchange of information and collaboration with patients, family members, and other health care professionals.[12] I acquired and improved upon the ability to communicate effectively once I returned to school to obtain my DNP degree.

**Table 9-1**

## ANESTHESIA HANDOFF CHECKLIST

**P A T I E N T**

- Patient identification (nameband check)
- Time in
- Allergies
- Surgical procedure and reason for surgery
- Type of anesthesia (general, total intravenous, regional)
- Surgical or anesthetic complications
- Past medical history and American Society of Anesthesiologists scoring
- Pre-operative cognitive function
- Pre-operative activity level (metabolic equivalent of tasks)
- Limb restriction
- Pre-operative vitals

**P R O C E D U R E**

- Positioning of patient (if other than supine)
- Intubation conditions (grade of view, airway, quality of bag mask ventilation, bite block?)
- Lines/catheters (IVs, a-lines, central venous lines, Foley, chest tubes, surgical drains, ventriculoperitoneal shunt)
- Fluid management
  - Fluids =
  - Estimated blood loss =
  - Urine Output =

**M E D I C A T I O N S**

- Analgesia plan (during case, post-operative orders)
- Antiemetics administered
- Medications due during post-anesthesia care unit (antibiotics, etc.)
- Other intra-operative medications (steroids, antihypertensives)
- Reversals used

# BUSINESS PLAN AND COST SAVINGS

A formal business plan was not utilized in this particular endeavor as there were no costs associated with implementation of the plan. There were no monetary gains from implementing the handoff checklist, but by allowing for decreased incidence of an adverse event, this created an opportunity for savings by prevention. A 2016 report from the Joint Commission indicated that communication errors resulted in 1700 deaths and a loss of $1.7 billion.[13] A breakdown in communication during a handoff is where safety may be compromised.[14]

# OUTCOMES AND INCORPORATION OF EVIDENCE-BASED PRACTICE

The creation of a handoff checklist brought this issue to light, and the staff became aware that ineffective handoffs and poor communication can lead to adverse events. Becoming aware of the problem and presenting the evidence were the first steps in creating a change in the environment.

Utilization of the checklist and identification of the problem led to immediate improvement in handoffs. We instituted this policy several years ago and have since hired new nursing and anesthesia staff. The handoffs have shown improvement since the problem was first identified and the change was implemented. It would be a good idea to provide an updated educational component due to the new staff and the tendency for long-term staff to fall into older patterns.

# IMPLEMENTING EVIDENCE INTO CERTIFIED REGISTERED NURSE ANESTHETISTS PRACTICE: OPIOID REDUCTION

An important component of anesthesia practice in today's world is the reduction of opioids. While opioids have been the mainstay of pain management, many factors have led to attempts to reduce their use both peri-operatively and in the post-operative period. The opioid crisis has been influential in this need to reduce their usage as patients often get their first exposure to narcotics following a surgical procedure. Indiscriminate prescribing of opioids can lead to addiction and associated complications such as overdose and death.[15]

The development of enhanced recovery after surgery (ERAS) is a multimodal pathway to improve patient outcomes after surgery.[16] There are pre-operative components of ERAS such as altering fasting requirements to allow carbohydrate-rich fluids up to 2 hours before surgery and avoiding bowel preps. Post-operatively, there is a movement to rid the patient of drains and promote early ambulation. During the peri-operative period of which the anesthesia provider has the most control, there is an attempt to reduce opioids and utilize non-opioid adjuvant medications along with regional anesthesia to control pain.[15] The reduction of opioids has been shown to improve patient outcomes by reducing complications such as nausea, vomiting, and post-operative ileus.

Reduction of narcotics is particularly important in the outpatient surgery arena as opioids can lead to respiratory depression and nausea/vomiting which can delay recovery and time to discharge. The number of outpatient surgeries has increased to more than 50 million in the past several decades.[17] Current recommendations for reducing opioid use include the use of non-steroidal anti-inflammatory (NSAIDs) drugs, cyclooxygenase (COX)-2 inhibitors, acetaminophen, and intravenous (IV) and oral alpha-2 agonists such as dexmedetomidine, glucocorticoids, and gabapentin.[18]

Limiting narcotic/opioid use was already an important part of my practice in an outpatient surgery setting. I often did procedures under monitored anesthesia care (MAC) or IV sedation. MAC involves the use of local anesthesia along with sedation and anesthesia. Airway reflexes and spontaneous breathing are maintained.

I utilized propofol and dexmedetomidine (an alpha-2 agonist) infusions with minimal narcotics. As I learned more about ERAS protocols and opioid-sparing techniques, I began to add some of the tools listed above to my regimen. For general anesthesia cases, I added magnesium sulfate, which is an N-methyl D-aspartate (NMDA) receptor antagonist, as well as sub-anesthetic doses of ketamine (0.3 mg/kg), another NMDA receptor antagonist.[18]

# INCORPORATION OF DNP ESSENTIALS

Utilization of DNP Essentials I and III were instrumental in educating other anesthesia personnel as well as nursing staff about ERAS and the changes being incorporated. The information presented is based on scientific principle, so DNP Essential I allowed for use of the theories based in research and then translation of this knowledge into a practice change.

DNP Essential III was utilized as ERAS, and the use of opioid-sparing techniques is rooted in evidence-based practice. DNP Essential III addresses the use of clinical scholarship and evidence-based practice. This Essential allows for the translation of research into practice. In the past few years, numerous studies have emerged on this topic, and it

**Table 9-2**

### OPERATIVE OUTCOMES BASES ON NARCOTIC USAGE

|  | N/V INCIDENCE | TIME TO DISCHARGE | PAIN SCORE |
|---|---|---|---|
| Fentanyl < 100 mcg total (n = 50) | 4%<br>2 out of 50 | 45 minutes | 48 patients = 0<br>2 patients = 4 |
| Fentanyl 100 mcg or > (n = 50) | 16%<br>8 out of 50 | 70 minutes | 48 patients = 0<br>2 patients = 4 |
| Patients N = 100 (50 patients each group) | | | |

is important for CRNAs to analyze the evidence and implement the data into clinical practice.[8]

## BUSINESS PLAN AND COST SAVINGS

This particular plan was implemented without a formal business plan. The cost savings associated with reducing opioids and utilizing ERAS protocols have been well documented. The cost savings are attributed to decreased length of stay and reduced readmissions and reoperations.[19] Different institutions have varying numbers, but a 2016 report from Johns Hopkins Hospital showed an annual total cost savings of $948 500.[20]

## INCORPORATION OF EVIDENCE-BASED PRACTICE: CLINICAL OUTCOMES

In my practice, I have personally reduced the amount of morphine and hydromorphone utilized during surgery. My experience with a reduction in longer-acting narcotics has been consistent with the research related to ERAS and reduced narcotic use. I am seeing less complications such as nausea, vomiting, and prolonged stays in the PACU.[21]

In a data analysis of 100 patients (n = 100), 50 patients were administered 0 µg to 100 µg of fentanyl along with other agents for pain control (IV acetaminophen, magnesium sulfate, ketamine, lidocaine, and dexmedetomidine). The other 50 patients only received fentanyl in doses of 100 µg or greater. The reduced fentanyl group had 2 incidences of nausea and vomiting (4%) vs the higher dose fentanyl group, which demonstrated a 16% incidence in nausea and vomiting. Both were less than the national average for nausea and vomiting for outpatient procedures, which is 30%.[22] All patients

received at least 3 anti-emetic agents preemptively to assist with nausea prevention.

The average length of stay for the reduced fentanyl group was 45 minutes vs 70 minutes for the higher dose group. There was no difference in pain scores. The vast majority reported a 0 pain score upon discharge. There were 2 patients in each group that reported a 4 in pain upon leaving the surgery center (Table 9-2).

Data collected by the surgery center independent of the above analysis showed a total nausea/vomiting rate of < 0.1%. This was significantly lower than what the analysis demonstrated in both groups. There are possible explanations for the disparity between the 2 data sets. The surgery center data included 495 total cases in comparison to the independent data analysis by the author of 100 patients. In the data analysis of the 100 patients, each one was asked if they were experiencing nausea or stomach distress. Affirmative responses regardless if the patients went on to have emesis, further treatment, or a prolonged stay, were counted as positive for nausea. In contrast, the surgery center only considered the patients positive for nausea if they required treatment for nausea and their discharge was delayed as a result. The extremely low rate in both the data analysis done by the author and the information collected by the center supports the assumption that decreased opioid use leads to less nausea and vomiting in the post-operative period.

## PROFESSIONALISM

Once I decided to pursue a DNP degree, I was asked by many why I was doing so and what my ultimate goal was. I did not have a definitive answer at the time, but truly believed the DNP degree would allow for achievement of skills that would assist me in rising to new levels as a CRNA. I often answered, "I believe it will open doors for me that I don't even know exist." This statement has been very true, particularly in the role of leadership and governance.

Prior to seeking my DNP degree, I became involved in leadership roles and state government affairs (SGA) advocacy with KyANA. I was ultimately elected to the Board of

Directors and during my pursuit of the DNP degree, I became the president of the state organization. I had also been appointed to the Public Relations Committee for our national association, the American Association of Nurse Anesthetists (AANA), during this time.

The combined efforts of these responsibilities, along with work on the DNP degree, led to a very busy life, but I knew I had discovered my passion: leadership and advocacy. The knowledge I was gaining from the DNP coursework was strengthening my ability to perform these roles.

I already had a strong interest in legislative and governance issues prior to pursuit of the DNP degree. Learning health care policy in the classroom only served to increase my interest in the topics. DNP Essential V: Health Care Policy for Advocacy in Health Care indicates that DNP graduates are prepared to design, influence, and implement health care policies. DNP graduates are well positioned to influence the content and quality of health care legislation.[6]

In 2011 to 2012, during my year as president of the state association, I had experience with key legislative issues. One was the introduction of legislation involving anesthesia assistants in Kentucky. An anesthesia assistant is an anesthesia provider trained in the administration of anesthesia who must always work under the supervision of an anesthesiologist. CRNAs are independently licensed in all 50 states and Washington, DC.[23] CRNAs may work independent of an anesthesiologist which leads to cost savings.[24]

Health care cost have continued to rise, with spending approaching 18% of the gross domestic product (GPD).[25] CRNAs have proven to be the most cost-effective anesthesia provider with a record of safe care.[22] This was the reason CRNAs were opposed to the anesthesia assistant legislation. In Kentucky, anesthesia assistants can practice if they are a licensed physician assistant. The legislation proposed removal of the physician assistant requirement. Another argument we were able to provide to legislators was that as CRNAs and APRNs we were raising requirements by changing entry level to a doctoral degree. The anesthesia assistants group was looking to reduce prerequisites. The stance of the Kentucky CRNAs was that we did not mind anesthesia assistants practicing in Kentucky, but we wanted them to maintain the standards that were currently in place.

The CRNAs of Kentucky were able to influence the legislators with strong arguments regarding access to care and cost savings. As CRNAs, we were able to practice independently and provide cost-effective care delivery in rural areas of the state where care was needed by the constituents. Anesthesia assistants were not the answer for access to care as they would always need an anesthesiologist supervisor, requiring 2 providers and, therefore, increasing cost. The CRNAs of Kentucky prevented passage of this bill with a strong grassroots lobbying effort. As president of the state association, I encouraged the CRNAs to call, write, and personally contact their legislators. Many of our legislators said their systems were overloaded with calls.

During this time, I was pursuing my DNP degree and had exposure to formal coursework in health care policy. I had learned the lobbying process in a very informal manner, though effective, the DNP degree gave me additional tools to work with, such as creating a policy brief to address the issue. A policy brief is defined as a brief report that addresses the interests and needs of policy makers through application of best evidence to produce a solution to a problem[26] (Table 9-3).

In 2012, due to the efforts of many CRNAs in Kentucky, Governor Steve Beshear sent a letter to CMS requesting the removal of physician supervision, making Kentucky the 17th state to opt-out of this federal Medicare and Medicaid requirement (Figure 9-1). Opting out of physician supervision refers to billing requirements set forth by the CMS. CRNAs were able to be directly reimbursed as a result of the Omnibus Budget Reconciliation Act of 1986.[27]

Though direct reimbursement for CRNAs (1986) was a victory, CRNAs began to lobby extensively to remove the supervision requirement. Eventually a compromise was reached where federal level supervision removal or opt-out was moved to the state level where the governor could make the decision in 2000.[28] My practice did not change drastically as a result of the opt-out. I had been working independently since 2007 under the direction of the operating surgeon without supervision from an anesthesiologist. Removal of the requirement did seem to bring some piece of mind to some of our operating surgeons as there were no requirements for their direction.

Being directly involved in the efforts to achieve opt-out in the state, in conjunction with the knowledge I had obtained from my health care policy courses during my DNP education, gave me expertise in this arena. I was consulted by the national organization, the AANA, to speak to this issue on several occasions.

Upon completing my term as president of the state association, I worked closely with the Government Relations Committee (GRC) for the state organization. We were fortunate not to face any difficult legislative battles during this time. My experiences with the legislative battles and my newfound knowledge gained from obtaining a DNP degree led to one of the most challenging endeavors I had ever encountered—that of running for public office.

# DNP Essential: Health Care Policy for Advocacy in Health Care—Campaign for State Representative

Spending time working with legislators on CRNA issues introduced me to the world of public policy. As I became more involved, I began to question if perhaps I could

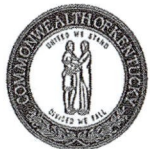

COMMONWEALTH OF KENTUCKY
## OFFICE OF THE GOVERNOR

STEVEN L. BESHEAR
GOVERNOR

700 CAPITOL AVENUE
SUITE 100
FRANKFORT, KY 40601
(502) 564-2611
FAX: (502) 564-2517

April 25, 2012

Honorable Marilyn Tavenner
Acting Administrator and Chief Operating Officer
Centers for Medicare and Medicaid Services
314G Hubert H. Humphrey Building
200 Independence Avenue, S.W.
Washington, D.C.  20201

Dear Administrator Tavenner:

Upon the recommendation of the Kentucky Cabinet for Health and Family Services and per the request of the Kentucky Hospital Association and the Kentucky Association of Nurse Anesthetists, I am exercising the option to exempt hospitals, critical-access hospitals, and ambulatory surgical centers in the Commonwealth of Kentucky from the requirement that certified registered nurse anesthetists be supervised by a physician, pursuant to 42 CFR 482.52(c), 42 CFR 485.639(e), and 42 CFR 416.42(c).  Having consulted with the Kentucky Board of Medical Licensure and the Kentucky Board of Nursing about issues related to access to and the quality of anesthesia services in Kentucky, and having determined that the opt-out is consistent with Kentucky state law, I have concluded that it is in the best interest of Kentucky's citizens to opt out of the current federal physician supervision requirement in order to improve access to critical services.

Sincerely,

Steven L. Beshear

**Figure 9-1.** Official Kentucky opt-out letter.

**Table 9-3**

## POLICY BRIEF DEVELOPMENT AND BASIC ELEMENTS

| POLICY BRIEF DEVELOPMENT | |
|---|---|
| *Overview* | • Make it brief and understandable for non–health care audience. |
| | • Know your audience and identify problem that needs solving. |
| | • Brief should be concise; 4 pages or less. |
| | • Present the brief efficaciously with appropriate timing. |
| **BASIC ELEMENTS** | |
| *Executive Summary* | • Strong introduction with overview of problem and a summary of why it needs to be addressed. |
| *Background* | • Identify the scope of the problem and why action needs to be taken. |
| *Author's Position* | • Discusses the advantages and disadvantage of policy implementation as well as alternatives. |
| | • Advocate for the desired solution. |
| *References* | • Provide data to support the policy and refute objections. |
| | • Demonstrate credibility and expertise in the area of concern. |

Adapted from DeMarco R, Tufts KA. The mechanics of writing a policy brief. *Nurs Outlook*. 2014;62(3):219-224. and O'Grady ET. The policy process. In: Mason DJ, Gardner DB, Outlaw FH, O'Grady ET, eds. *Policy & Politics in Nursing and Health Care*. 7th ed. Elsevier; 2016: 61-72.

contribute at a broader level by becoming a legislator. I found this role appealing and was approached by several people to consider this as an option.

I was accepted into a program called Emerge Kentucky, which is part of the national organization Emerge America. Emerge is an intense training program for Democratic women who wish to run for public office. During an intense 6-month training period, skills are taught that include fundraising, networking, campaign strategy, field operations, public speaking and communication, labor and endorsements, media and messaging, and cultural competency.[29]

After completing Emerge training in 2013, I made the decision to run for State Representative in the 36th district of Kentucky for the 2014 race. The district was newly created so this was an open seat. The Affordable Care Act (ACA) and health care were a hot topic at the time. I believed my background as a health care provider could be useful in correcting the problems associated with implementation of the law at the state level.

I also ran on the premise that I had education in health care policy and economics, obtained during my DNP education, as well as clinical expertise. I do not think I would have been confident enough to run for public office with the health care background alone. The policy and economic knowledge I obtained from my DNP degree gave me an added advantage in the arena as few people who run for office have any formal training in these areas.

Running for office took DNP Essential V to a different level than I had addressed it before. For APRNs and CRNAs to fully remove the barriers that exist, we must not only advocate for the profession but become the decision makers. As DNP Essential V states, "doctorally educated nurses will have the tools to engage in and serve as leaders in the development and implementation of health care policy."[6] My doctoral education gave me the tools and the confidence to pursue this goal.

I was unsuccessful in my run for state representative, but I learned valuable lessons during the process. I also gained access to some very important people in the legislative arena and I was able to increase awareness about the role of CRNAs. I am now encouraging other CRNAs to run for public office. It is no longer enough to have a seat at the table, we must have a seat that includes a vote when the practice rights of APRNs are in question.

## Chair of the Government Relations Committee for the American Association of Nurse Anesthetists

After my attempt at becoming a state legislator, I was elected to the AANA Board of Directors as the Region 2 director. I served 2 years in this capacity and gained valuable insight into the workings of the national organization. Upon completion of my term as an AANA Board member, I was still inclined to serve the organization, so I applied for a committee position.

I had served in this capacity before but thought the GRC was where my strength was. I was approached by the incoming president of the AANA with a request to chair the committee. Based on my government relations experience in my state and running for office, she believed I was the most qualified applicant to serve as chair.

The GRC works in conjunction with the SGA office of the AANA. The SGA office assists CRNAs through education regarding effective advocacy strategy and practice. The department also assists states in matters such as testifying at state legislative and regulatory hearings.[30]

The GRC provides input and practitioner perspective that assists the SGA division staff in their interactions with state associations regarding state legislative and regulatory issues. The committee is also responsible for developing tools, processes for enviro-scanning, state and issue specific research, and advocacy competence development.[29] The GRC also works with other committees to facilitate implementation of needed strategies.

As chair of the committee, I collaborate with the staff to prepare meeting agendas, conduct committee meetings, and make committee assignments as needed. My role also involves conference calls and meetings with other committee chairs when one or more committees are collaborating on a project. The committee receives charges from the AANA Board of Directors. I work with staff to make sure these charges are met and have quarterly conference calls with other committee chairs and the AANA president to update on our progress.

The role of the GRC and other committee chairs in the AANA have been served by many CRNAs who do not possess a DNP but all performed the job admirably. As with many situations that I faced since obtaining a DNP degree, I have found the degree to be valuable in this situation. DNP Essentials II and V are addressed in the role of GRC chair.

DNP Essential II, which addresses Organizational and Systems Leadership for Quality Improvement and Systems Thinking, is extremely important for the role of a committee chair. The AACN Essential notes, "advanced nursing practice requires political skills, systems thinking and the business, and financial acumen needed for the analysis of practice quality and costs."[2] As a DNP graduate, I am able to assess the impact of practice policies and procedures and their impact on the organization and, ultimately, patient care. The DNP education also provided the skills to assess risk and collaborate with others. My experience along with my DNP education have provided me the political skills, systems thinking, and organizational management to chair the GRC.

DNP education employs systems theory which recognizes the organization is an open system that exists as part of a larger network. Every decision made by the GRC committee affects the entire AANA organization, and ultimately can impact CRNA practice. The organization is basically an organism made up of numerous parts or subsystems that must work in harmony for the larger system to survive.[31] This theory was first proposed by Ludwig von Bertalanffy in the 1940s as general systems theory. The idea of viewing a system holistically goes all the way back to philosophers like Aristotle and Descartes.[31] When von Bertalanffy proposed his ideas, it went against reductionists belief that a system was nothing but a series of parts working in isolation.

The study of complex adaptive systems (CAS) and chaos theory, which I learned during my DNP education, are also applicable to systems theory and organizational leadership needed to chair a committee. A CAS says that a system is made up of interacting components whose interactions may be complex (ie, nonlinear) and whose components are diverse and have a capacity for learning that generates reactive or proactive adaptive behavior.[32] The description of a CAS is very applicable to an organization such as the AANA. We are made up of a diverse population with a lot of moving parts that interact and have a capacity for learning and adapting.

Chaos theory suggests there is order that emerges from chaos and it is necessary to creative ordering.[33] As a leader, being able to manage chaos to ultimately create order is an essential skill. Chaos tends to be an integral part of all organizations and can either lead to growth or disaster.

I entered my role as GRC with this systems theory knowledge, which stresses communication, setting goals and boundaries, and the use of feedback systems to improve the organization. This background indicated that as an open system, the GRC must continually interact with its surrounding environment and exchange information with AANA members, staff, and other committees. The advanced communication skills acquired in the DNP education have proved useful in this endeavor of interacting with others and managing the challenges of the organization.

The ability to design, implement, and advocate for health care policy as noted in DNP Essential V has been instrumental in the role of GRC chair. As this committee's primary role is to assist states with legislative and regulatory issues, the skills of analyzing the policy process and engaging in political action are critical.[2] Doctorate education prepares the graduate to demonstrate leadership in the development of policy; influence policy makers through participation on boards, committees, and task forces; critically analyze health policy proposals, health policies, and related issues; and advocate for the profession and all areas of social justice.[2]

Though I had been an advocate for the nurse anesthesia profession prior to obtaining a DNP degree, the skills obtained allowed me to translate evidence-based information and implement the knowledge while leading my committee.

Transformational leadership skills that are learned in DNP education are useful when chairing committees. These skills allow the leader to feel comfortable when engaging in the development and implementation of health care policy and allow for adaptation to change.[34]

Transformational leadership theory was developed by James McGregor Burns in 1978. This leadership style encourages others to not just follow, but become leaders also. The eventual goal is for the leader and the followers is to find meaning and purpose in connection to their work, growth, and maturity.[34]

As a leader, the goal is to motivate others. In my role as GRC chair, I do not want to be in charge and micromanage a group of people. I want them to feel empowered and excited about the work we are doing on the committee. I hope in my role as chair I have inspired others to step into leadership roles through encouragement, teamwork, and promoting self-esteem.

# Conclusion: Impact of the DNP Degree

As a result of obtaining a DNP degree, I have been able to rise to the challenge that the growing complexity of health care presents, and to manage the expansion of knowledge required.[1] The doctorate degree allows me to be involved in initiating real change, and to utilize strategy and vision to be a part of transforming health care in the United States. Advanced practice nurses have always delivered high-quality care to their patients. Now with DNP degrees in hand, we must lead the much-needed changes in health care and create a system that is both affordable and accessible.

With the complexity of health care continually growing, DNP-prepared APRNs face an incredibly challenging landscape that can be difficult to navigate. Demonstration of strong clinical skills and knowledge is critical, but DNP-prepared nurses in advanced practice must base this information on best practices and evidence. Through the implementation of ERAS and the reduction of opioids in my own practice, there has been an improvement in patient outcomes such as decreasing pain, nausea, vomiting, and PACU length of stay.

I now have the credentials to teach the next generation of CRNAs about the importance of becoming leaders in the health care profession. The students that I teach will become strong clinicians with a solid scientific base to support their practice. In addition to the clinical knowledge gained, the students will have expertise in topics such as informatics, health care policy, evidence-based practice, and leadership that are essential in today's health care environment.

When I began my DNP journey, I was already heavily involved with advocacy and health care policy. I knew I wanted to gain expertise and credibility in this field. Having earned my DNP degree, I have more credibility behind my name as an adjunct professor in a DNP program teaching courses such as leadership and health care policy. Whether I am providing testimony before a committee or being interviewed by a reporter regarding CRNA practice, the credentials of the DNP degree and faculty experience augment my endorsement as an expert.

It is a pivotal time in CRNA and APRN practice as legislators are making decisions that will affect our scope of practice and title recognition.[35] It is critical to be a nursing leader with the DNP skill sets that include collaboration and communication, being able to oversee interprofessional teams, and understanding fiscal, economic, and health care policy.

# Acknowledgments

I would like to acknowledge the staff from the State Government Relations division of the AANA, Senior Director Anna Polyak, and Assistant Director Jana Conover. They have been incredibly supportive during my tenure as the chair of the Government Relations Committee.

# References

1. Edwardson SR. Imagining a DNP role. In: Zaccagnini ME, White KW, eds. *The Doctor of Nursing Practice Essentials.* 3rd ed. Jones & Bartlett Learning; 2017.

2. The essentials of doctoral education for advanced nursing practice.American Association of Colleges of Nursing. Accessed May 7, 2019. https://www.aacnnursing.org/Portals/42/Publications/DNPEssentials.pdf

3. Peterson SW. Systems thinking, healthcare organizations, global health, and the advanced practice nurse leader. In: Zaccagnini ME, White KW, eds. *The Doctor of Nursing Practice Essentials.* 3rd ed. Jones & Bartlett Learning; 2017:39-63.

4. The future of nursing: leading change, advancing health 2010. The National Academies of Sciences. http://www.nationalacademies.org

5. CRNA fact sheet. American Association of Nurse Anesthetists. Accessed April 20, 2019. www.aana.com

6. Mund A. Healthcare policy for advocacy in health care. In: Zaccagnini ME, White KW, eds. *The Doctor of Nursing Practice Essentials.* 3rd ed. Jones & Bartlett Learning; 2017:189-230.

7. Riesenberg LA, Leitzsch J, Cunningham JM. Nursing handoffs: a systematic review of the literature. *Am J Nurs.* 2010;110(4):24-36. doi:10.1097/01.NAJ.0000370154.79857.09

8. Tymkov C. Clinical scholarship and evidence-based practice. In: Zaccagnini ME, White KW, eds. T*he Doctor of Nursing Practice Essentials.* 3rd ed. Jones & Bartlett Learning; 2017:67-130.

9. Potestio C, Mottla J, Kelley E, DeGroot K. Improving post anesthesia care unit (PACU) handoff by implementing a succinct checklist. Anesthesia Patient Safety Foundation. June 2015. www.apsf.org

10. Hetzler DC, Messina DR, Smith KJ. Conflict management in hospital systems: not just for leadership. American Journal of Mediation. http://www.americanjournalofmediation.com/docs/Conflict%20Management%20in%20Hospital%20Systems.pdf

11. Johansen, M. Keeping the peace: conflict management strategies for nurse managers. *Nurs Manag.* 2012;43(2):50-54. doi: 10.1097/01.NUMA.0000410920.90831.96

12. Standards and policies. Council on Accreditation for Nurse Anesthetists. http://www.aana.com/coa

13. High reliability healthcare. The Joint Commission. Accessed April 20, 2019. https://www.jointcommission.org/resources/news-and-multimedia/blogs/high-reliability-healthcare/

14. Improving patient handoff safety. Lippincott Solutions. Accessed April 20, 2019. http://www.lippincottsolutions.lww.com/blog.enter

15. Soffin EM, Lee BH, Kumar KK, Wu CL. The prescription opioid crisis: role of the anaesthesiologist in reducing opioid use and misuse. *Br J Anaesth.* 2019;122(6):e198-e208. doi:10.1016/j.bja.2018.11.019

16. ERAS society guidelines. ERAS Society. Accessed April 20, 2019. http://www.erassociety.org

17. Erhun F, Malcolm E, Kalani M, et al. Opportunities to improve the value of outpatient surgical care. *Am J Manag Care.* 2016;22(9):e329-e335.

18. Vo H, Clayton E, Stolyarskaya J. Opioid and non-opioid analgesia during surgery. American Nurse Today. Accessed April 20, 2019. https://www.myamericannurse.com/opioid-non-opioid-analgesia-surgery/

19. Pearl MA, Lloyd A, Higa K. ERABS leads to reduced opioid use among bariatric surgery patients. American College of Surgeons Bulletin. Accessed April 19, 2019. https://bulletin.facs.org/2019/01/erabs-leads-to-reduced-opioid-use-among-bariatric-surgery-patients/

20. Hospitals can save money with enhanced recovery program for colorectal surgery patients. American College of Surgeons. Accessed April 26, 2019. http://www.managedcaremag.com

21. Enhanced recovery after surgery. American Association of Nurse Anesthetists. Accessed April 20, 2019. http://www.aana.com/eras

22. Doyle C. Incidence of post-discharge nausea and vomiting higher than expected. Anesthesiology News. https://www.anesthesiologynews.com/Clinical-Anesthesiology/Article/11-12/Incidence-of-Post-Discharge-Nausea-and-Vomiting-Higher-Than-Expected/54223

23. State government affairs. American Association of Nurse Anesthetists. http://www.aana.com/sga

24. Hogan PF, Seifert RF, Moore CS, Simonson BE. Cost effectiveness analysis of anesthesia providers. *Nurs Econ.* 2010;28(3):159-169.

25. National health expenditure data. Centers of Medicare & Medicaid Services. https://www.cms.gov/Research-Statistics-Data-and-Systems/Statistics-Trends-and-Reports/NationalHealthExpendData

26. DeMarco R, Tufts KA. The mechanics of writing a policy brief. *Nurs Outlook.* 2014;62(3):219-224. doi:10.1016/j.outlook.2014.04.002

27. Larson S. *The Influence of Professions on the Development and Outcome of Federal Regulation That Affect Their Work.* Unpublished Thesis. The University of Illinois at Chicago; 2004.

28. Downey PM. Achieving the opt out for Medicare physician supervision for nurse anesthetists. *AANA J.* 2010;78(2):96-100.

29. About us. Emerge America. https://emergeamerica.org/about/

30. Committees. American Association of Nurse Anesthetists. http://www.aana.com/committees

31. von Bertalanffy L. *General Systems Theory.* George Braziller; 1968.

32. Cordon C. Systems theories: an overview of various system theories and its application in healthcare. *Am J Sys Sci.* 2013;2(1): 13-22.

33. Norberg J, Cumming GS. Practicing adaptive management in complex social-ecological systems. In: *Complexity Theory for a Sustainable Future.* 1st ed. Columbia University Press; 2008.

34. Smith MA. Are you a transformational leader? *Nurs Manag.* 2011;42(9):44-50.

35. Greenwood CB, Biddle C. Impact of legislation on scope of practice among nurse anesthetists. *J Nurse Pract.* 2015;11(5):498-504.

# CHAPTER 10

# The Role of the DNP in Reducing Health Disparities and Advocating From the Viewpoint of a Certified Registered Nurse Anesthetist

*Jorge A. Valdes, DNP, CRNA, APRN*

## Introduction

A Doctor of Nursing Practice (DNP) is the highest level of education for actual practice of a nursing discipline.[1] Nurse anesthesia is a subset of nursing leading to unique applications when implementing the DNP Essentials. The DNP Essentials provide a concrete road map of how the DNP degree functions. The 8 DNP Essentials are the foundational competencies required of all doctoral graduates. The following chapter will focus on the journey a DNP-prepared certified registered nurse anesthetist (CRNA) has taken to make a difference using the 8 DNP Essentials as a guide. The DNP Essentials often overlap in practice, as CRNAs usually address more than 1 competency at a time. There are 2 Essentials that will be discussed at length, Essential V: Health Care Policy for Advocacy in Health Care, and Essential VII: Clinical Prevention and Population Health for Improving the Nation's Health.

The Institute of Medicine's (IOM) report in 2002, "Unequal Treatment: Confronting Racial and Ethnic Disparities in Healthcare," was influential in setting the national agenda on health disparities.[2] CRNAs administer anesthesia in a variety of practice settings, including in hospitals, plastic surgeon offices, interventional pain management facilities, and ambulatory surgical centers. CRNAs are employed in rural and densely populated areas, including all major inner cities in the United States. CRNAs work in an acute care setting as opposed to a primary care setting. The vast majority of literature concerning advanced practice registered nurses (APRNs) role in reducing health care disparities points to primary care APRNs. However, CRNAs have established methods of reducing health care disparities and inequalities by adopting recommendations from the IOM report and developing ways to implement them. One way in which CRNAs are reducing health disparities among their patient population is by increasing minority representation within the nurse anesthesia profession. The American Association of Nurse Anesthetists (AANA) is one of the first APRN specialties to actively address the low percentage of minorities who are CRNAs through active awareness, education, and recruitment of prospective minority applicants to the nurse anesthesia profession.

Benson LA, ed. *The DNP Professional: Translating Value From Classroom to Practice* (pp 111-118). © 2021 SLACK Incorporated.

# The Advanced Practice Registered Nurse's Road Less Travelled: Becoming a DNP-Prepared CRNA

Growing up as a first-generation Cuban-American man in Miami, I had no idea what a CRNA was, much less what they did. Culturally, my initial perception of nursing was that it was a profession for women. Miami, unlike any other city in the United States, has been shaped by its proximity to Cuba and the number of exiled Cubans, which inhabit the city and surrounding areas. Cubans immigrated to the United States in large numbers beginning in 1959, due in large part to the fact that Miami is the closest large American city to Havana, which is just 330 miles away. However, South Florida is not as much a melting pot, but rather a peacock with an array of people from different cultures (feathers) and ethnic identities who work as one yet remain separate and unique. Melting pot refers to different cultures melting into one. According to the US Census Bureau (2011), the population of South Florida is comprised of approximately 13% White (non-Hispanic), 17.9% Black, 1.7% Asian, 69% Hispanic or Latino, and 0.9% other.[3] Growing up in South Florida with Latino, Haitian, and other Caribbean cultures represented shaped my view of the world and perceptions. Diversity became an everyday part of my life and was something I never questioned.

Upon graduating from high school, I knew I wanted to go into the medical field and stumbled upon the nursing profession where I decided to get my bachelor's degree and continue to medical school. Once I graduated from nursing school, I was hooked, and fell in love with the holistic approach to patient care that nursing offered. Knowing that I wanted to continue on to get a master's degree, I enrolled into a nurse practitioner program and during that time I shadowed a CRNA. The experience of caring for patients in the peri-operative theater inspired me to change my major to nurse anesthesia. I earned my master's degree in nurse anesthesia from the Mayo Clinic in Rochester, Minnesota. Yes, Minnesota! I was a foreigner in my own country as Minnesota is a northern land of the frozen tundra. After settling in, it was evident I was different almost immediately, because I was frequently asked questions about where I was from. I discovered to my surprise that I had an accent! Apparently, I always had a regional accent, but I never noticed it, partly because in South Florida, everyone speaks as I do. I was pronouncing vowels with Spanish sounds, making the accent obvious to anyone not from South Florida. Out of a class of 30, I was the only Latino and only 1 of 2 students of color in the program. I found myself explaining what a Cuban-American was and why I did not look Mexican. I

remember telling fellow colleagues that Latinos come in all shades of color, and that not all Latinos are from Mexico. I realized how unique my perspective on health care was, intertwining my cultural Latino norms with my knowledge of Western medicine. This different viewpoint and experience would serve me well in the future, as chair of the first-ever AANA Diversity and Inclusion Committee.

## Expanding My Role

Shortly after graduating from nurse anesthesia school, I did what the IOM report suggested. I moved back to a minority and medically underserved community. One of the recommendations from the 2002 IOM report on ways the United States can reduce racial disparities is to increase the number of minority health care providers, because minority providers are more likely to practice in medically underserved communities.[2] After moving back to South Florida, I began to practice in a large community hospital. Anyone working in health care in South Florida quickly realizes the importance of culturally competent care. It is not unusual to speak in Creole, Spanish, English, or Spanglish (a mix of both Spanish and English) when taking care of patients. Patients who communicated in their native language are more likely to give thorough health histories and therefore have less adverse effects.

After being a CRNA for 8 years, I decided I wanted to teach full-time and made the jump into academia. I enrolled in a PhD program as I was told I had to get a terminal degree if I wanted to continue to teach. Two semesters into my PhD studies, I began to learn about a new degree called a DNP geared for clinicians. I considered myself a clinician and not necessarily a researcher. The year was 2010, and nurse anesthesia schools had begun to mandate that all graduates graduating from accredited nurse anesthesia programs must have a practice doctorate or doctoral-level education by 2025. Therefore, the 2025 deadline was set for entry into practice. This deadline would make the CRNA specialty the first nursing specialty to mandate such requirements (Council on Accreditation).[4] The program I worked for at the time wanted to be the first to transition to an entry-level doctorate degree in Florida, and I needed my terminal degree in 2 years, so I went the DNP route. I attended the DNP program at the University of Miami, which at the time was an executive-style degree attending classes online and 1 weekend a month in person for a year. The program was rigorous and fast paced. I persevered and in December 2012, I graduated with my DNP degree.

## DNP Essentials

Armed with the 8 DNP Essentials, I was ready to change the world. Little did I know how quickly I was going to put my newfound knowledge to use. The DNP degree is centered on 8 DNP Essentials, including Scientific Underpinnings for Practice; Organizational and Systems Leadership for Quality Improvement and Systems Thinking; Clinical Scholarship and Analytical Methods for Evidence-Based Practice; Information Systems/Technology and Patient Care Technology for the Improvement and Transformation of Health Care; Health Care Policy for Advocacy in Health Care; Interprofessional Collaboration for Improving Patient and Population Health Outcomes; Clinical Prevention and Population Health for Improving the Nation's Health; and Advanced Practice Nursing.[5] Throughout the years, I have found implementing the Essentials in my everyday practice to be quite simple.

## DNP Essential: Health Care Policy for Advocacy in Health Care

This DNP Essential is one of the most important functions any practitioner can engage in. Advocating for your profession will allow you to be an active participant and become a change agent.

During the time I worked as a clinician in the hospital, I became involved in the AANA and the Florida Association of Nurse Anesthetists (FANA). I began to advocate for my profession and found I had a voice of unwavering activism. My involvement in FANA began in 2005 when FANA began to battle anesthesia assistant (AA) legislation in the state of Florida. AAs can be licensed or unlicensed practitioners. To be an AA, anyone with a bachelor's degree and 8 hours of documented shadowing experience can apply to a 24- to 28-month program to earn a master's degree. A CRNA can work independently, but an AA must work with an anesthesiologist at all times. Differences also exist in their training. To be a CRNA, you must be a registered nurse with a bachelor's degree and have a minimum of 1 year critical care experience before applying to a school. Nurse anesthesia school is typically a 28- to 36-month program that awards a DNP or Doctor of Nurse Anesthesia Practice (DNAP). When the Florida legislature began to consider allowing AA practice, it motivated me to advocate for my profession. Unfortunately, after a 3-year battle, legislation allowing AAs to practice passed and they were allowed to practice in Florida.

Three years later, I ran for a director position on the FANA Board of Directors, to which I was elected. Serving on the FANA Board of Directors, I learned how politics plays an important role within the nurse anesthesia profession. I developed a passion for my practice and urgency to protect nurse anesthesia. This passion drove me to run for president of the FANA, and I was elected as president of the FANA in October 2013.

Following my FANA presidency, I became even more involved in the AANA, and began to serve on the national AANA Education Committee and helped plan educational forums for CRNAs across the country. I continued to be involved in Florida, becoming the government and federal political relations chair, planning lobbying and advocacy days for CRNAs in Florida. In the summer of 2017, I was asked to chair a new committee for the AANA on diversity and inclusion by the AANA president at the time. I was honored and unsure as to what this committee would do, but I jumped at the idea of chairing a national committee. In my DNP studies, I learned the role diversity played in decreasing health disparities. I had read the 2002 IOM report, which was influential in setting the national agenda on health disparities.[2] As a nurse in South Florida, I had witnessed how health care could be different when there are language and cultural barriers. In my role as a nurse anesthesia program administrator, I wrote grants to the Health Resource and Services Administration (HRSA) and received nurse anesthesia training (NAT) grants to help recruit CRNAs to work in medically underserved communities. The HRSA grants I received have been to help offset the cost of training student nurse anesthetists from a nurse anesthesia school located in South Florida. South Florida is considered a medically underserved community. The grants were obtained because of the high number of students graduating from nurse anesthesia schools in South Florida and remaining in the area to work. Therefore, chairing a committee on diversity was an opportunity that I felt knowledgeable and comfortable taking on.

The AANA has led the way among nursing associations and with their role in diversity. They released a position statement in 2016 on Diversity, Inclusion and Equality.[6] Additionally, one of the AANAs core values includes diversity and inclusion. The precursor to the Diversity and Inclusion Committee was the Diversity and Inclusion Task Force formed in 2015. The task force was charged with developing diversity, cultural awareness, and competency initiatives for the association and for CRNAs. I was invited to join the task force in 2016, the committee was converted into an ad hoc committee, and I became the chair in 2017. Chairing the AANA Diversity and Inclusion Committee allowed me to help make a difference in population health and increase awareness of disparities. The Diversity and Inclusion Committee has several initiatives that were laid out by the AANA (Table 10-1).

## DNP Essential: Clinical Prevention and Population Health for Improving the Nation's Health

Nurse anesthesia as a profession is not representative of the current US population. It is projected that by the year 2050, 54% of the US population will identify themselves as a person of color with the largest growth occurring in the Hispanic population.[7] Currently, there are more than 50 000 CRNAs in the United States. Of those, 89% identify as White, 3% Hispanic, 1% Black, 3% Asian or Pacific Islander, 1% American-Indian, and 4% identify as Other.[8] The profession does not mirror the changing US population. Nurse

**Table 10-1**

## THE AMERICAN ASSOCIATION OF NURSE ANESTHETISTS DIVERSITY AND INCLUSION STRATEGIC FRAMEWORK

- Integrate diversity and inclusion into the work of the AANA board, committees, and staff through the AANA Strategic Framework.
- Initiate steps to ensure cultural awareness and competence in the nurse anesthesia community (including CRNAs and student registered nurse anesthetists).
- Focus on recruiting underrepresented groups into nurse anesthesia educational programs.
- Develop mentorship skills and activities for underrepresented individuals.
- Enhance patient-centered care and address health disparities with emphasis on cultural competency.

Reprinted with permission from the American Association of Nurse Anesthetists.

anesthetists lag behind the nursing profession as a whole, claiming a dismal 16.8% of nurses who consider themselves as non-White.[9] This gap in minority and ethnic representation can have severe implications on the health of the nation. One of the recommendations from the 2002 IOM report on unequal treatment was to increase the number of minorities in health care. Racial disparity in health care in the United States is very costly, ultimately leading to an increase in overall mortality. For example, White persons are significantly more likely to undergo revascularization, while Black persons are more likely to have unplanned procedures.[2] The average waiting time for Black patients needing kidney transplants is almost twice as long as that of White patients. Black women with breast cancer are 67% more likely to die from the disease than White women.[2] Hispanic and Black youth are substantially more likely to die from diabetes than White youths.[2] These are just a few of the countless racial disparities in our health care system. The IOM report makes several suggestions on ways we can reduce these disparities. The AANA has implemented many of the suggestions, including increasing minority providers, minority faculty, and educating future and current CRNAs on culturally competent anesthesia delivery.

The Diversity and Inclusion Committee gave me an open canvas from which to work, as being a new committee has its benefits. The committee came up with a myriad of ideas to increase awareness within the association. The initial Diversity and Inclusion Committee set a few long-term goals. These goals included to engage, recruit, and mentor individuals with different cultural backgrounds and perspectives into the nurse anesthesia profession, and increase awareness among members, instructing them on culturally competent materials. Cultural competency can be explained as practitioners who are able to set aside their beliefs, behaviors, attitudes, and biases and deliver care cross a variety of cultures. The Diversity and Inclusion Committee made

substantial strides toward their goals and contributed to achieving its objectives. The following are some of the deliverables the committee accomplished during the first 2 years:

1. The Diversity and Inclusion Committee developed PowerPoint presentations for use by CRNAs, student registered nurse anesthetists, and others to encourage high school and college students to consider nursing and nurse anesthesia as a career. The PowerPoint presentations use photos of health care professionals from all ethnic backgrounds.

2. The committee sends CRNAs to the National Association of Hispanic Nurses annual meeting and the National Black Nurses Association annual meeting where they exhibit and distribute information about the AANA and how to become a CRNA.

3. As chair, I had the opportunity to be interviewed by Nurses.com regarding racial disparities in health care.

4. The Diversity and Inclusion Committee launched a large public awareness initiative called "I Am Me" in April, which is known as Celebrate Diversity Month. The campaign used many social media outlets such as Facebook, Twitter, and Instagram. "I Am Me" campaign showcased different CRNAs and student registered nurse anesthetists from all backgrounds with a picture and 3 statements starting with "I Am Me…." If the practitioner spoke a foreign language, they were encouraged to translate and write in their native language as well. The marketing campaign was a huge success with the association, drawing unprecedented social media hits in the form of likes and views.

5. Articles were developed into a series in the AANA *NewsBulletin* and *Essential Anesthesia: From Science to Practice* to educate the membership about diversity and inclusion.

**Table 10-2**

## SWOT ANALYSIS

| STRENGTHS | WEAKNESSES |
|---|---|
| • Use evidence-based research to measure the impact that health care disparities have on the US population<br>• Intimate knowledge of the DNP Essentials<br>• Social-cultural enrichment<br>• Strong professional association support<br>• Changing population | • Anesthesia providers unwilling to participate in changes related to anesthesia practice<br>• Cost and time to develop new providers<br>• Disenfranchised members |
| **OPPORTUNITIES** | **THREATS** |
| • Inter-professional collaboration<br>• Social cohesion<br>• Collaboration among state and national associations | • Limited recruitment pool<br>• Cultural, religious, and ethnic biases<br>• Disenfranchised members |

6. I played a key role in developing 2 lecture series for the AANA named the Goldie D. Brangman Diversity & Inclusion Lecture and TAD Talk (Teaching, Anesthesia, & Diversity). Goldie D. Brangman was the first and only Black president of the AANA in 1973 to 1974. She remained the only minority for 42 years until Dr. Juan Quintana became president of the AANA in 2016 serving as the only Latino president of the association to date.

## SWOT ANALYSIS

To make change possible, a DNP-prepared practitioner needs support. Fortunately, the support and commitment the AANA has in support of Diversity and Inclusion Committee has led to the success of advancing the committee. As the chair of the Diversity and Inclusion Committee, I can say implementing diversity and inclusion strategies has been easy, however, there has been opposition from some members. Change and the perception of a need for change can be difficult for some. A SWOT analysis is often helpful in illustrating Strengths, Weaknesses, Opportunities, Threats that an individual may face when implementing different projects or even ideas. The idea of promoting and increasing diversity within the nurse anesthesia profession may sound simple, however, it is not. Many obstacles exist, the SWOT analysis in Table 10-2 illustrates potential impacts and failures such an endeavor may encounter.

The primary strength identified is the IOM report concerning health care disparities and also the recommendation made by the National League of Nursing for achieving diversity and meaningful inclusion in nursing education.[10] The Diversity and Inclusion Committee has created a great deal of buzz on social media platforms by promoting the "I Am Me" campaign and have begun to lay the foundation in establishing a more culturally enriched culture within the nurse anesthesia profession. Barriers, weaknesses, and threats have also been identified. Some practitioners have expressed concern as to why the association would spend time, money, and energy in promoting diversity when their community has a low number of minorities. Disenfranchised members feel the association's functions should not be expanded to recruit future practitioners but rather to protect the current status quo. Massive social media and public relations campaigns have been initiated to reassure some members, but ultimately, it comes to each individual's level of willingness to accept change. The AANA Public Relations Department has made a concerted effort to create and use photos and videos with an array of CRNAs from racially and culturally diverse backgrounds. One limitation for the association is the fact that there is a limited pool of prospective nurse anesthesia students from which to recruit nurses. Nursing as a profession does not have a high percentage of diversity within its workforce. This has created an opportunity to collaborate with undergraduate colleges and universities to attract minorities into the field of nursing. All promotional materials are made available to members to assist them with making presentations to high school and college students.

# INTEGRATING THE ESSENTIALS INTO PRACTICE

Upon graduation from a DNP program, the DNP Essentials are ingrained in all APRNs. The Essentials become part of the psyche of the newly minted DNP graduate, whereas they can be seen in common, everyday actions. Granted, some of the Essentials are easier to meet than others. The type of practice will also depend on the scope of the barriers that a DNP graduate may face.

Currently, my practice is somewhat different from the average CRNA. I consider myself lucky to have 2 simultaneous careers where I can incorporate the DNP Essentials seamlessly. On one hand, I am a practicing CRNA, practicing in an anesthesia care team model at a large teaching hospital. On the other, I practice autonomously in a plastic surgery setting and office-based surgery centers. I am also a clinical assistant professor in one of the largest state schools in the country.

## *DNP and the Clinical Setting*

As a clinician, there are a few Essentials that automatically apply and others that can prove to be a challenge. I employ many DNP Essentials without any thought or resistance in my role as an APRN, which allows me to deliver anesthesia in my capacity as a CRNA. My practice is guided by evidence-based practice (EBP). EBP is a conduit for improving patient care.[1] The use of EBP not only improves patient care through best practice interventions, but it can be used as supporting data to be an effective change agent.

Within the context of a hospital, there are many levels of bureaucracy a practitioner may encounter while practicing. Making positive and meaningful changes *must* be based on evidence using research to guide best practices and outcomes. Physicians and other health practitioners may impact a DNPs contribution in both positive and negative ways. For DNP's, the best defense is to arm themselves with evidence-based research to influence care delivery.

For example, when implementing DNP projects in hospitals I have found them to be either simple or extremely difficult. If the quality improvement/capstone projects are developed in conjunction with clinical partners, then the process becomes very simple. I had a student who looked at using the Caprini Risk Assessment Scale to determine if a patient needed antithrombotic therapy in plastic surgery centers. The DNP student worked for a large plastic surgery center and was able to develop his project in conjunction with the plastic surgeons at the center; therefore, implementation was straightforward. An example of a difficult project to implement involved the use of transverse abdominis plane (TAP) blocks in cesarean sections, although there is a large body of literature that strongly supports the use of the TAP block to reduce opioid use and hospital stay. The resistance from the hospital was primarily due to the cost of the medications used in the TAP block. A very detailed budget with a cost analysis and benefit risk ratio had to be developed in conjunction with the pharmacy department. The budget for the pharmacy was in addition to the budget for the proposed project, which had already been developed to implement the procedure.

## INTERPROFESSIONAL COLLABORATION

The AANA has collaborated and represented CRNAs on the national level by sending representatives from the Diversity and Inclusion Committee to the National Association of Hispanic Nurses and National Black Nurses Association. In addition, a video titled "Be a Nurse, Be a Nurse Anesthetist," which includes testimonials from CRNAs, student registered nurse anesthetists, and a diverse group of anesthesia providers, was made to encourage and educate viewers about becoming a CRNA. The video serves to increase the limited resources the profession draws from the registered nursing pool.

As a FANA board member and past president, I can speak to the actions I have been involved with that include interprofessional collaboration. As a state association, FANA is part of a statewide coalition of APRNs seeking to promote, educate, and advance APRN issues to the Florida legislators. In the state of Florida, the group lobbies in favor of numerous bills, helping to promote title change from ARNP to APRN, the APRN license compact, and prescriptive authority. The group meets regularly to discuss issues and concerns each independent association may be facing. There is power in numbers, and the more united voices become, the stronger the message can be.

## PROFESSIONALISM

I have learned many lessons about professionalism throughout my career. As a DNP graduate in the fall of 2013, shortly after being elected president of FANA, I was asked to speak before the Florida House of Representatives' Health Care Innovation Subcommittee in Tallahassee. A prominent state representative, who would later become speaker of the state's House of Representatives, asked me to come speak on behalf of Florida nurse anesthetists. The legislator told me I had 15 minutes to explain the training, practice settings, patient safety record, and outcomes of CRNAs in Florida. I agreed and used many of the things I had learned in my DNP program to prepare.

The testimony was held in the Capitol building. It was public and recorded, which proved to be a blessing and a challenge to me. During the testimony, I sat next to the president of the Florida Society of Anesthesiologists (FSA). I delivered a 15-minute testimony concerning nurse anesthesia practice. My testimony was followed by a 15-minute response from the FSA president. I was polite, modest, and presented myself with humility as I spoke about what current anesthesia practice entailed and what nurse anesthetists contributed to accessible health care. After the testimonies, the president of the FSA and I were asked follow-up questions for approximately 1.5 hours.

Once the subcommittee hearing was finished, I returned to South Florida. Over the course of several weeks, multiple media outlets from around the state began to publish editorials all authored by an anesthesiologist. I responded to some of the editorials that were written about me personally and the AANA with evidence-based research in a very professional manner. Eventually the controversy impacted my employment. Through this experience, I learned to always take the high road even at the height of a controversial situation. The overwhelming support from CRNAs was an unseen benefit of the testimony I provided. I found that in the mist of difficult times, if you do the right thing and stand up for what you believe in, people will come out to support you.

Another lesson in professionalism I would like to share occurred during my time as chair of the Diversity and Inclusion Committee. A large social media outcry by some members surfaced when trying to influence the committee to act and defend itself against a segment of the AANA membership regarding a contentious issue. I immediately reached out to the other committee members and asked them not to respond or use social media as an outlet for any negativity. Instead of airing any discussion on social media, I decided to write a letter to the members who had brought up concerns and address them privately, rather than in a public forum. Taking the high road, maintaining a sense of decorum, and urging others to follow suit will always result in a better outcome. Once the issue subsided, the Diversity and Inclusion Committee remained a positive, cohesive group that rose above name-calling and accusations. Maintaining calm when the sky is falling is difficult, takes practice, and years of experience, but is worth it not only to achieve a desired outcome and quell disputes, but also to protect your health.

## Pearls/Takeaways

All DNP graduates are taught in similar ways regardless of specialty. What differentiates each graduate is passion. Find your passion, something in life that moves and shakes you to your core and expand on it. You can use your degree to make a huge difference and touch many lives. The Essentials truly become second nature once you begin to practice. Involvement in any professional organization will give you a conduit in which to implement the Essentials. As a master's-prepared CRNA, I understood my role in providing anesthesia to my patients, my trade, and my practice. However, it was only after I went through my doctoral program that I fully understood how my profession was impacted by external and internal influences.

The American Association of Colleges of Nursing put forth the 8 DNP Essentials, with an incredible foresight, that a graduate only realizes years after they graduate. A good example is Essential I. The Scientific Underpinnings for Practice not only enable you to understand the theoretical aspect of practice, but also help an individual understand human behavior. A DNP graduates with an understanding of how to approach different scenarios. For the Diversity and Inclusion Committee, understanding the culture, constraints, and barriers that exists in society and the CRNA population is important to effectively bring about change.

When I think of my role as the chair of the Diversity and Inclusion Committee, I have used all the Essentials to meet the goals of the committee. The committee used EBP and clinical scholarship to help persuade change and guide solutions to the problem of diversity and inclusion. Bringing awareness to diversity and inclusion for the profession and leading efforts to recruit more minorities into the profession resulted in increasing minority health care providers, which improves the nation's health. This action is described in DNP Essential VII. This is a great example in how accomplishing one Essential leads to another. By serving as a health care advocate for patients and nursing, CRNAs can improve the health of the US population. The IOM report suggests that increasing minority providers will serve to reduce racial disparities.

# Conclusion: Impact of the DNP Degree

As a result of obtaining my DNP degree, I have been able to implement change and have an impact in my profession. By virtue of their educational process, DNP-prepared APRNs will be in positions to influence change by translating research into practice and creating new ideas based on sound research. My work on the Diversity and Inclusion Committee is backed by the IOM report and countless research studies on minorities and health disparities. Activism, for the sake of improving the nation's health, is not only a DNP Essential but it is a basic nursing function. I have been able to use my DNP education within my profession, in ways only possible because of my clinical doctorate. The road clinicians take to get a clinical doctorate is unique for everyone, as are the results. The DNP degree has truly changed my perception and the way I think about issues. Increasing the number of minorities going into health care and decreasing the barriers to practice autonomously for APRNs is only a small piece of tackling health disparities. My long-term vision is to continue to make advances in reducing health disparities in the United States, thus improving our nation's health.

I have been lucky enough to be involved at both the state and national levels of the nurse anesthesia profession and in a position to effect change. My training and education have led me to be successful in carving my own path. I believe DNP-prepared APRNs will be asked to be in positions of leadership and decision making. Using the DNP Essentials to guide your practice, advocating for your profession and patients, using EBP to guide practice changes, and collaborating with other health practitioners will become the norm. The DNP degree gives graduates the tools needed to improve patient outcomes and the overall population health.

My success with the Diversity and Inclusion Committee and advocacy for my profession is owed to those with whom I have collaborated. The countless hours of planning, failing, implementing, changing, and redirecting efforts are only worth your while if you do not do it alone. Support from colleagues and other interested parties is pivotal for success. I have always been open to ideas and trying new things even when they are out of my comfort zone. The saying "change is the only constant" is true because failure to change creates stagnation. For a profession to evolve and a society to progress, it must change and adapt. The DNP degree enables APRNs to shape nursing in all aspects of the profession and impact, not only the health of patients but the health of the nation. I am grateful for my profession and a doctorate degree, which have allowed me to follow my passion.

## ACKNOWLEDGMENTS

Marlene McDowell, MA, is the assistant director of public relations for the AANA. Ms. McDowell's dedication to the AANA and the diversity and inclusion committee has been paramount in making the committee a success. Her unwavering support and friendship has no limits.

## REFERENCES

1. Zaccgnini ME, White KW. *The Doctor of Nursing Practice Essentials: A New Model for Advanced Practice Nursing.* Jones & Bartlett Learning; 2011.

2. Institute of Medicine. *Unequal Treatment: Confronting Racial and Ethnic Disparities in Health Care.* Accessed August 22, 2019. https://www.nap.edu/catalog/10260/unequal-treatment-confronting-racial-and-ethnic-disparities-in-health-care 1999

3. QuickFacts. United States Census Bureau. Accessed August 22, 2019. https://www.census.gov/quickfacts/fact/table/miamidadecounty florida,FL/PST045218%202017

4. Position statement. Council on Accreditation. Accessed May 2, 2019. https://www.coacrna.org/about-coa/position-statements/

5. DNP essentials. American Association of Colleges of Nursing. Accessed April 19, 2019. https://www.aacnnursing.org/DNP/DNP-Essentials

6. Henrichs B, Thompson J. *A Resource for Nurse Anesthesia Educators.* American Association of Nurse Anesthetists; 2011.

7. 2017 national population projections tables: main series. United States Census Bureau. Accessed August 21, 2019. https://www.census.gov/data/tables/2017/demo/popproj/2017-summary-tables.html

8. Nurse anesthesia gender and ethnicity. American Association of Nurse Anesthetist Annual Membership Survey. Accessed August 22, 2019. https://www.aana.com/docs/default-source/exec-unit-my-aana-web-documents-(members-only)/member-surveys/membership-statistics-for-publication.pdf?sfvrsn=60e32899_4

9. US Department of Health and Human Services. *The Registered Nurse Population: Findings From the 2008 National Sample Survey of Registered Nurses.* HHS; 2010.

10. Achieving diversity and meaningful inclusion in nursing education. National League for Nursing. Accessed August 22, 2019. https://www.nln.org/docs/default-source/about/vision-statement-achieving-diversity.pdf?sfvrsn=2%202016

# SECTION V

## NURSE-MIDWIFE EXEMPLARS

# CHAPTER 11

# A DNP-Prepared Midwife's Role in Creating a Combined Prenatal/Substance Use Treatment Program

*Nancy Renn-Bugai, DNP, MSN, CNM*

## INTRODUCTION

The United States is in the middle of an opioid crisis. The rate of opioid overdose has risen out of control. Hedegaard et al[1] reported that "in 2016, the age-adjusted rate of drug overdose deaths (19.8 per 100 000) was more than 3 times the rate in 1999 and that between 2013 and 2018, the rate of overdoses increased by 88% per year." These statistics demonstrate that opioid use is continuing to rise and needs to be addressed. We are facing a health care issue that will not go away unless as a health care community, we come together to provide the help to people suffering with the disease of addiction and create better options for pain control, other than opioid medication (Figure 11-1).

Women as well as men are affected by opioid use disorders (OUDs), but when a woman with an OUD finds herself pregnant, her baby must also be considered. According to Krans et al,[2] "the United States has seen a 333% increase in pregnant women with OUDs in the last 15 years and from 1992 to 2012, the proportion of pregnant women admitted to substance abuse treatment facilities that reported a history of prescription opioid abuse increased from 2% to 28%."

In the 1990s, while working at a clinic in Grand Rapids, Michigan clinic, a special meeting was called to discuss the treatment of pain. All providers were told that "pain" was to be considered the "sixth vital sign" and that we would be held liable if we did not treat a patient's pain. Opioid prescriptions became the expected treatment. No longer were we as providers able to suggest other options without first offering pain medication. Krans and Patrick[3] state that between 1981 and 2012, the average price, per pure gram of heroin, dropped from $3260 to $465. The prescribing practices of prescription opiates and the decrease in cost of heroin have helped to create the current opioid epidemic we have today.

In 2017, the Kent County Needs Assessment[4] reported that Michigan had seen the number of opioid-related deaths in 2017 (93) exceed those in 2016 (70) and between 1999 and 2015 the drug-induced mortality rate (including deaths from any drug) increased nearly 4-fold, from 4.2 per 100 000 to 16.2. During that same time period, Western Michigan was rich with resources for many health care issues, but for a pregnant woman with an OUD, there were few.

It is difficult to discuss the effect the opioid crisis has had on women in Kent County without taking into consideration the newborns who also suffer due to this health care issue.

Benson LA, ed. *The DNP Professional:*
*Translating Value From Classroom to Practice* (pp 121-132).

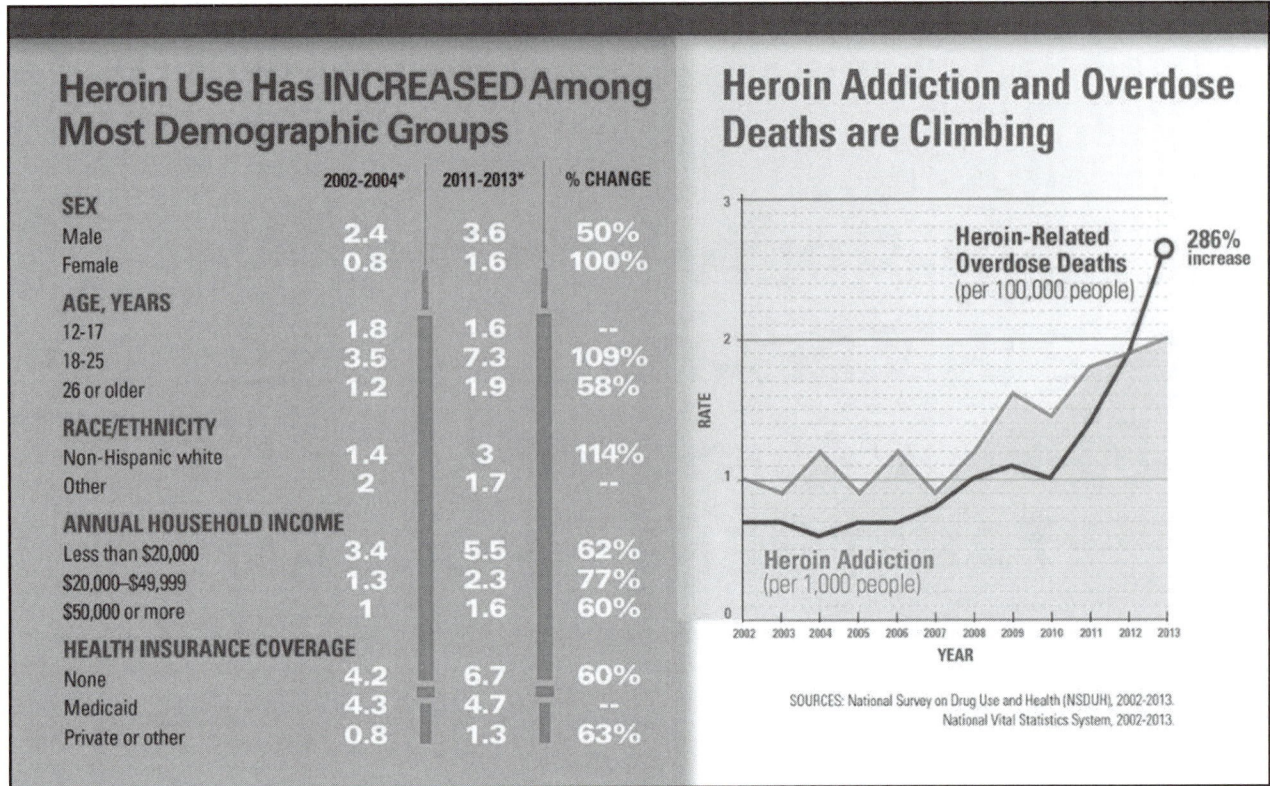

**Figure 11-1.** Opioid use is on the increase for most demographic groups. According to the National Survey on Drug Use and Health, from 2002 to 2013, the incidence of heroin overdose had increased by 286% and the use of heroin had increased by 100% in women of childbearing age (ie, 18 to 25 years old). (Reprinted from National Survey on Drug Use and Health (NSDUH), 2002-2013. National Vital Statistics System, 2002-2013.)

After birth, newborns whose mothers have an OUD, often go through a process of clearing opioids out of their system called *neonatal abstinence syndrome* (NAS). NAS is defined by signs and symptoms of withdrawal such as inconsolable crying, shaking, inability to sleep or eat, and poor weight gain. Typically, newborns will have signs of withdrawal 2 to 3 days after birth, but this varies with each newborn as some may never go through NAS. If a baby does go through NAS, many will only need comfort care, such as swaddling, keeping the baby in a dark room, and maintaining close contact with the mother. If comfort care is not sufficient, a baby may need to be treated with replacement opioids such as methadone or morphine and weaned from these medications over days to possibly weeks (Figure 11-2).

Just as we have seen an increase in OUDs, NAS has increased 5-fold from 2000 to 2012 in the United States.[5] This is not just a health care issue but an economic one as well. Nationally, the average length of stay for a baby with NAS is 16 days. This can cost $159 000 to $238 000 more than a healthy baby without health issues.[6]

Pregnancy is said to be one of the most important times in a woman's life and a time when women are vested in making healthy changes. When a woman finds out that she is pregnant, there is a realization that her baby will be affected by anything she does. The majority of women do not want to do anything that would hurt their baby. Many women in

treatment with an OUD think, "maybe I should just stop the treatment for my opioid use disorder." For those women not in treatment, they wonder if just going "cold turkey" and stopping opioids is the answer. Unfortunately, opioid detoxification or withdrawal in pregnancy is not recommended due to associations with decreased neonatal birth weight, illicit drug use relapse, and resumption of high-risk behaviors such as intravenous drug use, prostitution, and criminal activity. Therefore, treatment is the best option.[3]

The Centers for Disease Control and Prevention recommends that care given to women with OUDs includes care that is comprehensive, gender-responsive, trauma-informed, and family-centered. In her article on "Models of Care for Opioid Dependent Pregnant Women, Johnson"[7] states that evidence-based research has shown that pregnant women with OUDs often do better with more frequent prenatal and OUD treatment evaluations and visits, while pregnancy outcomes improved. Additionally, if a woman's visits for both prenatal care and medication for addiction treatment (MAT) were in one location, it also improved medication adherence related to her OUD. Women with OUDs need increased contact with providers to promote trust. Integrative systems of care for this health care issue are needed to address the complex needs of this population.

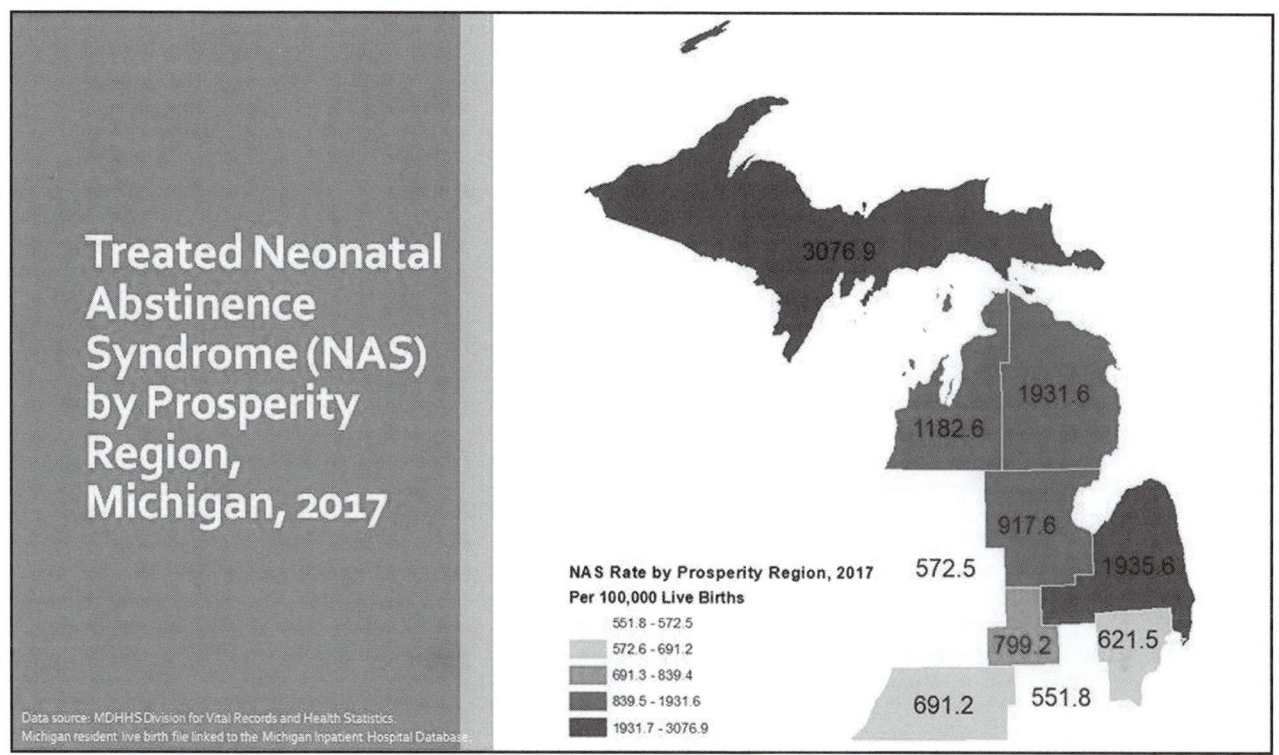

**Figure 11-2.** Treated NAS rate per 100 000 births by prosperity region in Michigan 2017. (Reprinted with permission from Michigan Health and Hospital Association.)

# THE GREAT MOMS PROGRAM

GREAT MOMs (Grand Rapids Encompassing Addiction Treatment with Maternal Obstetric Management) is a program that offers 1 location, with frequent visits for both prenatal care and OUD treatment. Before 2017, pregnant women in west Michigan who suffered with an OUD had no easy way to obtain care for their pregnancy and medication for their opioid use disorder (MOUD) in one location. Methadone, the preferred treatment before 2017 had to, by law, be given out at a federally monitored clinic. Pregnant women would need to go to daily or weekly visits to the methadone clinic and then find time and transportation to their obstetrician appointment in another location. Buprenorphine, the medication used in the GREAT MOMs program, can be managed in an outpatient setting and a woman, once stable, can be given a 4-week prescription. This, in our program, has proven to be an easier option for women.

In 2017, Michigan had limited resources for women with OUDs. Northern Michigan and the upper peninsula were especially impacted. There was only 1 physician in the upper peninsula who would treat substance use disorders in men and women, and there were no methadone clinics. Pregnant women only had 1 option for methadone and that was to move to the lower peninsula. In the upper part of the lower peninsula, resources were better, but limited. Most physicians that did manage with buprenorphine were reluctant to manage pregnant women. This led to high levels of NAS reported in those areas of Michigan due to women with no option for OUD treatment (Figures 11-2 and 11-3). Centers for Disease Control and Prevention–designated resources and strategies for addressing OUD among pregnant women are depicted in Figure 11-4.

The care available in Grand Rapids for women with OUDs was better, but previous to 2017, it was fragmented and required pregnant women to travel to many different locations for their prenatal care and OUD treatment. In 1 week, a woman may have had 4 different appointments at 4 different locations. The GREAT MOMs program was created to help solve this problem by bringing all of the services a pregnant woman would need to 1 location. The hope was that, by putting all of the woman's appointments in 1 location, she would have less missed appointments and this would lead to improved prenatal outcomes, better treatment for her OUD, as well as reduced days spent in the neonatal unit for NAS.

The GREAT MOMs program is located within the office of Spectrum Health Medical Group Maternal Fetal Medicine (MFM) and the Spectrum Health Medical Group Leadership. MFM is part of a larger physician medical group owned by Spectrum Health and is in located in downtown Grand Rapids, Michigan. Spectrum Health Medical Group is the largest multi-specialty physician group in west Michigan, spanning 13 counties, with 1600 physicians and advanced practice providers in more than 110 adult and pediatric specialties. This specialty program was created when an

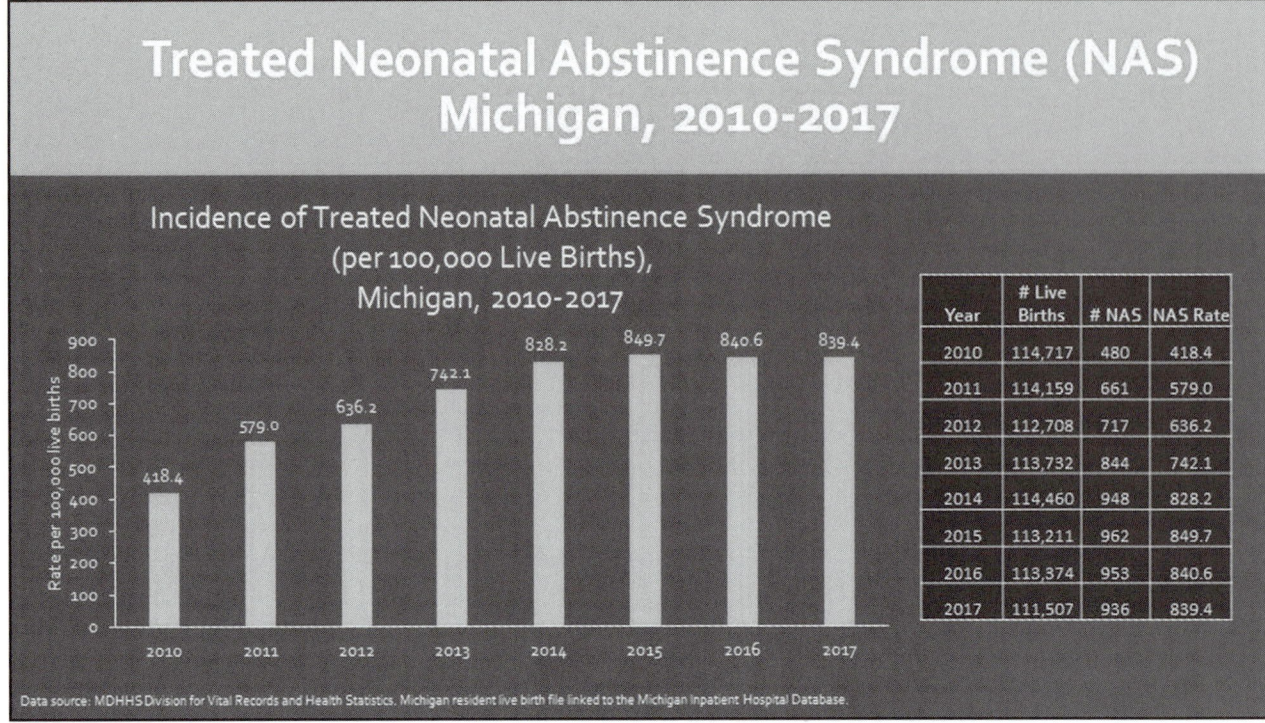

**Figure 11-3.** In Michigan, cases of NAS doubled between 2010 to 2017. (Reprinted with permission from Michigan Health and Hospital Association.)

addiction medicine physician and a certified nurse-midwife (CNM) came together with a common goal of combining MOUD and prenatal care in 1 location.

When considering where the GREAT MOMs should be located, it was determined that MFM would be the best location for the program because, not only did they support the dream, but they could offer comprehensive services related to a women's pregnancy. Services made available in the GREAT MOMs program are prenatal care, OUD management, ultrasound, lab, consultation with perinatologists, and collaborating care with community resources. Previous to the GREAT MOMs program, a woman with an OUD would need to travel to 3 to 4 different locations in the same week to obtain these services. Transportation was also a huge issue for many of the patients we serve, so having all of the services they need in 1 location was more convenient and more manageable.

The GREAT MOMs program is based on trauma-informed care and harm reduction principles. Jones and Karol[8] defined trauma-informed care to mean "that providers need to: (1) understand the role that violence and victimization play in the lives of women seeking substance use and mental health services, (2) design a service system to accommodate the vulnerability of trauma survivors, and (3) deliver services in a manner that would facilitate participation in treatment." Due to this principle, the goal of our program is to offer caring, supportive, and nonjudgmental care. We approach our patients with the understanding that many of them have experienced trauma in their lives. We try to support their

needs and try not to do anything that would cause them to be re-traumatized.

Harm reduction is the second principle we follow. This principle states that care should be offered in a non-judgmental way and that total abstinence from opioids is both impossible and unrealistic.[9] The principle of harm reduction is often used for women in our program who relapse. We understand that opioid use has been a big part of their lives and it is sometimes hard to change. We believe that meeting them where they are, in a nonjudgmental way, is important to their recovery. If a woman relapses, we continue to prescribe her medication but also increase the frequency of her visits to offer more support. If this does not work, we explain to her that she will need to be transferred to a higher level of care, which usually means transferring her to a methadone clinic where she will be seen on a daily basis until stable.

# MY ROLE AS A DNP-PREPARED CERTIFIED NURSE-MIDWIFE IN A MATERNAL FETAL MEDICINE OFFICE SETTING

MFM physicians are obstetricians/gynecologists who have completed an additional 3 years of training in high-risk pregnancy. They care for both women with medical issues

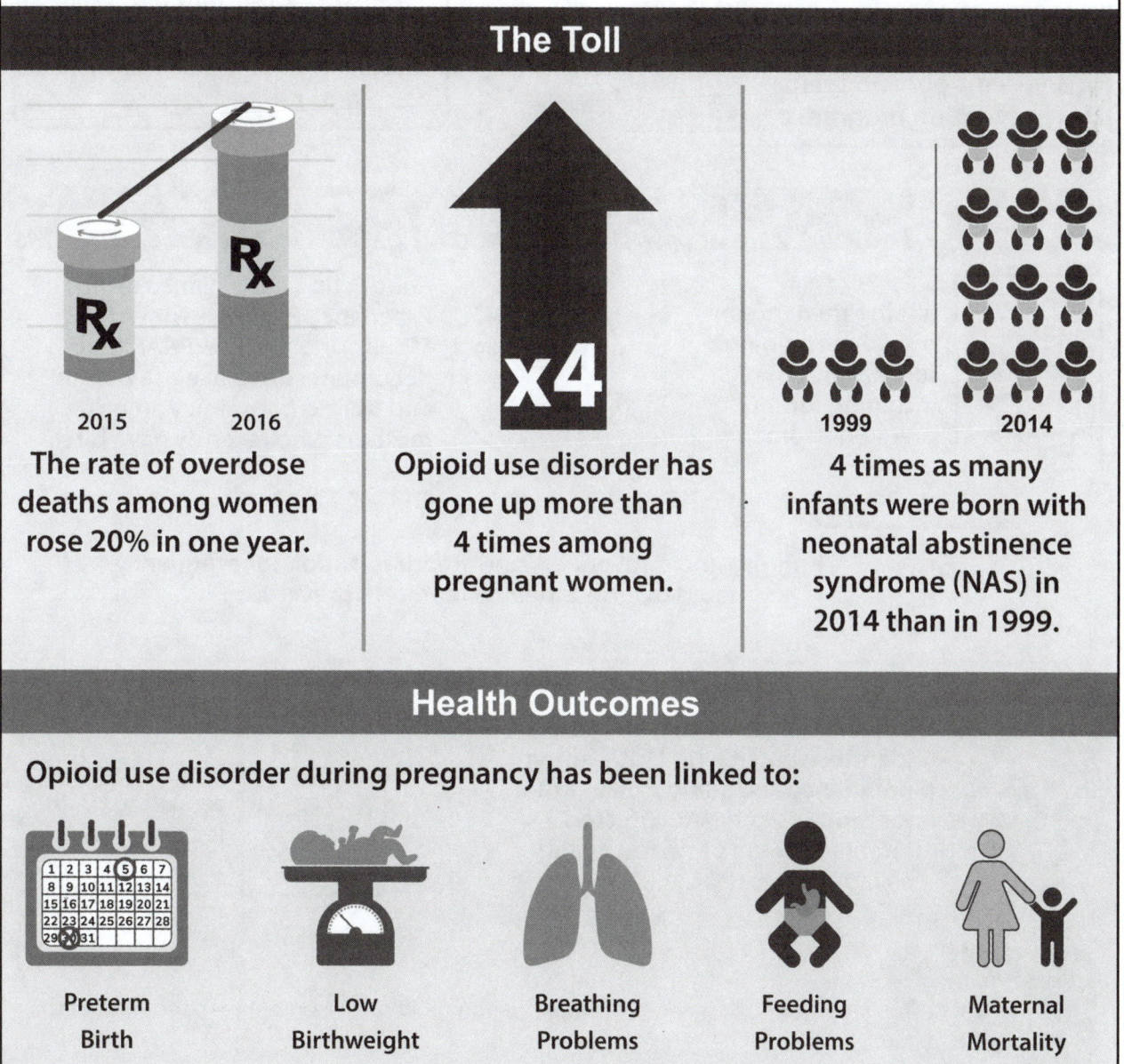

# US Opioid Crisis: Addressing Maternal and Infant Health

Opioid use disorder (OUD) can cause many negative health outcomes for mothers and their babies, both during pregnancy and after delivery. Infants can be born with breathing and feeding problems, and mothers are at risk of opioid-related overdoses. As part of its overarching five-point strategy to prevent opioid overdoses and harms, CDC is taking specific actions to prevent OUD among pregnant women and women of reproductive age and to make sure women with OUD get proper treatment.

## The Toll

**2015** **2016**
The rate of overdose deaths among women rose 20% in one year.

**x4**
Opioid use disorder has gone up more than 4 times among pregnant women.

**1999** **2014**
4 times as many infants were born with neonatal abstinence syndrome (NAS) in 2014 than in 1999.

## Health Outcomes

Opioid use disorder during pregnancy has been linked to:

Preterm Birth

Low Birthweight

Breathing Problems

Feeding Problems

Maternal Mortality

**Figure 11-4.** The maternal and infant opioid crisis in the United States. The toll, health outcomes, strategies for addressing OUD, and the Centers for Disease Control and Prevention response *(continued)*. (Reprinted from https://www.cdc.gov/reproductivehealth/maternalinfanthealth/substance-abuse/opioid-use-disorder-pregnancy/pdf/MMWR-Opioids-Use-Disorder-Pregnancy-Infographic-h.pdf)

## Strategies for Addressing OUD among Pregnant Women

Ensure appropriate prescribing.

Maximize & enhance prescription drug monitoring programs.

Ensure mothers with OUD receive adequate post-birth care, including substance use treatment and relapse-prevention programs.

Ensure pregnant women with OUD have access to medication assisted treatment and related services.

## CDC's Response

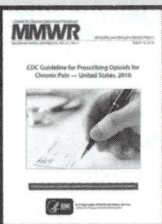 Issuing guidance on opioid prescribing for chronic pain, including for pregnant women

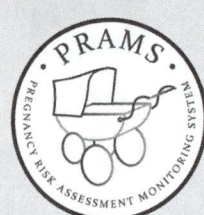 Conducting surveillance using the Pregnancy Risk Assessment Monitoring System (PRAMS) to document substance use before and during pregnancy among mothers who recently gave birth

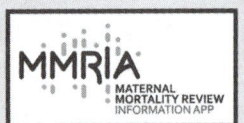 Improving data quality and standardization for pregnancy-associated overdose deaths to inform prevention

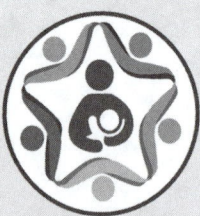 Building state capacity to better identify women with OUD during pregnancy and standardize care for mothers and NAS-affected infants through perinatal quality collaboratives (PQCs)

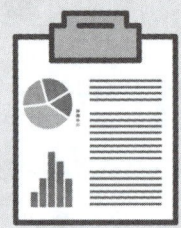 Monitoring and reporting on the incidence of NAS

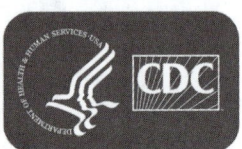 www.cdc.gov/reproductivehealth/opioid-use-disorder-pregnancy/index.html

**Figure 11-4 (continued).** The maternal and infant opioid crisis in the United States. The toll, health outcomes, strategies for addressing OUD, and the Centers for Disease Control and Prevention response. (Reprinted from https://www.cdc.gov/reproductivehealth/maternalinfanthealth/substance-abuse/opioid-use-disorder-pregnancy/pdf/MMWR-Opioids-Use-Disorder-Pregnancy-Infographic-h.pdf)

such as diabetes, hypertension, and cardiac disease, and/or babies with growth issues, birth defects, or genetic disorders. The typical pregnant woman is referred to the MFM office by their obstetrician provider due to issues related to their pregnancy that place them in a high-risk category.

Previous to starting the GREAT MOMs program, I was hired to work alongside the MFM providers, seeing women for their high-risk issues. A MFM physician and I would work together as a team. My job was to help carry out the plan created by the MFM physician after completing their consult. Some patients we saw became our "total care patients" so, in addition to following through with the plan created by the MFM physicians, I was also in charge of their prenatal care. Many of the patients would just come for ultrasounds and return to their obstetrician provider for their prenatal care, and it was my role to review their ultrasounds results with them.

While working with the MFM physicians, I expressed an interest in caring for women with substance use disorders. The director of MFM was supportive of my dream, was aware that there was a growing issue with OUDs in Kent County, and knew there were no programs that provided both prenatal care and MAT. We discussed the issue but were unsure how to put a program together.

Within 6 months of our discussion, Dr. Cara Poland, an addiction physician, met to discuss the opioid issue in Kent County and the work that was being done at Spectrum Health to help with this health care issue. While meeting with him, she expressed her interested in caring for pregnant women with an OUD.

Once we were given approval to start a program, Dr. Poland and I met on a weekly basis. We discussed what type of a program would improve care for pregnant women with an OUD and how it would be structured. She stated that during her training, she had done a rotation in a program that was similar to what we wanted to do but the program offered the MOUD but did not offer the same location for both prenatal care and OUD treatment.

# Program Planning

## The SWOT for GREAT MOMs

When we first came together to discuss what the program would look like, we created a SWOT analysis to help guide us:

- Strengths: Our program would provide 1 location for OUD treatment and all obstetrical services, such as MFM consults, antenatal testing, and ultrasounds. We would use interdisciplinary collaboration to improve outcomes. Both Dr. Poland and I and are connected to the community through committee involvement. Spectrum Health is a teaching institution, so research would be possible. In order to prescribe buprenorphine, the medication used to treat OUD, a provider needs to attend an 8-hour training and apply to the Substance

Abuse and Mental Health Services Administration (SAMHSA) for a special waiver. The majority of the MFM providers were willing to apply for their wavier, enabling them to treat the women both obstetrically and for their addiction if Dr. Poland or I were not available.

- Weaknesses: There is a lack of social workers in the office. Limited nursing support was available to assist with calls regarding patient appointments and medical issues. Not enough hours were allotted for the medical assistant (MA) to room patients, call for preauthorization of medication, and follow-up. There were limited office hours with the office being open only on Tuesdays and Wednesdays. Lastly, the program was given limited office space, with 2 rooms to operate out of in the back hall of the MFM office.
- Opportunities: When we first started, I was unable to obtain a buprenorphine waiver, which did not give me the ability to manage both obstetrician care and addiction management. Currently, babies are transferred to the neonatal intensive care unit (NICU) after the mother is discharged from the hospital. We saw the potential to keep moms and babies together and not have the babies go to NICU. This would improve both neonatal and maternal bonding and the breastfeeding rate, as well as decreasing neonatal inpatient costs. Other opportunities would be to add a pediatric services program, hire a social worker, and have additional postpartum visits for assessment of postpartum depression and relapse for up to a year.
- Threats: The women we serve need extra time and support, which is not paid for by insurance. Right now, the program is funded by the hospital, in kind, and grants. Costs are high and reimbursement is low. This issue could eventually close the program.

## Business Plan

We did not create a business plan for this program. The director of MFM was aware that Dr. Poland had worked in a program similar to the one we wanted to create, and he agreed that we needed to work fast to come up with a solution. Up to this point, the system was broken. Currently, pregnant women would see their obstetrician providers and their substance use providers in different locations. This led to missed obstetrician appointments and poor prenatal care, so he supported our idea and told us to start planning.

## DNP Essential: Scientific Underpinnings for Practice

In the past, methadone was the recommended treatment for women with OUDs during pregnancy. For this reason, the obstetrician providers in west Michigan would send all of their pregnant women to the methadone clinic if there was an issue with an OUD. Currently, there are only 2 clinics in west Michigan, 1 in Grand Rapids, and 1 in Muskegon.

Methadone clinics are run by private medical groups and regulated by the federal government. Methadone, for the treatment of OUDs, can only be given out at a methadone clinic. It cannot be provided in an outpatient or office setting. Typically, when a person starts their treatment, they are required to go to the methadone clinic every day. Once they prove (with urine drug tests) that they are not using any other substance and doing well in the program, they may get weekly "take homes" but only if they adhere to their treatment.

Recently, the American College of Obstetricians and Gynecologists (ACOG) has recommended treatment with buprenorphine as good or better for the treatment of OUDs in pregnant women. In the ACOG committee Opinion No. 711,[10] they cited a study that showed that, on average, babies required 89% less morphine to treat NAS, had a 43% shorter stay in the NICU, and a 58% shorter duration of medical treatment for NAS. Because of these findings, they now support buprenorphine as a potential first-line medication for pregnant women OUDs.

In our program, we offer MOUD with a medication that combines buprenorphine and naloxone. The trade name is Suboxone in the film form and Zubsolv in the tablet form. The medication is delivered sublingually because if used intravenously, naloxone will cause immediate withdrawal symptoms. We use this medication because it decreases the likelihood of diversion of the medication to other people with OUDs. The medication Subtext, which is buprenorphine only, is easily sold on the streets for intravenous use. Any of the buprenorphine formulations can legally be given out in an outpatient setting. Typically, patients can receive weekly to monthly prescriptions, depending on how stable they are in their treatment. Buprenorphine/naloxone works well in our program because women who are pregnant typically come for obstetrical prenatal care every 4 weeks at the beginning of their pregnancy, then every 2 weeks, and then weekly at the end of pregnancy.

# DNP Essential: Clinical Prevention and Population Health for Improving the Nation's Health

## Practice Outcomes

We have been collecting data since the start of the program, and so far, our patients have had good outcomes. As of May 2019, there have been a total of 27 patients who have been in the GREAT MOMs program. Out of these 27 patients, 2 had miscarriages before 20 weeks, 2 had to be referred to the methadone clinic due to noncompliance, and 1 transferred out due to the inability to engage regularly in the program. This left us with 22 GREAT MOMs women who have delivered while in our program.

One of the outcomes we were interested in was if patients would come for adequate prenatal care. In a normal pregnancy, the expectation would be to have a total of 14 visits throughout her pregnancy, at 8, 12, 16, 20, 24, 28, 30, 32, 34, 36, 37, 38, 39, and 40 weeks. Due to our patient's high-risk social issues, many are late to our care, so it is hard to determine for our statistics if they had adequate prenatal care. We can only determine if they were seen consistently after they came to us. In order to do this, missed appointments were tracked.

Of the 22 patients who remained in the program and have delivered, not one of them experienced a stillbirth. The average gestational age was 37.95 weeks, but this number was low due to 2 sets of twins, 1 delivered at 26 weeks and 1 delivered at 34 weeks. Both were high-risk twins due to issues not related to their Suboxone use. If we excluded these as outliers, our average gestational age would be 38.62 weeks and 96% of our patients delivered at term.

The length of stay for the babies delivered by GREAT MOMs patients to be observed for NAS, if we excluded the pre-term twins, was 6.54 days. Both of the twins stayed for an extended time, not due to NAS but due to prematurity related to the twin pregnancy. The mandated length of stay for a baby born to a women being treated for an OUD is 5 to 7 days, while the national average is 16 days.

Regarding treatment for OUD, there were no lapses in medication. If a woman missed an appointment, she called the office, her medication was sent in, and she was seen the next week.

Our 6-week postpartum visits had an excellent return rate at 81%. Per the ACOG committee Opinion No. 736,[11] as many as 40% of women do not attend their postpartum exam. This is important because postpartum is stressful even for a woman who has all of her needs met and does not have to deal with an OUD. There are many changes during this period, such as lack of sleep, breastfeeding issues, and postpartum depression, so the support we give when a women comes for her postpartum care is essential.

Dr. Poland is currently working with students from one of the colleges in Michigan to compare our program outcomes with women who were seen at an addiction clinic and had care with an obstetrician/gynecologist at a separate location. Her students looked at the data and compared our patients to a group that had prenatal care and MOUD in separate locations. In the group who had separate appointments for obstetrician prenatal care and MOUD, there were many missed obstetrician and MOUD appointments. We do not know the reason at this time, but we could surmise that their ability to go to multiple appointments in different locations was difficult for them.

# Cost Savings and Revenue Generation

The GREAT MOMs program operates at high cost to the state and the hospital in the outpatient setting. In a low-risk obstetrician/gynecologist office, an obstetrician provider would see 20 to 26 patients a day. In the GREAT MOMs program, the maximum we can see would be 8 to 10 patients. The cost of staff and operating costs are not reimbursed by insurance companies. The reason for the difference is that care for our patients is so involved, that most of the women need 30 to 45 minutes a visit, where normally a prenatal visit would take no more than 15 minutes. The cost of staff and operating costs are not reimbursed by insurance companies. As providers, we are the only staff that generates income. We soon realized that the GREAT MOMs program needed to be considered a community service program, and in order to survive, we would need to find funding in order to continue.

The grant department at Spectrum Health looked for grants that would fit our program and found one offered from Blue Cross Blue Shield (BCBS). The grant required that another funding source would match their grant. We contacted the Spectrum Health Foundation and they agreed to match the grant. As a requirement for our grant from BCBS, we also needed to create a toolkit for other providers to use if they wanted to model our program. Fortunately for us, Spectrum Health decided to support our program "in kind" until we could get the funding needed.

When caring for women with OUDs, there are both increased costs to care for the women, as well as increased costs of care for their babies after delivery. Patrick et al[12] stated that the average stay for a baby with NAS nationwide was 16 days and the average hospital charge, as of 2009, was $53 400. As of 2017, the state of Michigan estimates that the average stay for a baby with NAS is 15 days and the average cost for their stay is $28 413. This breaks down to $1894 a day per baby.[13] When we compare our 22 babies (with the average stay of 6.57 days, not 15 days), the total cost for a baby in GREAT MOMs was $12 444 per baby for each hospital stay. This comes to $286 212 for all 22 babies. If they would have stayed an average of 15 days, the cost to insurance companies would have been a total of $653 499. This demonstrates a cost savings of $367 287 to Medicaid and other insurance companies in Michigan.

## DNP Essential: Interprofessional Collaboration for Improving Patient and Population Health Outcomes

The GREAT MOMs program is an example of interprofessional collaboration at its best. The program started with a collaborative effort between 2 unlikely professions: addiction medicine and midwifery. On a daily basis, Dr. Poland and I work together managing the patients' care throughout the pregnancy. The interprofessional teams, from outpatient care to inpatient care, work together to make the pregnancy, delivery, newborn health, and the postpartum period as safe as possible.

## Interprofessional Collaboration for the Patients

Every 2 weeks our medical assistant Kristl, Dr. Poland, and I collaborated in the patients' outpatient care. Kristl works, not only to room the patients, but is basically the administrator of the program. She is an expert in managing the sometimes difficult task of assisting the patients with their medication preauthorization at the pharmacy and correcting any issues regarding their medications. She also helps to set up community support for women to ensure they have recovery coaches, counseling, and other support services. I am responsible for the patients' prenatal care and, at times, their addiction care. Dr. Poland manages the patients' medication needs and counsels them on the disease of OUDs. In addition to these professionals, the patient may need to see the MFM team of physicians who are in charge of any high-risk medical issues the mother or baby may need managed. The registered nurses in the MFM office are also very important to our work. They work 40 hours a week and answer any calls from our patients. They then take the responsibility to contact the person needed to help the patients if we are not currently in the office.

## Interprofessional Collaboration With the Community

Women who are in our program are required to have counseling to receive their medication. To fulfill this obligation, we partnered with one of the community mental health programs in west Michigan. The program we work with created a Specialty Assistance Program (SPA) for pregnant women, to help with issues regarding their substance use disorders and pregnancy needs. The program uses women who have had an addiction issue in the past and are now hired as recovery coaches to work with our women to support and guide them. The recovery coach will bring a woman to her appointments, support her through recovery, and even help her with daily chores around the house. They attempt to build a trusting relationship to encourage recovery during a woman's pregnancy. After the pregnancy, they work to make sure the patient is transitioned to the ongoing support she will need.

We also started a committee that includes all of the medical professionals involved in our patients' care. We meet on a monthly basis to address issues and create solutions so the patient is supported throughout her pregnancy, intrapartum, and postpartum care. Included in this team are neonatologists, social workers, neonatal nurses, labor and delivery representatives, community agencies, and our team. We all come together to discuss issues our patients may face and create solutions to make sure the women receive the care they need in the hospital and that the transition for the baby and family goes smoothly after the birth and at discharge.

## Interprofessional Collaboration With Inpatient Staff

During the pregnancy, all our patients go for a consult with the perinatologist and NICU social worker to discuss the baby's stay in the NICU. They are given a tour of the NICU and shown where their baby will stay after the mother is discharged from the hospital. This visit was created to decrease the anxiety the women may be feeling regarding their newborns' treatment after the birth. Babies are required to stay for 5 to 7 days after the birth to be observed and possibly longer if they need treatment for withdrawal symptoms.

As part of our ongoing work, we helped to developed a Save Plan of Care for the baby. The patient meets with the social worker to create a plan if she relapses and cannot care for her baby after they leave the hospital.

All practices inside and outside of the hospital have all come together to improve outcomes. My role as a DNP is to be involved in all these collaborative actions to see the big picture for my patients and to suggest other initiatives to improve practice. One of the accomplishments of our inpatient team was to create a brochure on NAS so the patient is aware of what to expect from her baby after the birth, and with the help of a DNP student, we developed a welcome brochure for patients new to the program. This brochure explains all of the patient responsibilities and what we offer in our program. As a part of my role, I am also involved in committees within the community to discuss substance use disorders and how to improve identification of women with addiction issues and care of the women, not just in Grand Rapids, but in all of west and northern Michigan.

## DNP Essential: Health Care Policy for Advocacy in Health Care

CNMs were not included in the Comprehensive Addiction and Recovery Act (CARA) of 2016. This law gave the right to nurse practitioners and physician assistants to obtain the special waiver that allowed them to write medication for the treatment of addiction. All of the other advanced practice registered nurses (APRNs) were left out of this bill, including CNMs. In an attempt to right this wrong, I spent hours writing my senators and to those at the Substance Abuse and Mental Health Services Administration (SAMHSA) to let them know that there were women out there that needed my help. As a CNM, I care for pregnant women with addiction issues but, due to the law, could not help them with mediation for their OUD. The legislators were not knowledgeable regarding the differences between physician assistants, nurse practitioners, and CNMs. Many of the legislators thought that CNMs had no formal education and were trained on the job so they were leery about voting yes to extend the right to have a waiver to write for buprenorphine to a CNM.

With the help of my professional organization, the American College of Nurse-Midwives (ACNM), the American Association of Nurse Practitioners (AANP), and many other midwives and nurses, the Substance Use-Disorder Prevention that Promotes Opioid Recovery and Treatment for Patients and Communities Act added all APRNs to the list of professionals that would be able to obtain the waiver.

I am happy to say that during the writing of this chapter, SAMHSA created the pathway for CNMs, certified registered nurse anesthetists, and clinical nurse specialists to apply for their waiver so all of our hard work paid off. It took a year to institute this law, but now I have my waiver and can manage medications for my patient's OUD.

## DNP Essential: Advanced Nursing Practice

After receiving the news about our ability to obtain our waiver, I reached out to the ACNM and asked that anyone interested in this work to apply for their waiver. As a team, we also sent an abstract to the ACNM National Conference in hopes of speaking and educating my fellow professionals about treating women with OUDs. Midwives are the ideal professional to take on this challenge. I plan to continue advocating for midwives and nurse practitioners to lead the way and continue to create programs for women who need help with OUDs.

# PROFESSIONALISM

I have always been involved with my professional groups on both a local and national level. I have served as the chapter chair for west Michigan ACNM and after the reorganization of the college to state affiliates, I served as member at large. Two years ago, I joined the AANP and recently, I joined the International Nurses Society on Addictions (IntNSA). I hope to become certified in addiction through the IntNSA in the future.

As a DNP, I participate in precepting both nurse practitioner and midwifery students. Recognition of the DNP is just starting in west Michigan. Currently, I am the only midwife in our medical group with a DNP. I feel that I have shown what a nurse with a DNP can do for patient outcomes but more education is needed.

I am very involved in the community. I sit on 2 committees, including the Kent County Drug Exposed Infants Team. This team consists of nurses from all the hospitals in Grand Rapids, public health nurses, social workers, and representatives from community resource associations. We meet monthly to discuss how we can educate women in the community as well as health care providers regarding all substance use disorders. This includes marijuana, alcohol, methamphetamines, and opioids. We have completed pamphlets to educate pregnant women on substance use, and we also use this time to discuss issues in Kent County regarding how all of the hospitals and community agencies can help solve these issues.

A second community coalition I sit on is the Region 4 Perinatal Alliance Collaborative. The state of Michigan is divided up into 10 regional collaboratives. We are region 4, which included the counties that feed patients into the hospitals in Grand Rapids. The goal of these collaboratives is to "ensure that mothers are healthy, and babies are healthy and thriving." Our region has decided to concentrate on (1) using a screening tool called the 5 Ps to screen for substance use disorders and (2) increase the utilization of home visiting programs. Our hospital system volunteered to start screening in one of our urban clinics and rural clinics to see if we could identify pregnant women with substance use disorders, smoking, and domestic violence.

Due to my involvement in this collaborative, I have also joined with one of my fellow nurses to create a research project that looks at the 5 Ps screening tool and compare women's answers to their toxicology reports. We want to see if women are forthcoming regarding substance use in their lives.

## Pearls/Takeaways

The implementation of the DNP Essentials is not well known in clinical practice. After practicing as a midwife for a few years, I became interested in women with substance use disorders. In my past, I was exposed to alcoholism in my family and friends. I always had the ability to look inside the person and see the good. I wanted to work with women who had substance use disorders because I knew they were good people with a difficult disease.

It was not easy for me as a midwife to work with this special population of women without the support of the leadership at Spectrum Health. As nurses, we work on the frontlines every day. We see what is working in practice and what is not working. As DNPs, we need to let others know what we have observed and keep persisting until someone listens to our ideas. Many times, we feel like we are powerless to change practice and it takes a lot of work to make others listen. In their review article on the impact of the role of the DNP, Edwards et al[14] point out that the DNP is prepared to "design and evaluate innovative patient care models, evaluate cost-effectiveness of patient care strategies, and influence health policies at various levels." We continue to lead and change patient care outcomes by altering and creating new clinical practice guidelines.

My advice to other DNPs would be, if you have an innovative idea, talk to everyone you can. Go as high up in leadership as you can until you find someone who will listen. Find a physician who shares your passion. The reality is that hospital administrators listen to physicians. They can be a valuable part of the solution.

It is also important to research your idea and find out if anyone else has put your idea into practice. Find support from other professionals in other states and see if they will allow you to use their work to help with yours. We have a great profession, and most nurses have the unifying goal of making the lives of their patients better. You can find someone to support you as long as you do the work to find that person.

I would also encourage the DNPs of the future to become political. I am sorry to say that our legislators only know what they hear from others. Let them hear from you.

## Conclusion: Impact of the DNP Degree

As a result of obtaining my DNP degree, I was able to implement a change in the health care delivery system for pregnant women with OUDs. Through interprofessional collaboration with addiction medicine, MFM, and midwifery, the GREAT MOMs program is creating a positive impact on pregnant woman and newborns. GREAT MOMs transformed a fragmented care system into one that not only resulted in improved outcomes but was designed to be patient-focused.

In my DNP program, preventive strategies using the IOM model were presented. It emphasized the role health care providers play in creating programs that target individual populations of patients at risk for poor outcomes. The IOM model identified 3 categories of risk: universal, selective, and indicated. Using this model, pregnant women who were enrolled in the GREAT MOMs program were identified as a group needing a selective intervention and prevention measures to improve outcomes related to their pregnancy and their substance use disorder. A gap analysis was performed to identify actual, as well as potential, programs to meet the needs of pregnant women with OUDs. It was determined that there were a limited number of programs available throughout the United States that focused on this issue, so we had an opportunity to develop a program that would address the poor health outcomes in this population of women. The knowledge on outcome assessment and program development I received in my DNP program gave me the skills to assist with the creation of the GREAT MOMs program.

Our program has been operating for 2.5 years and we have seen 2 significant outcomes. First, we have seen a decrease in the days normally spent in the NICU for NAS by more than 50%. This has resulted in a 50% savings to insurance companies with the major payor being Medicaid. Second, we have seen an increase in postpartum visits reach 81% as compared to the national average of 40%. This outcome is important because at the postpartum visit, the issue of depression and the need for birth control are addressed. The women we serve are at high risk for postpartum depression and unintended pregnancies, so discussing these issues are paramount to their future health status.

## ACKNOWLEDGMENTS

I would like to take this opportunity to thank all of the staff and colleagues that have worked so diligently on this program. First, I would like to thank Dr. Cara Poland, MD, MEd, FACP, DFASAM, for her support and hard work. The GREAT MOMs would never have come to fruition without her. I thank her for believing in me as a nurse-midwife and for supporting my passion to serve women with OUDs, when many others did not. I would also like to acknowledge Dr. David Colombo, director of Spectrum Health Medical Group MFM and the Spectrum Health Medical Group Leadership. Our program is expensive to operate, yet they continue to support our work. I appreciate the hard work and compassion that Kristl Smith, our program manager and MA, gives to this program every day. She has the broad base of knowledge regarding treatment of OUDs that keeps us going. To the nurses and MAs in the MFM office, I say "Thank you" for stepping in when we need you. Finally, thank you to the women we serve. You teach me every day what living with an OUD looks like and you let me into your lives. I am blessed to have been with you during these important times in your lives.

## REFERENCES

1. Hedegaard H, Warner M, Miniño AM. Centers for Disease Control and Prevention. Drug overdose deaths in the united states, 1999-2016. https://www.cdc.gov/nchs/products/databriefs/db294.htm

2. Krans E, Kim JY, James AE, Kelley D, Jarlenski MP. Medication-assisted treatment use among pregnant women with opioid use disorder. *Obstet Gynecol.* 2019;133(5):943-951. doi:10.1097/AOG.0000000000003231

3. Krans EE, Patrick SW. Opioid use disorder in pregnancy: health policy and practice in the midst of an epidemic. *Obstet Gynecol.* 2016;128(1):4-10. doi:10.1097/AOG0000000000001446

4. Kent county community health needs assessment 2017. Access Kent. https://accesskent.com/Health/CHNA/pdf/2017CHNA.pdf

5. Wachman EM, Schiff DM, Silverstein M. Neonatal abstinence syndrome: advances in diagnosis and treatment. *JAMA.* 2018;319(13):1362-1374. doi:10.1001/jama.2018.2640

6. Peltz G, Anand KJS. Long-acting opioids for treating neonatal abstinence: a high price for short stay? *JAMA.* 2015;314(19):2023-2024.

7. Johnson E. Models of care for opioid dependent pregnant women. *Semin Perinatol.* 2019;43(3):132-140. doi:https://doi.org/10.1053/j.semperi.2019.01.002

8. Jones HE, Kaltenbach K. *Treating Women with Substance Use Disorders During Pregnancy: A Comprehensive Approach to Caring for Mother and Child.* Oxford University Press; 2013.

9. Boyd SC, Marcellus L. *With Child: Substance Use During Pregnancy: A Women-Centered Approach.* Fernwood Publishing; 2007.

10. Opioid use and opioid use disorder in pregnancy. American College of Obstetricians and Gynecologists. August 2017. https://www.acog.org/clinical/clinical-guidance/committee-opinion/articles/2017/08/opioid-use-and-opioid-use-disorder-in-pregnancy

11. AGOG committee opinion no. 736: optimizing postpartum care. *Obstet Gynecol.* 2018;131(5):e140-e150. doi:10.1097/AOG.0000000000002633

12. Patrick SW, Schuamacher RE, Benneyworth BD, McAllister JM, Davis MM. Neonatal abstinence syndrome and associated health care expenditures: United States, 2000-2009. *JAMA.* 2012;307(18):1934-1940. doi:10.001/jama.2012.3951

13. The burden of neonatal abstinence syndrome (NAS) in Michigan. Michigan. December 2016. https://www.michigan.gov/documents/mdhhs/Burden_of_Neonatal_Abstinence_Syndrome_in_Michigan_548268_7.pdf

14. Edwards N, Coddington J, Erler C, Kirkpatrick J. The impact of the role of doctor of nursing practice nurses on healthcare and leadership. *Med Res Arch.* 2018;6(4). doi:https://doi.org/10.18103/mra.v6i4.1734

# CHAPTER 12

# ESTABLISHING A PRACTICE AS A NOVICE DNP-PREPARED CERTIFIED NURSE-MIDWIFE

*Michelle M. Davis, DNP, RNC-OB, NNP, CNM*

## INTRODUCTION

Maricopa Obstetrics and Gynecology Associates (MOGA) is part of Arizona OBGYN Affiliates, an integrated family of obstetrician/gynecologist (OB/GYN) physicians who are committed to excellent care of women and seeks to promote the safety and well-being of women and their families throughout pregnancy, labor, delivery, and the postpartum period. MOGA has 2 offices that serve women across the lifespan. Additional services offered by MOGA include ultrasound, breastfeeding and lactation consults, family planning, birth control, integrative medicine, gynecology, in-office surgery, well-women care, and overall maintenance of women's health.

MOGA's providers are affiliated with Banner University Medical Center Phoenix (BUMCP). BUMCP is a Level III perinatal and neonatal Magnet hospital situated in Phoenix, Arizona, where MOGA's physicians completed their OB/GYN residencies. MOGA recognizes the value of evidence-based models provided by OB/GYNs and certified nurse-midwives (CNMs) and seeks to enhance patient choice in the birth experience within their respective fields of practice and areas of expertise.

When I began my journey with MOGA, there were 7 physicians, 1 CNM, and 4 women's health nurse practitioners. During the past 6 months, 1 physician and 3 additional CNMs joined the team for improvement of its health care services. MOGA's model is firmly grounded wholly on the close collaboration of all health care professionals and providers. In order to maintain a high level of health care, one of the physicians is on a rotation schedule. This rotation is on call and in house at BUMCP. MOGA physicians are responsible for supervising residents in gynecology consultations for the well-being of women in the antepartum, labor, delivery, and postpartum periods to ensure that the residents successfully complete their postgraduate training in the field of OB/GYN. One of the more valuable and attractive features for myself and any new graduate is the 24/7 availability of at least one MOGA physician at the hospital. Having one as my supporting and backup physician is invaluable, as I am a newly graduated CNM. The availability of my physicians and their mentorship in the hospital and office provides me with a feeling of safety and security while providing excellent patient care.

Benson LA, ed. *The DNP Professional: Translating Value From Classroom to Practice* (pp 133-142).

# CREATING THE ROLE OF A CERTIFIED NURSE-MIDWIFE

A CNM is an advanced practice registered nurse (APRN) who has expertise in providing care to women of all ages. The type of care that CNMs provide includes primary care, reproductive, gynecological, well-woman care, newborn care up to 28 days of life (with emphasis on low-risk pregnancy), intrapartum, and postpartum.[1] CNMs are graduates of accredited graduate nursing programs. Additionally, CNMs may hold degrees such as the Doctor of Nursing Practice (DNP) or master of science in nursing (MSN). The DNP is a practice-focused graduate degree program whose purpose is to advance the education of an APRN.[2] The DNP prepares nurses for the highest level of clinical practice by teaching them to integrate evidence-based practice into daily patient care.[3]

Congruent with the scope of practice defined by the Arizona State Board of Nursing, a CNM's scope of practice is to provide primary care to women from adolescence to menopause, pregnancy and childbirth while utilizing the process of assessment, diagnosis, management, and evaluation to address the patient's needs in a clinical-based office and acute hospital setting.[1,4] The care provided by CNMs is comprehensive, continuous, and addresses the current needs of women's health care, assisting in the prevention of health-related problems that may arise in the future.[3] As a CNM, I am able to admit patients to health care facilities, order, perform, and interpret laboratory, radiographic, and other diagnostic tests, perform therapeutic procedures that the CNM is qualified to perform, prescribe treatments, and prescribe and dispense medications when granted authority by the Arizona Board of Nursing Section R4-19-511.[4]

"DNP graduates must be proficient in quality improvement strategies and in creating and sustaining changes at the organizational and policy levels."[2] Utilizing the hallmarks of midwifery, the CNM provides quality patient care, builds on the nurse-patient relationship, promotes health education and counseling, and contributes to the advancement of the CNM profession as an APRN. CNMs collaborate with other professionals within the health care team. Additionally, CNMs participate in the application and dissemination of research, further promoting the role of the CNM and the quality of the care that is provided.[5] Independent decisions are made after analyzing multiple sources of data and the current evidence, utilizing consultations or referrals as appropriate.[6] Creating clinical practice guidelines, designing evidence-based interventions, and evaluating practice outcomes are key skills that I have developed from my DNP education as well as from past working experience.

The term *midwife* is derived from a Middle English term, *mid-wif*. This term is thought to have the meaning of "with woman" (ie, "mid" refers to with and "wif" refers to a woman). In my opinion, this is the most appropriate understanding: to be "with [a] woman" during her care. Therefore, this meaning represents the voice of my heart. I love my patients and find providing their care to be one of the most beautiful things in my life. By considering the concepts of the hallmarks of midwifery, as an APRN, my main efforts are to provide an exceptional standard of care to my patients. For example, this includes quality care based on the relationship of the nurse and the patient, education, and counseling patients regarding healthy living, and contributions to the advancement and growth of the profession of CNMs.

Developing my professional life as a MOGA midwife was not an easy task. In fact, it was rather challenging. The more that patients sought my care, it became clear that midwifery was my passion and calling. First, and most importantly, MOGA had employed 4 CNMs prior to my employment. None of the previously employed, experienced CNMs developed any standards or processes for newly hired CNMs. In other words, there were no written practice guidelines for midwifery care at MOGA when I arrived. When I received and accepted an offer to work for MOGA, it was my understanding that an experienced and well-trained CNM would act as my mentor. She would be responsible for cultivating and enhancing my skills and knowledge as I advanced my career from the status of a novice CNM to, one day, that of an experienced CNM. Before I started my position at MOGA, however, the experienced CNM had already resigned her position. My physicians at MOGA were committed to training me, and I was precepted by CNMs that I admired while in school, however, there was no doubt that I would need extensive orientation and training as a newly graduated CNM. While working as a labor and delivery (L&D) registered nurse, I had worked with and developed a relationship with all 7 of the physicians at MOGA for more than a decade before starting work there. I was not aware of how challenging the role would be as the only midwife working with 7 physicians. Do not get me wrong, I admire every single one of them, but in comparison to my previous role, the new advanced practice role was a challenge. As a DNP-prepared CNM, I was not aware until now that most of the project-based work I am doing for MOGA and BUCMP are skills that I acquired during my education at Arizona State University (ASU). Projects that I have been involved with include developing health policy relating to maternal health and standards for MOGA midwifery practice that promotes a safe birthing experience for women. Additionally, I am currently developing educational programs for MOGA midwife patients to promote wellness during their pregnancy. This was followed by writing a blueprint for the MOGA midwife practice. The blueprint will be based on evidence that will increase utilization of midwifery care. My goal is to decrease maternal mortality by improving maternal and infant outcomes, decrease costs associated with interventions during birth, and develop additional care choices for our midwife patients. Requirements to build a collaborative practice include trust, communication, and the understanding that midwives serve an essential role in meeting the diverse needs of midwife patients.[7]

In a private setting, several points must be considered in developing a midwifery service. These points are as follows:

1. Financial and monetary issues
   a. Projecting the potential increase in patient volume
   b. Availability of the office space
2. Determination of operational issues
   a. The flow of patients in the health care setting
   b. Schedules and routines: According to the statements provided by the American College of Nurse-Midwives' (ACNM) scope of practice, CNMs have to work in close collaboration with all physicians whenever that is determined to be important.
3. Measures for evaluation and assessment
   a. The development of tools and questionnaires related to the Patient Satisfaction Survey
   b. The development of a data sheet for midwifery patients to aid in the quality improvement process

Previously, I worked in a hospital with well-established standard policies and procedures. I was extremely fortunate to have managers who mentored me and created an environment where I was able to continually grow as an L&D registered nurse. Every 3 months, I went through one-on-one evaluations as part of our professional development. The midwifery practice was new to MOGA. Therefore, policies and procedures had not been completely developed and documented. For example, applying for hospital privileges as a CNM was challenging, primarily because the administrative staff at MOGA were not aware of this process. After all, I was MOGA's first newly graduated CNM. Essentially, I took it upon myself to research and document the steps that were needed to apply for hospital credentialing and privileges. (The process for credentialing physicians is different.)

MOGA had policies and procedures that were separate from the CNM Collaboration Policies and Procedures, which were already created. I made sure both were congruent and provided feedback to the physician in charge of updating the document. I worked on increasing the compatibility of both policies and procedures, and after a thorough analysis, I provided feedback and suggestions to the physician who was in charge of updating the documents. In this regard, I also worked in collaboration with the office manager. This collaboration also helped me in developing a better understanding of the workflow in the office.

"DNP graduates are distinguished by their abilities to use information systems/technology to support and improve patient care and health care systems, and provide leadership within health care systems and/or academic settings."[2] I began providing input and suggestions about the ways in which I might be of value to the policies and procedures of MOGA that had not been previously shown by any CNMs at MOGA. I used my skills and acquired knowledge to redesign the MOGA website to include a section on MOGA midwife services. The MOGA website contains information about the practice, introduction of all the providers with our biographies, and services we provide such as obstetrics and gynecology, midwifery, family planning, in-office, integrative and function medicine, and gynecology surgeries. Furthermore, I took the initiative to develop and create patient educational materials to be posted on our website.

One of the most important elements in creating my role was to bring new midwife patients into the practice. Initially, as expected, there were no midwife patients on the books for me. I was reminded to bring my own midwife patients into the practice and to be cognizant of "stealing" established MOGA physician patients into the midwifery group. A majority of my patients were referred by others through word of mouth. Undeniably, my professional skills were evident when I delivered physicians' patients. My hospital orientation was different from that of midwives in a midwife practice, where they are oriented by other midwives. I was trained by my MOGA physicians (just as a reminder, there are 7 of them). I have mixed emotions on this topic. I am truly and immensely grateful for each one of them, however, attempting to learn from 7 different providers, each having their own preferences in how they provided excellent patient care, was challenging to say the least. Initially, I kept asking myself, "Michelle, what did you get yourself into?" On the upside, I was able to take something from each one of them to make it my own and integrate it into my service.

I was on call every Monday with an on-call physician and worked as the physician's resident for approximately 6 months. I was diligent in showing up for my shifts regardless of whether there was a patient in labor or not. I was extremely dedicated and motivated in enhancing my skills. I was fearful of disappointing my physicians. My goal was to exceed their expectations of what a newly graduated CNM could be. During my 6-month orientation, many of the MOGA patients I had the privileged to deliver hired doulas. My meeting these doulas was among the more important reasons why midwife patients started coming to MOGA based on the referrals of other patients.

Doulas are certified by Doula Organization of North America International, the Childbirth and Postpartum Professional Association, the International Childbirth Education Association, or ProDoula organizations. The doula's role is to provide support to women at the time of labor by encouraging them to utilize techniques they had learned during their childbirth-preparation classes, but not limited to non-medical comfort techniques, hydrotherapy, positioning, and breathing in the labor and delivery. Doulas advocate for their patient's wishes in the birth plan. This does not mean that the doula speaks or answers questions instead of the patient. Doulas cannot diagnose medical conditions, interpret medical treatment, or clinical results. They are not able to make decisions for the birthing mother or give medical advice. Most important, doulas cannot have access to the patient record and cannot deliver the baby.

# SWOT Analysis for Maricopa Obstetrics and Gynecology Associates

MOGA has numerous strengths. They choose top-notch providers to offer excellent patient care. The working environment associated with the medical assistants (MAs) is amazing. Without these women, my workflow would be in chaos. Most importantly, MOGA's physicians recognized that the increase in midwife patients was not sustainable for 1 midwife and hired 3 additional CNMs. Increasing to 4 CNMs allowed MOGA's midwifery service to expand. My working relationship and support network with the physicians are impeccable. They truly consider my best interest. They perform postpartum rounds for me when I must be absent, and I can also depend on them as my backup if I am unable to make it in time for a delivery (which does not happen often, but knowing that they are present gives me a sense of assurance that CNM patients will receive great care). Every physician at MOGA mentors me in a unique way, thereby helping me to learn new things and apply them in my professional life. The other beneficial points associated with MOGA include the physicians' prompt support for management of non-reassuring fetal heart tracings, hemorrhages, third- and fourth-degree laceration repairs, and medical conditions or complications including diabetes, hypertension, preeclampsia, and other comorbidities.

From a patient's point of view, barriers to midwifery care at MOGA include their lack of knowledge of the benefits and availability of midwifery care. Many patients lack the knowledge of how midwifery care is similar to or differs from regular obstetric care. The care provided by midwives during a low-risk delivery has fewer interventions leading to higher-quality care. Even with this knowledge, there is a percentage of patients who may choose the physicians' group. Another barrier to midwifery acceptance is a lack of continuity of care spanning the 4 midwives for the patients. However, in retrospect, having 4 CNMs can also be a benefit. Knowing a provider is important to many patients. The trust that has been built between the patient and the provider allows for more productive visits and of course a better outcome.

An important weakness associated with working at MOGA includes contradictions of directions given from the different physicians working at MOGA. For example, the physicians have different preferences regarding how they would like to be informed of the CNM patients in labor, regarding their presence in the room, and the performance of cesarean delivery. Furthermore, in the case of charting, for example, I may get ordered to perform a procedure from one physician that may not work according to the standards of all providers, including the nurse practitioners. This lack of consistency can eventually cause a general lack of motivation and positive strength. Absence of adequate support in the office management is also an important weakness. Computer systems are not up-to-date in such a way that they would be able to clearly identify CNM patients.

# DNP Essentials: Outcomes of Evidence-Based Knowledge and Its Incorporation in Practice

The evidence-based practice project that is close and dear to my heart was completed for my DNP project at ASU, which is related to my role at MOGA. The title of the evidence-based practice project was "Implementing Skin-to-Skin Contact in the Operating Room Following a Cesarean Delivery," and I implemented this project at BUMCP, where I currently deliver patients for birth.

## *Background and Problem Statement*

Cesarean delivery is the most common major surgical procedure in the United States, representing 38.2% of live births in 2012.[8] Infants delivered by cesarean delivery may face a more difficult transition to extrauterine life due to retained fluid within the alveoli.[8] Skin-to-skin contact (SSC) and breastfeeding have been shown to help these newborns. However, BUMCP did not have a policy to support immediate SSC and breastfeeding after cesarean delivery. This was a barrier to obtaining Baby-Friendly hospital status,[9] despite being a Magnet hospital accredited by the American Nurses Credentialing Center for excellence in patient care with a Level III perinatal and neonatal unit. BUMCP is a busy urban academic medical center with 5847 infant deliveries in 2013.

## *Purpose*

An evidence-based practice pilot protocol was designed for the implementation of SSC in the operating room soon after cesarean delivery at BUMCP. This protocol was designed to gather clinical data. SSC followed by a cesarean delivery facilitates newborns in getting adapted to extrauterine life and helps infants and parents in developing close bonds and success in breastfeeding. SSC can also assist with decreasing the quantity of time spent by the infants in the neonatal intensive care unit (NICU), which leads to a reduction in working hours of nurses and eventually an overall reduction in financial burden related to both the patients, their families, and the hospital.

## Procedure

The evidence-based practice project was conducted with approval from the Institutional Review Board at ASU with reciprocal agreement from BUMCP. The 7-step Iowa Model of Evidence-Based Practice guided the evidence-based practice project:

- Step 1: Topic selection (discussed previously).
- Step 2: Evidence-based practice team was formed and met biweekly, with members including project lead (L&D nurse and DNP student), L&D nurse manager, surgical scrub technician, OB, nursing representative from the nursery team, and anesthesiologist.
- Step 3: Systematic evidence retrieval to support the "triggering" question.
- Step 4: Evidence-based practice team critically appraised the evidence to build obstetric section stakeholder buy-in.
- Step 5: Development of standards for the pilot SSC protocol.
- Step 6: Three-month implementation of the pilot SSC protocol for all mother-infant dyads admitted for scheduled or repeat cesarean delivery with a live, singleton fetus greater than 37 weeks' gestation, with no preexisting medical complications or fetal anomaly (n = 193). Nursery staff tracked neonatal outcomes including temperature, respirations, glucose, and disposition during the 2-hour transition after birth. These data were compared to historical data for mother-infant dyads meeting protocol inclusion criteria in the 3 months prior to protocol implementation (n = 302). A double-entry process was used to verify the data. Data were analyzed using chi-square test to compare rates of SSC application, infant disposition, and paired $t$-test to compare pre- and post-protocol neonatal outcomes including temperature, heart rate, respiratory rate, and blood glucose.
- Step 7: Evaluation of the overall SSC procedure, including process review, outcomes data, and staff feedback for protocol evaluation and modification.

## Outcomes

There were no baseline demographic differences between pre- and post-intervention groups. Neonatal outcomes were significantly different for infant temperature (SSC = lower), heart rate (SSC = lower), respiratory rate (SSC = lower), and blood glucose (SSC = higher) between pre- and post-intervention groups. Notably, SSC resulted in statistically and clinically significant reduction in hypoglycemia ($P = .002$). Additional outcomes included an increase in exclusive breastfeeding by 38.3% ($P = .000$) in the intervention group, and an 84% decrease in NICU admissions ($P = .000$) in the intervention group.

SSC in the operating room is a valuable, safe, and feasible intervention following a cesarean delivery, with no additional expense to the facility and potential for significant cost savings due to deceased NICU admissions. This evidence-based practice outcome supports the American Academy of Pediatrics' (AAP) recommendation for SSC in the first hour after birth[10] and promotes exclusive breastfeeding, which is one of the Joint Commission's mandated initiatives.[11]

## Implication for Practice

NICU admissions in the case of normal term infants with hypothermia and hypoglycemia cost, on average, $76 164 per infant.[12] The evidence-based practice SSC strategy helped reduce admissions to the NICU by approximately 84% in the case of normal term births that occurred through cesarean delivery. This reduction in admissions represented a cost saving of approximately $2 million to the hospital in just 3 months.

The findings of this evidence-based practice project became the reason for BUMCP to include the intervention of SSC, not only in its training of newly hired health care providers, but also in the required training for annual competency of skills for experienced employees. This additional training was a useful strategy, as it required scarcely any resources and no additional staffing or costs. The SSC intervention has also been added to the present charting system of BUMCP.

This evidence-based practice project has been disseminated in different forms on different occasions, as follows:

- Poster at the Arizona Nurses Association conference, October 2014
- Presented in the *Chief Nursing Officer's* weekly journal, October 2014
- Selected as one of the parts of BUMCP's Magnet documentation
- BUMCP's Poster Walk Showcase, November 2014
- Selected as the "Best Practice" innovation for BUMCP
- Podium presentation at Banner Shared Governance conference, April 2015
- Podium and poster presentation at the Advanced Practice Neonatal Forum held in Washington, DC, May 2015
- Evaluated by the Magnet recertification evaluators for BUMCP, July 2015

- Invited as a podium presenter at the National Phoenix Perinatal Associates Challenges in Obstetric Care conference, April 2016

# BUSINESS PLAN: FACILITATING THE DEVELOPMENT OF NEW REVENUE STREAMS FOR MARICOPA OBSTETRICS AND GYNECOLOGY ASSOCIATES

In order to facilitate new revenue for MOGA, I began offering diabetic and self-administration of insulin instruction to our pregnant patients. These patients were usually referred to a maternal fetal medicine office to receive instruction on managing their diabetic nutrition and treatment. In this regard, I created the proper handouts for education and teaching. Furthermore, I provided support for lactation and its management to our patients rather than sending patients elsewhere for lactation-management support.

I also improved the operational aspects in the office and marketing strategies for MOGA. During my third month of working at MOGA, I attempted to improve the clinical forms. In this regard, I redesigned the intake forms that were commonly used in the office. The design was developed to improve the workflow for both health care providers and the MAs. Additionally, I am designing educational brochures for patients, including management for labor and information on newborn medications.

While seeing the physicians' patients, I became aware that many patients did not know that MOGA had a midwifery service. In order to market the midwifery services provided by MOGA, I designed a midwife banner for MOGA that was placed in both the offices. I scheduled events to take place at MOGA primarily for the free marketing. Events that MOGA hosted and paid for included prenatal yoga and lactation-education classes. These were free events for all MOGA patients.

In the realm of marketing myself, managing the MOGA Midwife Facebook page and continuing to work side-by-side with doulas has brought numerous midwife patients to the practice. Nonetheless, word of mouth has helped in moving forward and fulfilling the objectives of the health care practice. Eventually, the midwifery service at MOGA became too busy for 1 midwife. The MOGA physicians saw that the number of patients I was seeing and delivering was not sustainable. I was averaging at least 18 to 20 deliveries per month from August 2018 to October 2019. The MOGA financials are not shared with me, so I can only assume I was growing the midwifery practice because we hired 3 more midwives to work in collaboration with me.

MOGA lacked any supporting structure for midwifery care. Developing an appropriate support structure for midwifery care became a primary goal for me in the first year at MOGA. I had very limited resources or metrics to work with. The practice lacked the ability to track patients who came for the midwifery service. Therefore, I started tracking the midwife patients on my own, and started conducting my own research and analysis.

From February to December in 2018, I attended a total of 150 deliveries. Of the 150 deliveries, 93% (constituting 139 deliveries) were related to spontaneous vaginal delivery (SVD), 3% (constituting 5 deliveries) were related to primary cesarean delivery, 3% (constituting 5 deliveries) were related to vaginal birth after cesarean delivery (VBAC), and 1% (constituting 3 deliveries) were related to forceps-assisted vaginal delivery (FAVD). Approximately 71% were CNM patients (constituting 107 patients). From this cohort, the percentage of physician patients that eventually moved toward CNM care was 23% (constituting 34 patients), the percentage of newly admitted patients who requested for CNM care was 22% (constituting 33 patients), and the percentage of transfer of patients and their care from other clinics and departments to the department for CNM care was 19% (constituting 29 patients).

The percentage of deliveries I attended during the time when I was on call as a resident was about 29% (constituting 44 deliveries). The percentage of patients who showed their desire to continue their health care services with a CNM and showed interest in having a different experience of labor as compared to the conventional model of medical care was nearly 19% (constituting 28 patients). Furthermore, referrals and word of mouth calculated to about 3% (constituting 6 patients) of cases.

The benefit to having 8 physicians and 4 CNMs in a group is that there will always be physician backup for the CNMs. For patients with comorbidities that need to be co-managed, a physician in the same practice who knows both the patient and the CNM will provide a better outcome in the patient's care. To some patients, knowing who their providers are is extremely important. When a deviation from the normal occurs, a referral, consultation, and or collaboration may be warranted, and a mutual agreement may be arranged between the OB/GYN physician and the CNM to collaboratively manage the care of a woman who has developed medical or obstetric complications. A patient who has developed a medical diagnosis beyond obstetric complications may warrant a referral for the management of a particular aspect of the patient's care or for assumption of total management of the patient's care. The scope of collaboration may encompass the physical care of the patient, including delivery by the CNM according to a mutually agreed-upon plan of care. When the physician must assume a dominant role in the care of the patient due to an increased risk status, the CNM may continue to participate in physical care, counseling, guidance, teaching, and support. Effective communication between the CNM and the physician is essential for ongoing collaborative management. Patients with a history of (or who are currently experiencing) certain medical, surgical, or obstetrical conditions or complications may require consultation and/or collaboration.

# BUSINESS PLAN: CERTIFIED NURSE-MIDWIFE INCOME

The income that a CNM receives is strongly correlated with the amount paid by the patients for a CNM visit. Nevertheless, the cost related to the employment of a CNM in a company includes several elements besides salary, such as malpractice insurance, health insurance, federal insurance contributions in line with the Federal Insurance Contributions Act, the 401(k) pension plan, continuing education, licenses, connections with professional organizations, and overhead charges. However, the probable income earned by a CNM is based on office working hours (eg, 36 working hours per week; two, 24-hour call shifts in a week; and a minimum of 10 deliveries in a month).[13] Furthermore, the salary structure is based on the experience and the degree qualification of the CNM. Apart from salary, there are also periodic bonuses and incentive programs that are based on quality, productivity, patient satisfaction, and profit.[14]

Some of the most important services linked to generating the highest revenue in a private practice are those related to new patients of gynecology, newly admitted obstetric patients, and technical procedures, such as the use of the intrauterine device (IUD), Nexplanon insertions (Merck & Co), ultrasounds, and endometrial biopsies.[14]

# INTERPROFESSIONAL COLLABORATION AT MARICOPA OBSTETRICS AND GYNECOLOGY ASSOCIATES

Interprofessional collaboration takes many forms, such as externally facilitated interprofessional activities, rounds, meetings, and checklists.[13] Interprofessional collaboration means that several members of the health care profession may take part, including physicians, MAs, office managers, schedulers, lab personnel, and front and back office leads. Interprofessional collaboration in our setup involved health care team members from almost all of these categories. For instance, we developed job descriptions for all the members and associated certain responsibilities with them. Interprofessional meetings were also regularly held, in which the participants were asked to give suggestions for the improvement of the health care offered. This interprofessional collaboration might be described as externally facilitated interprofessional activities. Interprofessional rounds also took place, in which all the members of the health care team spent 5 to 10 minutes discussing every patient, and identified and addressed the problems that could be experienced by the patients. Interprofessional checklists were also considered, in which the team members were asked to review the history of a patient before performing a cesarean delivery. During all these types of interprofessional collaboration, physicians were of considerable help, and, after the appointment of more CNMs, they also showed significant interest and involvement in the health of the patients.

One of the most important factors in successful interprofessional collaboration is communication, both among health care professionals, for the discussion of problems, and in exchanges with patients and their families in a manner that is understandable.[15] In our health care setting, we developed an environment that was conducive to better communication, and it was also due to effective communication that word of mouth became one of our key means of marketing.

# PROFESSIONALISM

After obtaining my DNP, I attempted to promote the nursing profession in different ways, such as speaking at several conferences and enhancing my network to increase the level of engagement of people in my DNP project, as well as winning the national American Association of Colleges of Nursing (AACN) award for Outstanding DNP Project. Furthermore, participation in the American College of Nurse-Midwives (ACNM) local chapter conferences (along with their planning and operation meetings) and their national events also helped both to promote the nursing profession and allow me to present my point of view regarding nursing and midwifery practice.

During the year that I was a solo midwife, I taught myself how to be a midwife in a physicians' world. I connected with the local ACNM Phoenix chapter and stayed in close contact with my CNM preceptors. The CNMs who attended the meeting were all amazing. They assisted me when I had questions and guided me through my anxiety. I was extremely active with the ACNM Phoenix chapter to gain knowledge and awareness and, most importantly, to connect with fellow CNMs.

Presently, I am working as an assistant clinical professor, which requires that I teach OB residents. I have been invited to give lectures and present information regarding midwifery practices to the OB residents and medical students. I have also been invited to give mini-lectures for new L&D nurses. Apart from my regular work, I take part in various committees of the hospital, such as the Women's Health Clinical Consensus Group (CCG) Committee, the Advanced Practice Credentialing Committee, and the OB Committee.

I am committed to using my DNP in numerous ways to help bring positive changes in the hospital. My membership on committees, such as the OB Committee and the CCG Committee, has allowed me to introduce a change of policy that provides for doulas to attend deliveries for their clients if a cesarean delivery is warranted. This means that doulas are now able to be a second support for our patients in the operating room, as well as in the OB triage settings in which they previously did not have access to their clients, and BUMCP policy had specified only 1 support person for the patient was allowed. I wrote the Doula Agreement for BUMCP, the official agreement that allows the doulas to attend cesarean deliveries as explained in the previous comments. Additionally, I have been working on a policy to allow CNMs to acquire admission and discharge privileges for the hospital with which we are affiliated. In this regard, I have helped rewrite the delineation of privileges and the hospital bylaws for CNMs. Furthermore, in order to fulfill the different aspects of my upcoming projects, I have collaborated with a BUMCP physician. These projects will benefit midwife patients. It is also relevant to mention that I am a co-chair of the planning committee of the ACNM Phoenix chapter winter summit.

I am extremely passionate about integrating midwives, doulas, and low-risk labor techniques to enhance the laboring woman's birth experience. In a tertiary L&D unit that specializes in high-risk obstetrics care, staff will expect that laboring patients may eventually develop a high-risk condition that requires intensive and invasive care during their admission. It is equally important for a labor nurse to have knowledge of how to care for low-risk patients desiring a non-pharmacological birth. High-risk patients can benefit from a few alternative comfort measures to assist them with the discomforts of labor. Knowledge of the use of low-technical labor interventions is just as important a skill as caring for an OB with comorbidities.

When BUMCP realized there was a desire from patients in the community to have a midwife and/or doula to assist in the delivery of their infant, I assisted in creating a workshop and invited community doulas. Nurses/OB providers and doulas do not always have positive views of one another. Conflicts can occur because of overlapping roles in providing continuous labor support. An integrated culture that fosters collegial, interprofessional collaboration can benefit patients and families. The workshop day had breakout sessions, tours, and discussions of guidelines for working together for the best outcome for mother and baby.

## Pearls/Takeaways

My fellow DNP students, while moving on a path that will eventually change your life, it is imperative to know the different aspects of the journey and the destination of that journey. First, it is important to look at the midwifery service. In my case, while working at MOGA, I realized that the physicians there were used to training only other physicians and had very little experience in training a newly graduated CNM. Furthermore, the absence of an adequate structure created a non-supportive environment for a midwifery service. For these reasons, it took approximately 1 year to

develop an appropriate structure that aligned with midwifery care and practices.

Though there was no structure or metrics in place to address the challenges of developing a midwifery service at MOGA, I utilized my years of registered nurse experience from BUMCP and my DNP training to successfully develop the practice. For example, there was no tracking system for midwife patients, so I developed my own tracking tool as a means of assessing my own outcomes. I am extremely resourceful and there are a plethora of resources around me that I have no hesitation in using. I have reached out to other CNMs that I have networked with in the past, and they helped by sharing their model of care for their clinic. I presented the information I gathered to my physicians to assist us in developing a midwifery service that aligned with MOGA's model of care. I found it important to develop this structure before attempting to utilize the DNP Essentials.

There are many challenges involved in bringing on midwives, whether they are newly graduated or have several years of experience, and first and foremost is cost. How will MOGA pay for our salary? The answer is easy: seeing patients in the office, of course. The answer may be easy, but the logistics are not. It gets complicated when the new midwives in the practice are not credentialed with insurance companies, which means they are limited to the type of patients they are able to see. This also includes deliveries at the hospital, as a MOGA-credentialed person must be present so that they can bill for the services.

I have found the addition of new resources may not always increase the efficiency of the practice, as new resources can require existing staff to teach the new team members, thereby slowing down day-to-day processes. In this regard, newly graduated individuals need constant guidance and mentoring, orientation, clinical training, and training in the use of the office electronic medical record (EMR) system. Moreover, experienced midwives who have newly started in the practice may need help with the EMR system, along with an orientation to midwifery practice in the new setting, where policies and procedures may differ from those that were applied in their previous setting. For a novice CNM, the challenges may seem large, but with dedication and persistence, these challenges can be overcome.

## Conclusion: Impact of the DNP Degree

As a result of obtaining my DNP degree, I was able to implement the evidence-based hallmarks of midwifery into practice in order to focus on the provision of quality patient care. I also increased my interprofessional collaboration with other staff members in order to make use of all the information obtained from their experience for the betterment of the health care services. Furthermore, I brought in new patients to the practice related to the profession of midwifery to enhance the profile of this field.

The ideal midwifery model focuses on empowering women to understand their bodies during the birth process. Systematic reviews and case studies have shown that the care provided by CNMs is safe and effective when compared to that provided by physicians, with lower cesarean delivery birth rates and adverse perinatal outcomes.[7,16-18] Interprofessional collaboration between OBs, CNMs, and nursing staff is the key to providing high-quality maternal, improved neonatal care, and helping women achieve their goal of having a non-invasive birth experience with increased satisfaction.[19]

The American College of Obstetricians and Gynecology[19] supports using evidence-based practice techniques that are associated with minimal interventions for low-risk patients in spontaneous labor. Common obstetric practices such as continuous fetal monitoring and routine amniotomy may not be necessary for all patients in labor.

My DNP training allowed me to bring scientific underpinnings and new knowledge that created a different perspective on how to care for pregnant patients among my MOGA physicians and L&D registered nurses. I implemented an evidence-based practice project that is currently being used throughout the United States. SSC was implemented in the operating room following a cesarean delivery. SSC resulted in statistically and clinically significant reduction in hypoglycemia ($P = .002$), an increase in exclusive breastfeeding by 38.3% ($P = .000$), and an 84% decrease in NICU admissions ($P = .000$). Cost savings because of the reduction in NICU admissions was estimated to be $2 million in just one quarter.

In the future, I would like to evaluate the effects of low-risk modalities and midwifery outcomes in the low-risk patient population. Ongoing education related to non-pharmacological labor interventions provided to the OB residents and nursing staff is required.

MOGA is a well-known, respected, and reputable practice. Working for MOGA has been a beneficial growth experience in my professional career. My DNP education allowed me to be able to evaluate and implement evidence-based practice to improve patient outcomes, develop standards and protocols for the practice through interprofessional collaboration, redesign the practice website, develop tools and questionnaires related to the Patient Satisfaction Survey, and create a data sheet for midwifery patients to aid in the quality improvement process.

# Acknowledgments

Most importantly, I am very thankful to God for blessing me and helping me at every step of the way, not only in my personal life, but also in my professional life. I am also very grateful to Kyle Davis, my husband, without whose constant support I would not be able to meet the challenges of the different phases of life. He has been at my side, unconditionally loving me and making sure I excel in everything I attempt to accomplish.

I am highly obliged to the staff at MOGA, especially Dr. Celeste Pottorff, Dr. Laura Mercer, and Dr. Michael Urig, whose guidance and support, both in the clinical setting and emotionally, have helped me progress. I thank you for believing in me as a new graduate CNM.

I wish to also thank Dr. Heather Ross, my ASU DNP mentor, who exemplifies the definition of a true mentor. The success of my evidence-based practice project is primarily due to her support and continuous assistance. I am thankful for her deep dedication to making sure I would be successful. She eliminated all the barriers I encountered during my DNP journey and I would not have been able to overcome them alone. She was also a huge help in decreasing my stress and enhancing my experience at ASU by making it less overwhelming.

I am also grateful to Chris Tussey, MSN, CNS; Krysia Gaisor, BSN, RNC-OB; Brittany Saenz, BSN, RNC-OB; Jalyn Rheinhardt, BSN, RNC-OB; and many more wonderful people at BUMCP. This group of people are my family away from home. Without them, my first year as a CNM would have been a disaster. They are continually making sure I am well and supported.

# References

1. Definition of midwifery and scope of practice of certified nurse midwives and certified midwives. American College of Nurse-Midwives. http://www.midwife.org/acnm/files/ccLibraryFiles/Filename/000000007043/Definition-of-Midwifery-and-Scope-of-Practice-of-CNMs-and-CMs-Feb-2012.pdf

2. AACN position statement on the practice doctorate in nursing. American Association of Colleges of Nursing. https://www.aacnnursing.org/DNP/Position-Statement

3. Joel LA. *Advance Practice Nursing: Essentials for Role Development.* 2nd ed. FA Davis Company; 2017.

4. Article 5: Arizona administrative code. Arizona State Board of Nursing. Accessed July 1, 2017. https://www.azbn.gov/sites/default/files/2018-12/ruleseffectivemay232018.pdf

5. Nurse Practitioners in Women's Health. *The Women's Healthcare Nurse Practitioner: Guidelines for Practice and Education.* 5th ed. 2002.

6. Buppert C. *Nurse Practitioner's Business Practice and Legal Guide.* 3rd ed. Jones and Bartlett Publishers; 2008.

7. Hutton EK, Reitsma AH, Kaufman K. Outcomes associated with planned home and planned hospital births in low-risk women attended by midwives in Ontario, Canada, 2003-2006: a retrospective cohort study. *Birth.* 2009;36(3):180-189. doi:10.1111/j.1523-536x.2009.00322.x

8. Boyle A, Reddy U, Landy H, Huang C, Diggers R, Laughon K. Primary cesarean delivery in the United States. *Obstet Gynecol.* 2013;122(1):1-8.

9. The guidelines and evaluation criteria. Baby-Friendly. http://www.babyfriendlyusa.org/get-started/the-guidelines-evaluation-criteria

10. American Academy of Pediatrics. Breastfeeding and the use of human milk. *Pediatrics.* 2005;100(6):1035-1039.

11. Implementing the joint commission perinatal care core measure on exclusive breast milk feeding. United States Breastfeeding Committee. http://www.usbreastfeeding.org/tjc-measure-ebmf

12. Special care nursery admissions. March of Dimes. https://www.marchofdimes.org/peristats/pdfdocs/nicu_summary_final.pdf

13.  Reeves S, Pelone F, Harrison R, Goldman J, Zwarenstein M. Interprofessional collaboration to improve professional practice and healthcare outcomes. *Cochrane Database Syst Rev.* 2017;6(6):CD000072. doi:10.1002/14651858.cd000072.pub3

14.  Pottorff C. Personal interview. July 4, 2017.

15.  Busari JO, Moll FM, Duits AJ. Understanding the impact of interprofessional collaboration on the quality of care: a case report from a small-scale resource limited health care environment. *J Multidiscip Healthc.* 2017;10:227-234. doi:10.2147/jmdh.s140042

16.  Johantgen M, Fountain L, Zangaro G, Newhouse R, Stanik-Hutt J, White K. Comparison of labor and delivery care provided by certified nurse-midwives and physicians: a systematic review, 1990 to 2008. *Womens Health Issues.* 2012;22(1):e73-81. doi:10.1016/j.whi.2011.06.005

17.  Tracy SK, Hartz DL, Tracy MB, et al. Caseload midwifery care versus standard maternity care for women of any risk: M@NGO, a randomised controlled trial. *Lancet.* 2013;382(9906):1723-1732.

18.  McLachlan HL, Forster DA, Davey MA, et al. Effects of continuity of care by a primary midwife (caseload midwifery) on caesarean section rates in women of low obstetric risk: the COSMOS randomised controlled trial. *BJOG.* 2012;119(12):1483-1492. doi:10.1111/j.1471-0528.2012.03446.x

19.  ACOG Committee Opinion No. 766: Approaches to Limit Intervention During Labor and Birth. *Obstet Gynecol.* 2019;133(2):e164-e173.

# CHAPTER 13

# FROM MID-LEVEL MIDWIFERY TO HIGH-LEVEL HUSBANDRY

## A RURAL CERTIFIED NURSE-MIDWIFE'S DOCTORAL JOURNEY

*Dixie Shaheen Rasmussen, DNP, MSN-Ed, CNM*

## INTRODUCTION

I was stereotyped a "mid-level" practitioner after graduating as a master's-prepared certified nurse-midwife (CNM). I cowered, practicing under the auspices of inferiority within a rural hospital's all-male physician staff. I was the first mid-level practitioner, midwife, and woman to practice at this facility. At the age of 56, after practicing for 18 years as a CNM, I returned to the University of Utah to obtain a Doctor of Nursing Practice (DNP) and a master's in nursing education (MSN-Ed) degree. I wanted and needed to have a seat at the table as a doctoral-prepared nurse. This extraordinary journey propelled my mid-level standing into a new role of high-level husbandry (Figure 13-1).

Husbandry[1] is defined as manager of domestic affairs, head of household, conserver of resources, and one who uses the application of science, skill, or art when cultivating agriculture. Through DNP preparation, I have privileges in 2 rural-area hospitals, practicing in a main office and 2 outreach offices while managing an extended staff. This pioneer nurse-midwife is now a manager, practicing a husbandry of sorts.

On my first day in the doctoral program, I took notes with pen and paper, obviously old-fashioned compared to the young whippersnappers who were simultaneously taking notes, shopping, and looking at Facebook on their laptops. Three years later, this senior practitioner was recognized by the American Association of Colleges of Nursing for the university's and nation's top DNP capstone project. My intention with the preceding sentence is not to be boastful but rather to highlight the impact the doctoral experience can have on an individual. This chapter can provide insight and inspiration to those who are embarking on the doctoral path.

### Personal Introduction

I was born and raised in rural central Utah. I graduated from high school with 31 other students. I married my high school sweetheart. We left home to gain an education at Brigham Young University. This rich foundation prepared me to return home and become a rural nurse. A rural nurse requires a jack-of-all-trades foundation, as they work in emergency room, medical/surgical, obstetrical, pediatric, and even surgical nursing realms.

Benson LA, ed. *The DNP Professional: Translating Value From Classroom to Practice* (pp 143-153).

# DESCRIPTION OF PRACTICE SETTING: FAMILY PRACTICE

Precepting during midwifery school placed me back in my rural area. In that area, at that time, family practice physicians provided all obstetrical services. During my precepting experience, I was approached by 2 family practice physicians to pioneer midwifery and women's health services. I was offered a space in their clinic to create a women's health clinic. The success of this venture was seeded by women who already knew me. I had been a labor and delivery nurse for 17 years and a prenatal teacher for 15 years. The hospital that "raised" me was again my home as an advanced practice clinician.

I continue to practice in rural central Utah. I offer obstetrical, gynecological, women's, and infants' primary care health services. Patients who have entered my care live in an approximately 460-square mile area. Many patients travel to the outreach clinics or to our main office. My practice partner and I deliver at 2 rural hospitals approximately 32 miles apart. About 60% of the population I serve is on Medicaid and about 40% have private insurance or access health care on a self-pay basis. The main occupations in this geographical area are in agriculture and coal mining. The largest city in this service area has a population of about 8000 people. Most communities in the area range from 1000 to 6000 people. Both hospitals have about 30 beds. We have provided or currently provide care for patients in more than 40 communities in this service area. In the home clinic, I currently practice with a family practice physician, family nurse practitioner, physician assistant, and newly graduated CNM/women's health practitioner. We also collaborate with 3 other physicians in the other rural hospital.

# ROLE EXPANSION

My transformation from midwife to husbandry-type manager evolved as the original women's health clinic prospered. My education and career took me away from family and family-related functions. My husband picked up all the loose ends in home, family, and society. He has been my main example, teaching me to how to exercise the ideals of husbandry and fulfill the obligations of my practice.

Similar to when a husband has more children, his work and responsibilities grow. So, as my practice grew, it required a higher level of leadership and management. In the book *The Doctor of Nursing Practice*,[2] Lisa Astalos Chism explains that a leader becomes a manager as they recognize that change is needed. She explained that transformation takes place as leaders/managers can have inspiration and create for their constituents the vision necessary to enact and sustain the change.

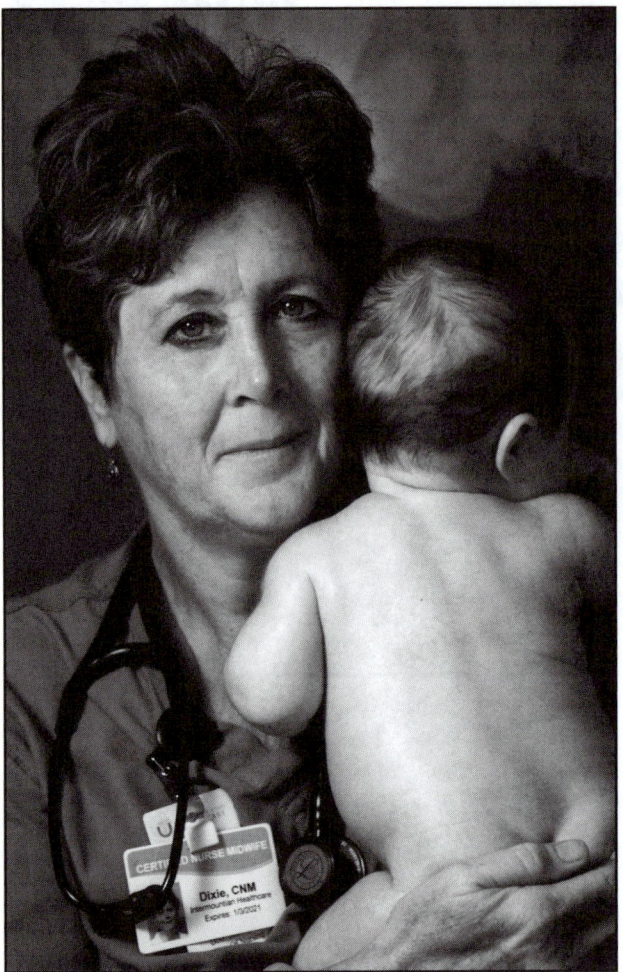

**Figure 13-1.** Nurses uphold the future.

During the first years of my career as floor nurse, I learned to navigate patient care and establish clinical experience. I earned a baccalaureate degree in nursing through an outreach program at Westminster College in Salt Lake City, Utah. I was recruited to teach in the local technical college's practical nursing program. This allowed me to have weekends, nights, and holidays off as my husband and I were trying to raise 5 children. This amazing 9-year excursion enhanced my intellectual nursing knowledge and skills. Teaching unleashed a passion for continual learning; however, I missed direct patient care and could feel my hands ache for my true passion of obstetrics. Again, travel and an innovative nurse-midwifery outreach program at the University of Utah allowed those humane hands to gain the proficiencies needed to catch infants and care for their mothers. I am blessed to have been a nurse for 37 years.

# SWOT Analysis

A SWOT[3] (Strengths, Weaknesses, Opportunities, Threats) analysis about yourself and your work/culture environment reveals how you might transition toward becoming a leader/manager. The Biblical story of King David[4] may give insight to an advanced practice clinician striving to develop the ability to expand their role and explore the importance of a SWOT analysis. Michelangelo's beautiful sculpture of David depicts, not a scrawny shepherd boy, but a beautiful, muscled, masterpiece of a man's physique. Again, those years of physical work "in the trenches" mentally and physically prepared a man who became a great king. Those years, most of them alone, shaped David as he gained strength and prepared himself to meet threats. Yet, his weaknesses did negatively affect his leadership and management. I think as managers/husbandry-type leaders, we are never above ethical reproach.

# DNP Essential: Scientific Underpinnings for Practice

In a rural hospital, the middle of the night is a fearful time. There are a limited number of staff in-house, and birth does not always present itself at convenient, well-staffed times. Birth emergencies are also not respecters of optimal circumstances. Surgical crews are at home with a 20-minute response time. An American Congress of Obstetricians and Gynecologists (ACOG)[5] evidence-based standard states that "decision to incision time" (DIT) for an emergency cesarean section (ECS) should be less than 30 minutes. Birth asphyxia,[6] with the terrible malady of cerebral palsy, results in the biggest payouts in obstetrical malpractice. There is a physician in-house for the emergency room; however, many physicians do not practice obstetrics and could not initiate an ECS. The inability to have all key players immediately present for an ECS is like watching an apneic patient in anaphylactic shock deteriorate in front of a locked crash cart stocked with epinephrine. The realizations of helplessness spawned my capstone project, which the American Association of Colleges of Nursing ultimately recognized as the top DNP project in 2018. The quality improvement (QI) project was entitled "Pit Crew for Emergency Cesarean Section."[7] The project's purpose was to develop a rapid response team to enact a multidisciplinary process within the hospital prior to the arrival of the surgical services team. The DNP project was titled "Can a Rural Hospital Reliably Preform an Emergency Cesarean Section in 30 Minutes or Less?"[7]

Using scientific underpinnings and scholarly research, this QI project, using the plan-do-study-implement (PDSI)[8] cycles, reduced the DIT cycle by 7 minutes overall.

Disappointingly, however, DITs remained prolonged during evening and weekend shifts.

This project has now triggered system change, as labor and delivery nurses are being considered for training in surgical responsibilities along with the Code OB rapid response team process. Training labor and delivery nurses to scrub and circulate during all cesarean sections seems like such an easy fix; however, the larger system is in strong opposition. Their position is that our cesarean section numbers do not support the need for labor and delivery nurses to safely exercise these skills, thereby keeping the operating room and its staff as the responsible service. My challenge to the larger system has been to develop a competency training with simulation, preparing the rural nurse that experiences a low volume of emergencies to be trained in a high-risk skill set. This will remain an issue as 18 million women of reproductive age live in rural America, and more than half a million babies are born in rural hospitals every year.[9]

# DNP Essential: Organizational and Systems Leadership for Quality Improvement and Systems Thinking

The clinic I work for is independent of the larger hospital system to which all the other obstetrical physicians belong. The hospital's location is rural; however, it belongs to a robust organization. Leadership with the quality improvement project was painstaking. The rural hospital realized that DIT was the standard of care but felt that we were all doing the best we could. I could see ways to improve the situation, yet I lacked any political power to do so. A SWOT analysis of myself and the system was an essential component to the process. I questioned whether the system could and/or would initiate change and whether I had the leadership skills to maneuver within it. In doing so, I identified that rural staff were overburdened with responsibilities that were weighing down all individuals and programs. A new electronic medical record (EMR) system also overwhelmed the hospital and the larger corporate system. I had to stop the project and slowly resurrect it 8 months later because of the staff's reluctance to change or expand any system or any individual's workload. Kurt Lewin's[10] theories guided my leadership to become an effective force in this system change. Another game changer was using the University of Utah's support and my dynamic project leader's name (Barbara Wilson, PhD, RNC-BC). Her association added validity to this rural caretaker's plight. Dr. Wilson's research reputation and previous important leadership positions prompted action and respect. I attribute the opening of doors at the system level and during the Institutional Review Board's review process to her. Whenever

I encountered a roadblock, Barbara gave me evidence-based information to jump the hurdle or guide me in the push and pull (give and take) at the barricade. Referring to my example of King David, Barbara (figuratively) placed the sling and stone in my hand and coached me to keep swinging until I was confident and trained to aim.

The change was slow, yet "near misses" with ECSs prompted the staff to want to improve and change the process. Being a key member when an ECS was needed, without having immediate system support or needed operating room skills, created fear, and staff members started to jump on board. After one case with a near miss, the nurse involved was invited to provide information for a root-cause analysis. One labor and delivery nurse changed the local system's direction when she tearfully and emotionally explained that she never wanted to be in the fearful situation again of not knowing how or being trained on how to circulate or scrub. She was upset that the local and larger system had not prepared her for an ECS, where many labor and delivery emergencies might lead. The night and weekend staff members were mostly on board with the ECS QI project, while the daytime staff were apathetic because ECSs during their shifts were usually supported with operating room staff and nurse leadership in-house. The DNP program and the Essentials classes lent foundation that prompted me to push forward rather than abandon the project. I often related to the leadership video about "herding cats,"[11] and like the cat cowboys, continued to push forward because of my devotion to the "cats" or frontline staff. I found that reevaluating my individual SWOT analysis was improving my leadership skills. I focused on the weaknesses and had to calm my exuberance, seize opportunities, and eliminate threats.

## DNP Essential: Clinical Scholarship and Analytical Methods for Evidence-Based Practice

Dissemination of my capstone project included local, state, regional, and national presentations. After finishing your project and degree, there is such a relief that it is done, that you may become complacent about continuing to share your project. I implore you to take your "dog and pony show" out to help others and utilize the project's findings while still valid.

For me, the most intimidating audience was the local medical and nursing staff. They had ownership in the project, and it was difficult to present scholarly outcomes demonstrating that the standard of care was not consistently being met. This left the groups frustrated, yet did lend impetus to continue the project and ponder the findings. Analytical methods of the DITs were never studied prior to the capstone project. I had studied ECS DITs 2.5 years before, and 2.5

years after implementation of the QI project. After dissemination of the project, I was given permission to continue following DIT analytical findings. I have also noticed that DIT times are mentioned and noted by staff after every ECS. The ongoing DIT times are still prolonged in the evenings and weekends when the operating room staff are not in-house. I hope this information will jolt the labor and delivery nurses' training to circulate and scrub for all cesarean sections. This is the key to enabling the in-house staff to effectively and speedily respond to an ECS.

I also precept nurse-midwives, family nurse practitioners, physician assistants, and medical students. It slows your clinic day and tends to increase the mental and physical demands of your practice; however, I feel it is my duty and honor to pass along the efforts of the fine and selfless preceptors who provided my foundation and powered my passion. At times, student nursing can be difficult for patients. When I precepted a student who was difficult, I would allow time for the patients to regain our personal relationships prior to having another student begin. By allowing time to pass, the newer student is also afforded the opportunity for a stellar experience.

## DNP Essential: Information Systems/ Technology and Patient Care Technology for the Improvement and Transformation of Health Care

From black pen and paper to "click, click, click." Over the past 37 years, I have been honored to see the information technology revolution. There were absolutely no computers in my rural hospital in January 1982 when I started as a registered nurse. We did have electric typewriters to print patients' names on charts! Just like libraries without books, hospitals are now without medical record chart rooms. That was initially intimidating for this experienced nurse; however, computer systems have enabled significant improvements for the health care worker. In the following section, I discuss the top 4 technology systems that have improved patient outcomes.

First, neonatal telemedicine is currently the most important patient care technology for rural newborns.[12] Dr. Stephen Minton, a neonatologist at Utah Valley Hospital, pioneered this process for rural hospitals. When a newborn is experiencing serious problems after birth, within minutes, a neonatologist from a tertiary center can view a 180-degree live image of the infant and hear auditory sounds from the newborn. This can provide immediate guidance to the rural staff and may be paramount to newborn stabilization. Proctored emergency care of the infant has sparked excellence in our Level 1 nursery. Stabilization prior to transport has become orderly and has improved neonatal outcomes.

Second, the ability to have wireless fetal monitoring has freed the prisoners! For more than 35 years, we have leashed women to the bed for the sake of monitoring.[13] As a nurse-midwife, it has been difficult to monitor for safety while allowing women to walk and to use different positions and hydrotherapy. Just during the past 5 years has this luxury been available in my rural labor and delivery unit. It has revolutionized how I support patients in labor. My patients are happier when they can get out of bed. Less labor dystocia or difficult births affected by immobility have ensued since a wireless telemetry system has allowed movement.[14] These systems are welcome partners on the labor and delivery units. Many of these systems still have flaws; however, I have faith that competition in the integrated technology world will continue to bring about improvements.

Third on the list is the smart phone. I reach for it several times a day, right in front of patients, to immediately connect to the information I need. I have a full page of apps at my fingertips that direct my clinical decisions and increase my knowledge. I can view active fetal heart strips from 2 different hospitals, and consulting physicians can readily access them and give recommendations from wherever they are.

Fourth, telelactation[15] was brought to our rural hospital because of the capstone project of the DNP student who is now my practice partner. Telelactation has since supported hundreds of patients with breastfeeding advice and taught them hands-on skills. The service has also expanded to other rural hospitals. The large television screens in each room have given patients privacy to bare their breasts and have the lactation specialist give advice and support. The lactation specialist can use the camera to focus right on the infant's latch and can then guide our staff to help at the bedside.

# DNP ESSENTIAL: HEALTH CARE POLICY FOR ADVOCACY IN HEALTH CARE

Husbandry responsibilities include becoming an advocate for those you are responsible for and for your neighbors. I recently witnessed my son taking out the garbage for his neighbors. They had a family member with a medical emergency and had gone out of state. My son also parked his truck in their driveway to make it look as if someone was home. I know this was a simple act, yet it exemplifies our responsibility within and beyond our practices. It takes energy, forethought, and time.

There does not seem to be enough time to take care of my patients and practice and be active in local, state, and national organizations. I tend to depend on others to represent me. Attending state meetings would entail about 6 hours of travel. Telecommunication for these meetings has not been offered. I realize that through email messages and phone conversations, I could do more; however, just like David out in the fields, I am exerting all my energy in taking care of the local flocks.

I believe it is important to attend your organization's national meetings yearly (or at least every other year). I go to political action committee meetings, pay membership dues, and donate to the cause. This helps me stay informed and try to help those fighting for my rights. I also pay dues to many local, state, and national organizations and trust they are representing me. I would like to do more in the state rural health organization.

# DNP ESSENTIAL: INTERPROFESSIONAL COLLABORATION FOR IMPROVING PATIENT AND POPULATION HEALTH AND OUTCOMES

This DNP Essential specifically relates to the important task that the DNP graduate performs as they interact with multidisciplinary members. The goal of this process is to provide patient-centered care that is safe and efficient. I have already explained how painful it was to lead my scholarly project. The project required a team approach in an ECS. The staff did not want to change. It was relaxing to remain in the old culture doing things the old way. The new constituents of the multidisciplinary teams would follow their leaders rather than buy into changes. When some of the older leaders were sold on the project, the younger staff settled into the new process. Interprofessional collaboration can be difficult, yet, in order to improve patient and population health outcomes, it is imperative.

# DNP Essential: Clinical Prevention and Population Health for Improving the Nation's Health

I had practiced as an CNM for 17 years before returning to school for my DNP degree. Population health near our clinic has improved, and I am now able to analyze data and enable implementation to improve community health. Administering the Edinburgh Depression Scale[16] (EBDS) throughout pregnancy and at postpartum visits gives evidence to focus on preventing postpartum depression. By using the questionnaire tool only for postpartum, I missed the opportunity to implement treatment and counseling during pregnancy. Now, this tool is administered at the first obstetrical visit and then at 28 and 36 weeks of pregnancy. The tool is also administered after birth at the hospital and again at the clinic at 2 and 6 weeks postpartum. This awareness also energized me to contact a local psychologist to set up a support group. Patients who had suffered with postpartum depression have also volunteered as peer advisors. The clinic EBDS scores have been informally studied and have demonstrated that communicating on the specific EBDS visits heightened awareness and has improved patient, family, and staff relationships. One of our patients recorded her struggle and story about postpartum depression. She was interviewed on a local podcast. We had worked with her and her family as she was struggling with functioning as a mother of 2. She was utilizing medications and counseling networked from our practice. One of the concerns that continued to haunt her was her perception that she had not created an attachment to the infant. When the infant was 4 months old, she just casually walked out into her garage and saw a rope and then her mind and eyes fixated on a wooden beam. She stated that she did not have a plan for suicide and had never marked on the EBDS that she had thought of it. Yet, at that moment, she instantly decided to hang herself. She stated that she immediately felt better just knowing she could end the pain she was feeling each day. She called her grandmother to see if she could drop off her children. Her plan was to take the children to her grandmother and to come back to the garage and throw the rope over the beam. Her grandmother did not answer. She was devastated that she could not carry out her plan and knew she had to get help. She stated that she was crying and found herself driving to the clinic. She just walked in and asked for our staff. The one medical assistant that was a postpartum depression peer advisor immediately dropped everything when she realized that the patient was in crisis. The clinic staff folded the clinic day to take care of her. She expressed that because of the constant communication, acceptance, and transparency our clinic demonstrates regarding postpartum depression and anxiety, she felt that the clinic and staff created a safe haven for her and her children.

Starting locally and disseminating grassroot efforts has augmented other preventive programs. I would like to further investigate outreach prenatal and postpartum depression telehealth visits.

# DNP Essential: Advanced Nursing Practice

As a DNP, I am trying every day to expand my knowledge about the services I provide. Chism[2] explained that a DNP develops expertise in her or his own area of specialization. She suggested that we should prepare and continue to gain knowledge. I read the ACOG's headlines every day. I have the app on my phone and try to open it prior to opening social media. If I miss a day, I go back and try to catch up. This habit has extended my clinical credibility when working with physicians, peers, and preceptees. Recently I had a radiologist remark that performing a 37-week ultrasound did not yield important information. I immediately opened the recent headlines from a reputable site about a prospective study that included more than 50 000 pregnancies. The study reported that a high proportion of fetal anomalies were detected for the first time at ultrasound examinations at 35 to 37 weeks' gestation.[17] The radiologist reviewed the study and shared it with staff.

Knowing people at local businesses and being transparent, approachable, and friendly wherever you are also advances nursing practice. Remembering and acknowledging others' stories has enlarged my ability to care for them. Visit their homes and attend their celebrations and family funerals. In one of the DNP classes, it was recommended that we make cards about the patients to remember their stories. I have been blessed with a good memory, and it has blessed me as I have met them on the street. I might not remember their names; however, I remember their stories. I start every patient interaction by getting to know him or her and always start the next interaction with something I learned on the first appointment. This is easy for me because I love people and love talking. Most patients come back because we have connected. I know social media can seem unprofessional; however, I use social media to find out about their lives so we can send cards, offer support, and improve care. I do not often give written comment, yet I often leave a red heart. I think that the compassionate nursing approach, which differs from many medical approaches, is the reason patients adapted and appreciated it when nurses became advanced practice clinicians. Patient satisfaction scores are compiled by the hospital. I have had high satisfaction scores throughout the years. The remarks that accompany most of the scores have reflected the caring methodology of nursing. The remarks that were mentioned most centered around themes that the midwife stayed with me and gave emotional support and physical comfort measures.

## BUSINESS PLAN

The practice needs to be solvent, which means it needs to make a profit. The business plan that I was offered after finishing school was designed to generate profit when I was productive. I was offered a base pay compared to state statistics for a new graduate that was 20% of my intake after overhead was paid. Overhead was defined by the clinic, and each year this was recalculated as staff, benefit packages, and clinic needs changed. Bonus pay was also provided when production numbers were achieved. Our clinic offers after-hour and weekend shifts. The family nurse practitioner and physician assistants often achieve bonus pay, especially in the cold seasons. A bonus is also paid at the end of the year if feasible. The bonus is equally divided among the providers and changes every year. Provider meetings are important to review clinic operations.

Chism,[2] when writing "Shaping Your Brand: Marketing Yourself as a DNP Graduate," discussed the "Four Ps"—product, price, place, and promotion—as a strategy to enhance your worth. Product represents the service you can render, price represents the price you would charge for the service, place is the area that you will be serving, and promotion is continuing to market yourself, with increasing worth during your career.

- Product: Assisting first-time mothers (product) seems to take longer during the weekends and at night. An hourly wage would have been nice!
- Price: After 10 years with variable pay, I requested a salary. I accidently found out that I was making much less than the nurse leaders in the hospital. The clinic ran calculations that included a cost-benefit analysis and felt confident that the salary I asked for was reasonable. I was underpaid for years; however, it was only my fault because I was too busy taking care of the practice to investigate the changing wages in nursing and midwifery. When you work for a larger institution, raises, incentives, and base salaries are set. When you work for a smaller organization, you might have more freedom to negotiate; however, you need to sharpen your business skills and the organization's profit margins in order to ask for a raise.
- Place: With the place of my practice being a rural area, I was greatly disappointed that I should not expect the same pay as my urban counterparts working in group practices.
- Promotion: The salary I receive does not pay for the massive number of management (husbandry) hours that are required for the households to be functional yet profitable.

## COST SAVINGS/REVENUE GENERATION

I did not learn how to code diagnoses or patient interaction levels in school. The full business realm of clinic operations and revenue generation was a problem for this new graduate. I wanted to leave all the financial obligations to the clinic operators. I soon realized that needing to do charge sheets on every patient was perplexing. I had spent 10 years in school to know how to diagnose; however, to now use that code to initiate insurance, self-pay charges, and Medicaid/Medicare reimbursements seemed senseless. So many rules and modifiers! In 2011, our clinic invested in an EMR that had a coding and diagnosis program. If the government had not issued Medicaid/Medicare mandates for clinics to have EMRs, I do not believe we could have afforded to move away from written charts. There were monetary programs to allow independent clinics to be able to afford this upgrade. Electronic charting has sharpened my skills and increased the clinic revenue. The EMR codes the encounter for payment; however, we have personnel who also review the diagnosis codes and negotiate with third-party payers. I have found it helpful and informative when the coding specialists meet with me regarding certain charges. This has helped me improve documentation that might improve reimbursements.

Chart reviews are conducted quarterly to enhance correct coding and diagnosis charting. This process has increased revenue. Through these charting reviews, I came to learn that many tests and functions within the clinic are not reimbursable. I have learned to sharpen my diagnostic skills rather than overuse clinic staff and resources that are not billable. When working for a larger system, you also need to increase revenue and use correct coding behaviors, but you feel comfortable that the bottom line has a large financial base. In a smaller clinic, you need to "nickel and dime" your costs and revenues. This is where the husbandry responsibilities increased for me as our midwifery services were recruited by the outreach community clinic and the neighboring hospital. The burden of these business responsibilities is still on my shoulders today, and it is my responsibility to run the outer households efficiently and productively. The EMR has also allowed the clinics to easily run reports on cost savings and revenue. This has improved the clinic's day-to-day management.

I have noticed that in some advanced practice nursing programs, students are learning to code. They are doing SOAP (Subjective, Objective, Assessment, Plan) notes with diagnosis codes for every patient they see. They are memorizing codes and have apps on their phones to help them find correct International Classification of Diseases (ICD) codes. I hope more educational programs are taking this important step to help the student be successful in practice.

Long-term husbandry has taught me that nothing is free. Money talks. In managing new clinics, I have found that the honeymoon period ends abruptly if there is no profit and no compensation for those who collaborate. We made the mistake of being conservative and not offering the physicians who covered us at the new hospital practice any monetary incentives. We did not compensate them for phone consultations. They charged the patients for formal consultations, and we thought that would suffice. The honeymoon period has now ended, and those physicians do not feel that interruptions to their home and professional lives are worthwhile without compensation. I totally agree with them and realize I took for granted their initial willingness.

# OUTCOMES AND EVIDENCE-BASED PRACTICE

In the late 1990s when I finished the midwifery program, the master's degree earned entry to practice if all requirements and licensure was successful. I remember in the classroom the saying "research says" meant taking that statement as literal proof. Classroom research classes taught us to decipher research articles for validity and the ability to generalize findings. Out in practice, I reasoned that experience, knowledge of pathophysiology, and the ability to learn from more experienced practitioners would generate good outcomes. I was fortunate to start my practice under the auspices of 2 family practitioners who were proficient patient teachers. I was so busy, that I would not take the time to stay current with emerging theories and research findings. I was so intent on making it though the clinic day and laboring nights that I would not stay current and be like the wise lumberjack who would take the time to sharpen his axe! During these years, conferences and journals started to circulate new verbiage named "evidence-based medicine and/or practice." This new phrase was intimidating to me because I felt I could not find books that could stay up with the newest findings. As soon as some texts were written, they were out of date. The original computer searches were difficult and internet entities like "Up to Date" were not developed. When I returned to school 17 to 20 years later to obtain the DNP degree, the didactic paradigm changed to "evidence-based practice and/or best practice." In those 20 years, research exploded! Good outcomes, high-quality patient care, and current best-practice evidence can now be easily and quickly found. The DNP educational experience taught the ability to explore recent literature in a critical manner by analytical and methodological processes.

Perineal lacerations are common after vaginal birth. Lacerations can also occur to the vagina, vulva, labial, periclitoral, and periurethral areas. A severe perineal laceration called a third-degree laceration is an injury to the perineum that involves the anal sphincter complex. A fourth-degree laceration injures the perineum involving the anal sphincter complex (external and internal) and the anal epithelium. These lacerations can cause pelvic floor dysfunction and bowel incontinence. Obstetrical anal sphincter injuries (OASIS) are a quality measure reported as a Core Measure

Set (CMS). The Joint Commission included OASIS in 2002 as reportable. Each quarter, the hospital gives statistics on each obstetrical provider concerning third- and fourth-degree lacerations. Personal, system-wide, and national statistics are reported. The goal is to reduce pelvic floor dysfunction by implementing best practice during labor and the second stage of labor. During one delivery, I had a father upset at me that I had not cut an episiotomy. This mother did experience a fourth-degree laceration. She had a very short perineum and the infant had a large head. He felt that if I would have cut the episiotomy, the fourth-degree laceration would have been avoided. I tried to explain that the surgical cut of an episiotomy is not evidenced as best practice. I was fortunate that I could pull up on my phone and quickly print the current practice bulletin from ACOG. The practice bulletin was also in alignment supporting the other measures that he had witnessed that I had done to try to avoid this laceration. I was also able to show him my personal scores from the CMS statistics that demonstrated that I had less third- and fourth-degree lacerations when compared to system and national percentages. Since that time, I have delivered 2 more of his infants and the mother experienced an intact perineum after each birth.

# DATA MINING

If the clinic genie granted me 3 wishes, I would ask for a clinical nurse specialist, a clinical nurse specialist, and a clinical nurse specialist. Many rural clinics that are not funded by the government and some larger systems do not have clinical nurse specialists and/or managers. Sylvia and Terhaar,[18] in their text on clinical analytics and data mining, specifically expressed how the DNP is juxtaposed as problem solver, analyst, and translator. A DNP-prepared clinical nurse specialist could greatly aid in this plight. In our rural clinic, run charts, data analysis, and risk reduction are not transparent. Our providers informally recognize deficiencies and strategies for better outcomes rather than depending on data-mining techniques. Using data and measures to improve clinic operations and patient outcomes can be accomplished by the providers using EMR reports. The EMR that we utilize will generate many reports; however, we are overwhelmed with patient care. I plan to start reviewing nulliparous, term, singleton, and vertex statistics as a focus to reduce cesarean sections. Using data-mining techniques, I have started to track data to reduce first-birth cesarean sections. This is important husbandry housework that would directly benefit maternal/child outcomes in our clinic.

The lunchroom at the rural outreach community health center has a huge white board. My practice partner and I travel to this clinic 3 times a month. This is a rural health clinic that is required to report Uniform Data System (UDS) measures in order to operate. The clinic is funded by a Health Resources and Services Administration (HRSA) grant. The lunchroom board has the past year, year to date, and clinic goals posted by percentages. The statistics are extrapolated from their EMR. The clinical nurse specialist supervises the data mining. She has medical assistants in the clinic to champion a measure. The items on the board include hypertension, colonoscopy, depression, adult body mass index (BMI), diabetes, tobacco, asthma, Pap smear, childhood BMI, coronary artery disease, ischemic vascular disease, and immunizations. The champions' responsibilities are to watch monthly percentages and track proper documentation and patient outcomes. The registered nurse has noted that the champions have ownership and encourage clinical adherence. If goals are not met, then a "ticket to fix" is generated to the department and/or provider. Data mining is also used for quarterly reports to the providers. The reports generate information to the providers about the UDS measures. Their individual compliance and QI processes are then required. This clinic also has other clinical sites, and they compare these measures to reduce risk, remain solvent, and improve patient outcomes.

## INTERPROFESSIONAL COLLABORATION

In his book *The Conservative Heart*,[19] Arthur C. Brooks gave advice on how to build a "fairer, happier, and more prosperous America." He explained that it is important to go where you are not welcome. David met Goliath by taking lunch to his soldier brothers. His father gave him the job each day to take lunch to the frontlines of the Hebrew army. His brothers were physically large, important soldiers who defended the Hebrews from the Philistine army. The Philistines were at their borders and had a large soldier named Goliath. Goliath and the Philistines were harassing and pillaging the Hebrew villages. Simple service from a lunch boy is how the king and important officials first met David. Young and small-statured David witnessed the carnage that Goliath was inflicting and was inspired to take the giant down—something the whole army could not do.

Can you image what Goliath thought as he saw this scrawny, young boy approach him? This story leads back to the advice from Arthur Brooks[19] as he explained how we try to collaborate with 3 different groups:

1. True believers: those who are already with us
2. Persuadables: those who are not yet with us
3. Hostiles: those who will never be with us

Brooks went on to explain that it is important to rally the true believers by encouraging, supporting, and fostering happiness in their professional and personal lives. In this endeavor, it is important to forget negativity. Next, it is important to collaborate with those who are neither with us nor against us, specifically the persuadables. This group is looking for solutions and usually will give all sides a chance. They are attentive in their personal interactions with you. They are watching your character and behavior behind the scenes.

Most importantly, they are intensely interested in how you interact with the third group, namely, the hostiles. Taking the sling and flinging the stone at the hostile's forehead is not productive. I know we want to take the hostiles out of our environment and we do not want them in our midst. Conversely, Brooks encouraged us to walk among them and to understand them. This is where Brooks' advice is in sharp contrast to what David did. It is inconceivable how David could have walked toward Goliath without encountering his 300-pound sword. Hostiles are not friends, and they may never be; however, the persuadables will notice and might defend you when the hostiles are once again at your forefront. Brooks encouraged us to meet the hostiles' anger with love and compassion. By doing this, we might realize what might be motivating their actions against us. This is not meant to persuade them or change them into true believers, it is only to find if there is some common ground.

Agitation from the hostiles can also sharpen our axes. We work harder and smarter when hostiles refuse to cooperate or are impolite when we try to collaborate with them. Competition from the hostiles also encourages you to strengthen your relationships with the true believers and persuadables. True believers and persuadables can be rallied in order to maintain support and respect in a hostile environment. Figure 13-2 shows an example of interprofessional collaboration.

## PROFESSIONALISM

In the previous section, I discussed collaboration. I provided information about becoming the ideal professional. I had witnessed a doctoral-prepared nurse who wanted to be addressed as "doctor" in the clinical setting. Physicians targeted her and destroyed her professional credibility. I hope that your generation of DNPs and future DNPs can break this pattern of behavior. The "mid-level" stereotyping also continues, and I hope we can be brave nurses and batter down this designation as well. After recently graduating with the DNP, I chose not to allow myself to be called Dr. Rasmussen. It was confusing for patients who thought I had gone back to medical school and became an obstetrician/gynecologist. I also knew this would cause resentment among the medical staff.

To promote professionalism, I continue to contribute, attend all midwifery meetings, and attend to responsibilities. I accept new challenges and opportunities to disseminate knowledge to all groups through presentations and publications.

I fully try to be a professional and a personal example to the youth and encourage them to reach out and dare to educate themselves. Remember, I live in a small hometown where the high school has fewer than 200 students. One of my most rewarding experiences was volunteering to be this small high school's advisor to the Health Occupations Students of America Club. The high school came home with

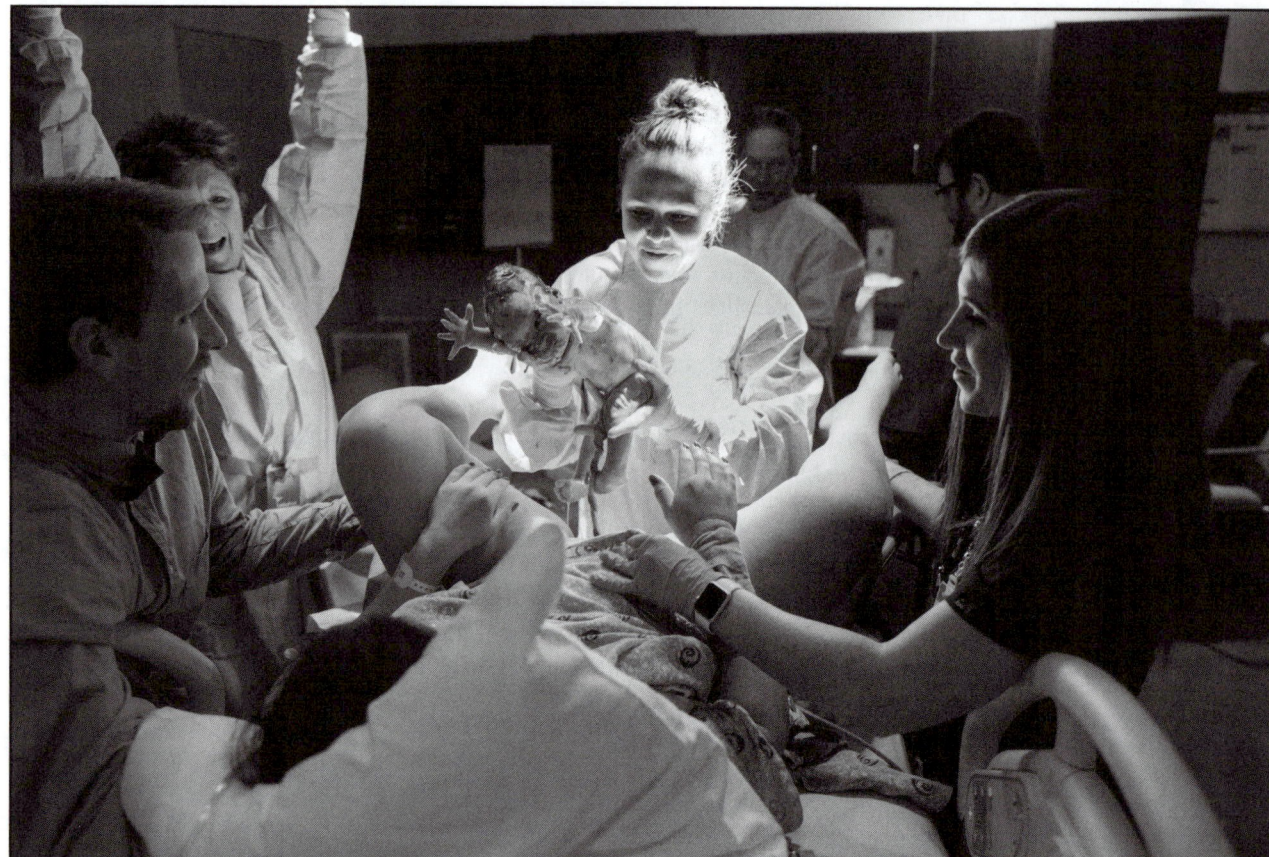

**Figure 13-2.** Birth circle.

many student state winners and club awards. We now have students across the nation as health care workers.

I think professionalism comes by being a good shepherd, doing little things each day that are known to be the right things. By exerting "husbandry" efforts in protecting the flock. To encourage civility and compassion among those within our realm, while pushing toward success, is something the head of the household should strive for. Our professionalism is also is defined by how we treat the predators, Goliaths, and hostiles.

## Pearls/Takeaways

You have had the repetitive themes and analogies of husbandry, shepherding, King David's leadership, and Goliaths throughout this chapter. Brooks'[19] "The Seven Habits of Highly Effective Conservatives" encircles and gives counsel for all these examples. Please accept these suggestions for improving humanity without political bias:

1. Be a moralist.
2. Fight for people, not against things.
3. Get happy.
4. Steal all the best arguments.
5. Go where you are not welcome.
6. Say it in 30 seconds.
7. Break your bad habits.

I wish you success and happiness as you set out on or continue to travel this exciting path in your life and career. For at least the past 30 years, I have displayed this quote from Ralph Waldo Emerson[20] in my home and offices. Most of my presentations and speeches end with this quote. It is currently on my fridge and is planned for my funeral announcement. It defines the meaning of success for me:

*What is Success?*
*To laugh often and much;*
*To win the respect of intelligent people and the affection of children;*
*To earn the appreciation of honest critics and endure the betrayal of false friends;*
*To appreciate beauty;*
*To find the best in others;*
*To leave the world a little bit better, whether by a healthy child, a garden patch or a redeemed social condition;*
*To know even one life has breathed easier because you have lived.*
*This is to have succeeded.*

# Conclusion: Impact of the DNP Degree

As a result of obtaining my DNP degree, I have obtained an overview look to better evaluate evidence. This innovative practice degree has allowed me to gain a "Google Earth perspective." The educational process has provided me an elevated viewpoint to solving health care dilemmas by investigating evidence-based findings and translating to direct patient care.

My husband thought if he irrigated his crop more effectively he would gain higher yields than the surrounding fields. On the ground, he noticed no-growth areas in what he thought were poor irrigation techniques by his neighboring farmers. Recently, he pulled up Google Earth to view our field. Much to his surprise, he discovered that several of the neighboring acreages have scars that showed historically flooded landscapes. It was blatantly apparent that narrow bands of gravel-type soils were fanned out across approximately 1000 acres. What he thought was poor irrigation was gravelly soil that produced poor crops. The pattern clearly demonstrated how the floods created random courses of flood-plain patterns into the Sevier River.

The DNP degree, like Google Earth, has prepared me to investigate, decipher, and enact visionary management. The DNP's foundation has given me an elevated view of evidence. It enables me to navigate imaginary drones to study, evaluate, and further advance the professional role of the nurse. Just like seeing the historical flood damage, the DNP can use studies and historical patterns in preventing further disparities in health care and continue to serve an important role in preventative health care. Becoming a DNP has prepared me to become an overseer, a leader, elevated from mid-level midwifery to high-level husbandry.

# Acknowledgments

A lifetime of love and support has allowed me to actualize my goals. From an early age, my mother encouraged me to be a nurse. My father also worked hard to help finance each step. My husband, Kreig, and children have been flexible and understanding as I have juggled professional and personal responsibilities. My husband is my foundation and lends daily strength.

DeAnn Brown, DNP, CNM, and I accomplished our bachelor's, master's, and doctorate degrees together. We traveled many miles and endured long hours. Without her, I would not have had the strength and fortitude to accomplish home, educational, and professional responsibilities.

Two educational mentors stand out in my journey. Dr. Joyce Foster and Dr. Barbara Wilson, both from the University of Utah. Joyce allowed DeAnn and I to live with her family when we traveled for the midwifery program. Joyce believed that rural Utah needed midwives. Barbara exuded enthusiasm and gave tremendous support as my DNP project chair. Barbara continues to demonstrate genuine love and devotion to every student she meets.

Sevier Valley Hospital and staff have allowed me to learn and serve. Dr. David Pope and Dr. Jeffery Chappell, along with Mountain Utah Family Medicine staff, have supported the methodology of midwifery.

I was born, raised, and blessed to stay in my own hometown. I appreciate the support I have been given from the rural communities that I love. I am now delivering the babies of the babies and am honored to be a part of their lives.

# References

1. Simpson J, ed. *Oxford Dictionary of English.* 3rd ed. Oxford University Press; 2010.
2. Chism L. *The Doctor of Nursing Practice: A Guidebook for Role Development and Professional Issues.* Jones and Bartlett; 2019.
3. SWOT analyses. Strategic Management Insight. http://www.strategicmanagementinsight.com
4. Coogan MD, ed. *The New Oxford Annotated Bible.* Oxford University Press; 2007.
5. Boehm FM. Decision to incision: time to reconsider. *Am J Obstet Gynecol.* 2012;206(2):97-98. doi:10.1016/j.acog.2011.09.009
6. Lie K, Growbolt E, Eskild A. Association of cerebral palsy with Apgar score in low and normal birthweight infants: population-based cohort study. *BMJ.* 2010.341; c4990.
7. Rasmussen D. *Can a Rural Hospital Reliably Perform an Emergency Cesarean Section in Thirty Minutes or Less? Power Point Presentation-Pit-Crew For Emergency Cesarean Section.* Doctoral Project. University of Utah; 2017.
8. Edwards D. PDSA cycle. Accessed August 5, 2019. https://deming.org/explore/pdsa/
9. Delivering rural babies: maternity care shortages in rural America. National Rural Health Association. Accessed August 30, 2019. https://www.ruralhealthweb.org/blogs/ruralhealthvoices
10. Lewin K. The Kurt Lewin change management model. Change-Management-Coach. Accessed August 5, 2019. https://www.change-management-coach.com/kurt_lewin.html
11. Herding cats. YouTube. Accessed August 10, 2019. https://www.youtube.com/watch?v=Pk7yqlTMvp8
12. Albritton J, Maddox L, Dalto J, Ridout E, Minton S. The effect of a newborn telehealth program on transfers avoided: a multiple-baseline study. *Health Aff.* 2018;37(12):1990-1996.
13. Association of Women's Heath, Obstetrics and Neonatal Nurses. *Fetal Heart Monitoring: Principles and Practices.* 5th ed. Kendall Hunt; 2015.
14. Dekker R, Bertone A. The evidence on fetal monitoring. Evidence Based Birth. Accessed August 12, 2019. http://www.evidencebasedbirth.com/fetal-monitoring
15. Dalhsrud S. *Can Telehealth Lactation Services Provide Effective Breastfeeding Support for Rural Areas?* Doctoral Project. University of Utah; 2018.
16. Edinburgh postnatal depression scale (EPDS). Perinatology. Accessed August 12, 2019. http://perinatology.com/calculators/Edinburgh%20Depression%20Scale.htm
17. Schwartz, B. Should ob/gyns perform ultrasound examinations at 35-37 weeks gestation? Contemporary OB/GYN. October 2019. https://www.contemporaryobgyn.net/view/should-obgyns-perform-ultrasound-examination-35-37-weeks-gestation
18. Sylvia M, Terhaar M. *Clinical Analytics and Data Mining for the DNP.* Springer; 2018.
19. Brooks A. *The Conservative Heart: How to Build a Fairer, Happier, and More Prosperous America.* HarperCollins; 2015.
20. Emerson RW. *Essays and Poems.* Barnes and Noble; 2005.

# SECTION VI

## NURSE EXECUTIVE EXEMPLARS

# CHAPTER 14

# THE DNP DEGREE

## A FUNDAMENTAL REQUIREMENT FOR THE CHIEF NURSING OFFICER

*Janet Hunt Davis, DNP, RN, NE-BC, CPHQ*

## INTRODUCTION

Tampa General Hospital (TGH) is a 1009-bed four-time Magnet-designated, teaching hospital located in downtown Tampa, Florida. TGH is a Level 1 adult and pediatric trauma center, burn-verified center, 82-bed neonatal intensive care unit, and transplant center. It is the primary teaching hospital for the University of South Florida College of Medicine, and serves more than 800 students a month in nursing, therapies, pharmacy, and other clinical roles. TGH employees more than 3000 registered nurses in multiple roles and has more than 400 advanced practice providers on staff. The chief nursing officer (CNO) is directly responsible for more than 2500 team members, a $250 million budget, care of more than 1000 patients per day, and responsible for the practice of more than 3000 registered nurses and 400 advanced practice providers.

The Doctor of Nursing Practice (DNP) and Doctor of Philosophy (PhD) nursing roles contribute in creating evidence that enlightens and influences nursing practice. The DNP and PhD functional domains of education are best compared by the terms *research scientist* which is the PhD,

and the *research translation professional*, who is DNP prepared. The DNP curriculum was established to identify gaps in professional practice within the complex health care system and to develop new knowledge, practices, and skills that improve nursing care delivery.[1] Doctorate programs are focused on the progress of the specialized practices and identity. It is a vehicle that defines the distinct characteristic of that practice with pertinent theory and develops innovative solutions for challenges in the workplace environment. Throughout history, nurses have a very strong commitment to their professional identity being guided by practice standards and competencies. Today, like other health care professionals, nurses are practicing in a fast-changing environment with significant regulatory and oversight requirements, and an ever-expanding interprofessional team.[2] The DNP is essential for the CNO with this scope of responsibility. The DNP program prepares nurses to develop as leaders influencing policy at the highest level of the organization, as clinical experts with practice innovations, and as advanced practice providers or executive leaders who have the opportunity for specialty tracks.[3]

Nursing is a comprehensive science interwoven with a complex art to advance the well-being of individuals and

Benson LA, ed. *The DNP Professional:
Translating Value From Classroom to Practice* (pp 157-165).
© 2021 SLACK Incorporated.

society. Advancing well-being includes all aspects of life from encouraging breastfeeding with a new mother whose infant is in critical care, to supporting a family's decision of providing comfort measures for end-of-life care, to ensuring a newly transplanted organ remains perfused. Doctorate-prepared nurses with diverse skills and knowledge are required to meet the challenges of our constantly changing and complex health care environment and advancing nursing practice at all levels. Nurses with doctorate nursing degrees have the skills to influence the health care system, policies, teams, and organizations. The future of nursing practice requires nurses with DNPs and PhDs to inspire, stimulate, and lead innovation.[4]

In reflection of pre- and post-doctorate education I am able to identify differences in my practice. Pre-doctorate, I would describe my practice as being an authentic, transformational leader and collaborator with interdisciplinary and interprofessional teams. I was constantly busy, successfully inspiring teams to work hard to accomplish challenging goals and being able to implement change to reach goals using a consistent approach regardless of the change. I was challenged with identifying strong evidence and challenged with sustaining positive change. Nursing practices would change, outcomes would improve, but when we moved onto the next priority, the previous practice would revert to old ways and outcomes would slide back to previous results.

# Incorporating the DNP Essentials Into the Chief Nursing Officer Role

The DNP CNO should be incessantly challenging current practices and evaluating the value of such practices. They should be a catalyst for innovation where underachieving departments or systems are reconstructed with enhanced and innovative practices and processes. The DNP-prepared nurse should be an expert architect of change and innovation. This advanced knowledge should be used to develop ideal leadership models that perform at high levels of excellence.[5] The CNO role is a long-standing role at this organization, although it has grown in responsibility over the past 10 years with the significant growth in census, complexity, and technology. Completing a DNP 2 years into the CNO role improved my skills in the areas of evidence evaluation, data analysis, strategic planning, prioritizing, execution on goals, operational efficiency, change management, and gaining significant respect from my medical partners, executive team peers, and practicing nurses.

Evidence evaluation is best reflected in my work through a partnership with our advanced nurse specialist in research. We consistently review evidence tables when addressing new challenges, evaluating current practice, and contemplating practice changes that others bring to our attention. When practice changes are brought to my attention, I will request a meta-analysis or have the individual discuss the strength of the peer-reviewed, non-vendor sponsored evidence. Data analysis improvement is best reflected by the understanding of trends vs common variation. One example is best described in our work with central line infections. Our practice to prevent infections from maintenance was controlled until a substation cap was introduced. Within 2 months, the data demonstrated a special cause variation, which we were able to point back to the cap change and action was taken promptly to bring the practice back to controlled.

Strategic planning, prioritizing, execution on goals, operational efficiency, and change management can best be reflected in the process of developing and communicating the organization's nursing strategic priorities. In the past, these changed annually, were not clearly communicated, and progress was inconsistent. One of the most significant changes I made was in the decision to require a DNP for the hospital's quality nurse specialist role. Together, we developed a plan aligned with the organization's strategic plan, a process for consistent, daily communication, and a commitment to keep the plan prioritized on nursing sensitive indicators. By this work we have demonstrated significant improvement or controlled process to keep our patients safe. Obtaining my DNP was formally recognized by the leadership team at the hospital and the medical and nursing team during our conversations or when introducing me as Dr. Davis. Developing ourselves is the first step in obtaining the skills required for excellence in leadership. The need for nursing administrators who have advanced preparation is evident as we look to the future complexities of health care.

Actions taken based on knowledge gained in the DNP program varied in complexity. One of the earliest actions I took occurred during the DNP program when we were evaluating nursing leader competencies. In comparison to nationally published competencies for nursing leaders, it was determined ours could be improved. We aligned the organizational nursing executive's, director's, and manager's competencies with nationally published competencies. This is a critical first step in that nurse leader competencies include fundamental skills that are vital for fulfilling one's responsibilities. It is important to clearly define nurse leader competencies to establish a foundation for nursing practice at all levels. The competencies identified the need for additional leadership education programs and the expanded team evaluated the new competencies. Examples include a 10-year cultural change project that I led, which improved team pride and patient and team experience. But we were unable to sustain the improved outcome and quality improvement initiatives demonstrated normal variation and positive trends, but there was no movement of the organizational mean with infections and injuries. Post-doctorate education improvements have been sustained and organizational means moved, team engagement improved, and I became more effective and worked less hours.

Incorporating the DNP Essentials in to the CNO role first occurred during the program when I shared the American Organization of Nurse Executives' (now the American Organization for Nursing Leadership) Nursing Executive Competencies with the TGH nursing executive team (NET). The team decided to update nursing competencies, peer-review tools, job descriptions, and annual competencies to align with the documented professional nursing competencies. The most significant change I made while still in the DNP program was the decision to hire a doctorate-prepared nurse to serve in the role of quality nurse specialist, which was previously held by a master's-prepared nurse. Within the first 5 minutes of the interview with a doctorate-prepared nurse, the research nurse specialist and I knew that we had the perfect candidate, and we were not wrong.

Upon her start at TGH and my completion of the DNP program, the quality and research nurse specialist and the CNO developed an annual Nursing Strategic Priorities that aligned with the organizational strategic plan. The strategic priorities would include process and outcome goals that nurses could directly impact with their practice. The initial draft was shared, revised, and approved by each of the Shared Governance Councils, until a final document was agreed upon. On an annual workshop, the NET and other key organizational leaders meet to review and revise the Nursing Strategic Priorities.

The progress toward the strategic priorities are reviewed monthly with all of nursing leadership at the Nursing Leadership Update led by the CNO with reports by the quality nurse specialist, research nurse specialist, and other nurses throughout the organization. The idea of a monthly Nursing Leadership Update was obtained during my DNP clinical hours shadowing a CNO at another Magnet-designated hospital in western Florida.

The required clinical hours of the DNP program were a great investment of time for my professional growth and development. I had the opportunity to shadow 2 amazing chief nurses: Jan Mauck at Sarasota Memorial Hospital and Kathy Boyle at Denver Health. Both were very generous with their time, open with the information they shared, and remained mentors post-graduation. I also used the clinical time to shadow our chief informatics officer and chief technology officer. During this time, I gained a new approach to project evaluation, planning, defining resources needed, and process mapping. This time has also been critical to the change in my personal practice and success as a CNO. Other clinical hours included time obtaining a black belt in Lean Six Sigma and earning certification in quality. The clinical time, aligned with the academic courses, combined to advance my individual knowledge and skills to address the ever-changing and complex health care environment.

# EVALUATING THE ESSENTIALS OF THE DNP

DNP education prepares a nurse to have advanced skills with clinical care, performance improvement methodologies, translating research into nursing practice, evaluation of care, clinical education strategy and application, assessing sustainability, defining performance metrics, and fiscal impact. Other skills of the DNP include health care leadership, health policy development, cost-benefit analysis, interprofessional collaboration, and dissemination of improvements through publications and professional presentations.[3] In 2010, the Institute of Medicine (IOM) published a report on progress toward the initial report on the "The Future of Nursing."[6] Their recommendations were to double the nurses with doctoral degrees to improve nursing's competence to partner with providers and other interprofessionals to lead health care changes. These recommendations are critical as the care needs of society escalate and health care systems endure fundamental changes.[7]

Evaluating the role of a CNO and integrating the DNP Essentials into practice can best be described with a SWOT (Strengths, Weaknesses, Opportunities, Threats) analysis. The strengths associated with daily operations of a large, complex medical center include the required elements of: Scientific Underpinnings for Practice; Organizational and Systems Leadership for Quality Improvement and Systems Thinking; Clinical Scholarship and Analytical Methods for Evidence-Based Practice; Information Systems/Technology and Patient Care Technology for the Improvement and Transformation of Health Care; and the Interprofessional Collaboration for Improving Patient and Population Health Outcomes. The chief nurse of an organization is responsible for nursing practice across the continuum. This requires a broad breadth of knowledge incorporating the state and federal regulations regarding the practice of nurses, the organizational policies, and procedures that involve nursing practice; professional organizations approach to nursing care; and individual's interpretations of each of the areas. The CNO is continually educating providers, administrators, nurses, and the interdisciplinary/interprofessional teams on the scope of practice for a nurse. Communication regarding the standards of practice must be provided to elicit collaboration and understanding vs creating a divisive environment giving the impression nurses are being difficult or refuse to help.

Other critical DNP Essentials for the CNO include the Organizational and Systems Leadership for Quality Improvement and Systems Thinking. This DNP Essential is interwoven with the Scientific Underpinnings for Practice constantly in daily operations. Daily operations include all shifts and all days of the week, including holidays. The CNO must be visible and present, advocating for the team working all shifts. In an acute care hospital, the majority of leaders are physically present 30% of time. Ensuring consistent care requires the CNO and key nursing leaders be present, provide education, offer meetings, and share face-to-face communication for evening, nights, and weekends. In describing my role as the CNO, I often describe it as 5% fiscal responsibility and 95% nursing practice and system-level performance improvement. The Scientific Underpinnings for Practice require the constant redirection of team members to remain focused on the priorities of the division when there are so many competing interests.

The CNO role requires that nurses are involved in almost every aspect of patient care in an acute care hospital requiring nurses to have constant vigilance and advocacy for the patient and can provide many levels of care. The CNO must constantly and consistently evaluate practice with the goals of continuous improvement. The improvement elements of the CNO are aligned with the 2001 IOM report "Crossing the Quality Chasm" which defined the improvement goals of care to consider safety, timeliness, efficiency, effectiveness, equity, and patient-centeredness. Since first published in 2001, CNOs have aligned nursing priorities with these aims and vary focus areas within each element based on identified organizational risks and goals. One example of a revision to the aims is the current understanding of the value of the work environment on patient outcomes and the need to revise patient-centered to people-centered, to include the team members of an organization.

Three other DNP Essentials strengths critical for an effective CNO include Clinical Scholarship and Analytical Methods for Evidence-Based Practice; Information Systems/Technology and Patient Care Technology for the Improvement and Transformation of Health Care; and Interprofessional Collaboration for Improving Patient and Population Health Outcomes. Advancing the practice of nurses at all levels can only be accomplished when the CNO and team members have a keen skill in review of evidence. Evidence tables are helpful to present data and findings in a systematic format which demonstrates the weight of the evidence, and the required resources, knowledge, communication, tools, and critical steps. Working with our nursing team, I consistently request evidence tables when considering new projects, changes in practice, and in revising policies and procedures. The CNO must critically evaluate all high-risk steps since nurses provide hands-on care, which make check lists and 2-people interventions challenging and not always possible due to constant interruptions, constantly changing workloads, novice to expert nursing levels, and many competing priorities. Reality is key in this area and requires a CNO who can communicate without being perceived as complaining or having a lack of interest.

Information Systems/Technology and Patient Care Technology is as critical as electricity in a large medical center. The CNO who has a strong skill in the use, understanding, process development, and implementation of technology will be better able to support their teams in practice and their own individual efficiency and effectiveness. CNOs or nursing leaders who are not actively using and understanding technology are dependent on others to evaluate nursing

practice, understand workflow, and identify opportunities. Many examples are evident in my work since entering the DNP program. One of the largest projects has been our biomedical device integration plan. Partnering with the information technology (IT) and facilities teams, the CNO led the project, which provided standard physiological monitoring in critical care and telemetry for the acute care facility, integration of equipment with the electronic medical record (EMR), and the smartphone technology carried by all clinical team members. This project was presented to the board of directors by the CNO and was granted more than $20 million. Another critical role for the CNO is ensuring the EMR system is efficient and effective for the end users, primarily nurses. As the CNO, I serve as the executive sponsor by attending all meetings with our nurse practice council, which includes a bedside nurse from each department. At the council meetings, nurses described the challenges and extensive time they spent documenting. In response, I partnered with our finance and process engineering departments and one of the schools of nursing to document the exact time nurses spent in the EMR. This review identified that nurses spent more than 180 minutes per shift in the EMR. Together with IT, the regulatory manager, and clinical nurses, we have been able to decrease documentation by more than 20 minutes per shift and continue to work to decrease this time to allow nurses more time with their patients. Technology is critical today and continues to be one of the top 5 critical skills for nurses at all levels to continually advance nursing practice and ensure a safe environment.

The fifth DNP Essential for the CNO is the Interprofessional Collaboration for Improving Patient and Population Health Outcomes. The DNP curriculum provides strong skills for innovation with care delivery, interdisciplinary and interprofessional improvement projects, and influencing community health programs and societal health. Hospital and health system administrators should be enthusiastic about the contribution of the DNP nurse leaders in new and reformed roles. The health care environment will improve with the integration of the DNP graduate competencies and systems approach to improvement. DNP-prepared nurses need to demonstrate and document their value to executives by presenting their work and improved outcomes.[8]

There is nothing a nurse can do without other members of the health care team. All areas of operations, from support services and facility operations, to finance, technology, regulatory, process engineering, to the entire hands-on care team including providers, therapists, pharmacists, licensed and non-licensed team members. This required collaboration with open, transparent, and genuine communication, always assuming good intent of each other, is the first step to improvement work. Academic programs in the field of communication should include at a minimum for health care: using and determining the most appropriate communication tool or method for the situation; technology communication; conducting effective meetings; encouraging healthy banters; managing conflict resolution; and public speaking. These are all elements in this DNP Essential and should be clearly documented on the DNP curriculum for practitioners, leaders, and educators.

The DNP Essentials are interwoven in the practice of the CNO. One example in my practice that addresses all of the areas would best be reflected by the work we have done to improve care of adults with significant development and physical disabilities (SDPD). The medical director of a home for adults with SDPD shared her concerns for the care these adults received at all acute care organizations in our community. I visited the center with the chief operating officer and medical social worker and learned about their care practices and the challenges faced during admission to acute care facilities. Understanding their challenges, the CNO championed for their care and led the formation of an interprofessional team. The team reviewed the evidence, conducted sited visits, evaluated current care, and developed an action plan. The plan was implemented and included team education, daily interprofessional team huddles with each patient/caregiver, revisions to the EMR, care protocols, family communication tools, and designation of specific units to ensure competency maintenance. Through these efforts, improvements we were able to significantly improve care as measured by more than a 50% decrease in length of stay, retainment of individual's adaptive equipment, improved nutrition, decreased pressure injuries by 80%, and improved communication with the patient and caregivers.

The DNP Essential that is the most significant weakness for my practice is closely aligned with the lack of time to dedicate to Health Care Policy for Advocacy in Health Care and a lack of the CNO being able to communicate this Essential to practice to other executives. Improvement in this area is necessary since nurses are the largest population of employees in most acute care facilities. One DNP Essential opportunity to continually improve and advance is the Clinical Prevention and Population Health for Improving the Nation's Health. The holistic practice of nursing would offer significant value to the national effort with population health.

The most threatened DNP Essential is the Advanced Nursing Practice role. Over the past 10 years, this role has aligned more with the medical staff at acute care organizations in part due to the medical staff and the advanced practice registered nurse's (APRN's) request, state rules associated with the lack of autonomy for the APRN, and the frequent interchange and lack of practice delineation with physician assistants. Another more obvious but often overlooked threat to the DNP Essential of Advanced Nursing Practice is also evident in the challenge many DNPs experience in the acute care environment using the title "Doctor."

The DNP Essentials or aspects of these elements and competencies are applicable to many nursing leadership roles. We have promoted the need for a DNP with succession planning for associate CNO roles, nursing vice presidents, and nursing directors by including them into job descriptions, requirements for positions, educational opportunities, and performance competencies and evaluations. Nurse managers seeking to advance their careers have also sought DNP degrees. In addition to the value for nurse leaders in designated leadership roles, the DNP program is also critical for nurse specialists who guide nursing practice and quality, and for nurse educators who are responsible to support nurses at all levels to continue to advance their practice at the bedside.

# BUSINESS PLAN USED IN DELINEATING THE DNP-PREPARED CHIEF NURSING OFFICER ROLE

A business plan was not used to support the DNP-prepared CNO role. Tuition prepayment is an organizational benefit to a lifetime maximum. The organization program supported 50% of the tuition for the DNP program. Only medical staff team members require a doctorate, so there was no salary increase with obtaining the degree. Various scholarships are available but competitive, so as an executive I did not feel it was appropriate to seek these limited funds. There was not a financial benefit, but since obtaining the degree I have been more productive, had easier access to opportunities, and have perceived an increased respect from medical and nursing team members.

Cost-benefit analysis of the CNO role with a DNP has not been officially reviewed by the organization. The previous 2 CNOs for the organization had an average tenure of less than 2 years. The skills obtained in the DNP program has helped me manage the stress of the role, be more efficient, and be effective with reaching and sustaining goals. Although the degree itself cannot be directly tied to financial impact, the DNP project during my course of study have helped the organization save more than $4 million annually. The organization implemented video monitoring to replace in-room sitters in 2008. The practice was revised in early 2009, which demonstrated consistent outcomes for falls with injury and self-harm events. We did not have evidence to support the program but consistent outcomes from in-room sitters. The DNP project was a quasi-experimental, 4x8 design series with non-randomized, consecutive sampling. The study identified no statistically significant variance in patient self-harm events or falls when using video monitoring with a statistically significant lower cost per patient a day. This study was used in consultation with state and federal regulators during organizational visits. This DNP project helped to change health care policy and organizational practice.

DNP-prepared nurses served as nursing role models have channeled their efforts to change care delivery, improve team outcomes, increase team engagement, and lower staff turnover. DNP-prepared nurses demonstrated an impact on patient outcomes by leading initiatives that addressed clinical care challenges such as infections and injuries or patient populations improvements with self-care and medication compliance.[9] Nursing is a vital element to ensuring access to value-based health care. The Health System Leadership–prepared DNP serving as a CNO will be a key informer and influencer of decisions concerning health care delivery, communicating the value of patient-centered care, ensuring high reliability and integrity of nursing practice with effective use of resources.[10]

# INCORPORATION OF EVIDENCE-BASED PRACTICE, DATA MINING, AND OUTCOMES

Incorporating evidence into practice is essential for all CNOs. The DNP in a leadership role has competence to develop new concepts by restructuring and leading innovative practice changes that improve the care provided while ensuring fiscal responsiveness. When facilitating innovative changes, the DNP is able to connect these changes with the goals of an organization and more importantly with the health of the community.[11] A CNO with a DNP degree has extensive experience reviewing and determining the strength of the evidence and identifying the best evidence for the work environment requiring change. Once evidence is evaluated, the DNP has extensive experience with performance improvement methodologies, change management theories, and data analysis tools. One key to success with performance improvement work is understanding common and special cause variations with control charts to support a comprehensive analysis of actual improvement. This knowledge and experience gained through the DNP program is how I have been able to be more effective and efficient as the CNO. Doctorate-prepared nurses often work on system projects, impacting the organizational outcomes and recommending new models of care delivery. DNP-prepared nurses have demonstrated success using available data to assist leadership with options to achieve or exceed organizational goals.[9]

Effective evidence-based practice is available through a number of examples. As explained previously, the nursing team identifies what needs to change to support the organizational strategic plan, how they will measure that change, and document it as the annual nursing priorities. The goals and metrics are reviewed and revised by all levels of nurses through the Shared Governance councils. Evidence is reviewed to identify the best structure and processes to obtain the nursing sensitive outcomes. Literature reviews are conducted prior, throughout the process change timeline, and post-improvement to ensure the nursing practice remains on the cutting edge and provides the safest patient care.

Over the past 6 years, the nursing priorities focused on preventing patient harm from pressure injuries, falls, urinary catheters, and central line catheters. Evidence is reviewed annually and documented on an evidence table for each of the teams. Interventions to incorporate into practice are identified at the unit or organizational level and with interprofessional team members, including pharmacy, nutrition, therapies, security, and the medical staff. The most significant change implemented was the individual case reviews of all harm events. This started with pressure injuries and is now conducted for falls with injury, central and urinary catheter infections, sepsis cases, and deep vein thrombosis. A review document has been developed for each event and is completed by the team closest to the event. The team conducts a gap analysis by sharing a brief summary of the patient's case and focusing on the barriers they experienced with ensuring patient safety. Identified opportunities have been from minor to system-wide and resulted in sustained change with more than a 90% decrease in pressure injuries, consistently exceeding national benchmarks for falls with injury, and initial improvement with urinary and central line catheters, currently demonstrating a controlled practice. The CNO and other nursing leaders attend these meetings and work to promptly implement changes the team request to eliminate barriers

Data analysis and evidence review has also helped in discussion to support increased staffing. During discussions with the chief executive officer, the CNO was able to articulate the nurse-to-patient ratio as aligned with national benchmarks, but the challenge was with certified nursing assistants (CNAs)-to-patient ratios. He requested more information and a cost-benefit analysis. The CNO was able to promptly provide staffing evidence, increases in staff members and costs of $1.7 million, and expected outcomes with patient experience, and reduction in falls with injury and pressure injuries. Rapid hire of more than 80 CNAs was supported by human resources, patient experience, and the nurse managers. To improve success with retention and meeting metrics, the CNO met with the vice president and nurse manager of clinical education to revise the CNA onboarding program. The program was revised based on published and nationally presented program success and included simulation. Performance improvement is constant for an effective CNO and takes on many forms.

Another example of using evidence and performance improvement science to improve outcomes was in relation to team engagement. The CNO identified that clinical nurses and nurse manager engagement was not improving although many interventions were implemented. The CNO conducted a literature review and identified that the manager's span of control was directly related to team engagement. Literature demonstrated that managers with less than 15 employees had the best team engagement, while managers with less than 40 employees also had better team engagement. In review of my nurse managers span of control, almost all had more than 40 employees and a number had more than 100. The nurse manager responsibility for patient engagement is also critical for patient outcomes. As a CNO with a DNP degree, I applied the team member engagement evidence to patient engagement. I added the team members and average daily census together to better reflect the nurse manager true span of control. A cost-benefit analysis was developed with expected measurable outcomes.

The information was presented to nurses, nurse leaders, the patient experience officer, the chief financial officer, chief human resource officer, and the chief executive officer. Support was obtained to decrease the nurse manager span of control with the requirement that if expected change in patient engagement, patient safety, team member engagement, and registered nurse turnover was not reached, span of control would return to previous ratios. To effectively and promptly onboard multiple new nurse managers, the CNO, clinical education, and a graduate nursing student developed a 65-hour program taught by successful nurse managers and leaders throughout the organization. Improvements have been demonstrated and sustained in all areas since this change. Registered nurse turnover was 3% above the state average prior to the change and has improved to more than 2% less than the state average and continues to trend down.

The DNP education provided a comprehensive foundation with data analysis, performance improvement, and change management for the CNO to be effective and efficient incorporating evidence into practice to improve outcomes for patients and the team. Results of the improved outcomes are celebrated by nurses on an ongoing basis with unit celebrations, Shared Governance council's full-day conferences, and during our fourth consecutive successful Magnet appraiser visit. Based on the continuous improvement practices of nurses at all levels annually, the CNO presents to the Board of Directors Quality Council.

# Interprofessional Collaboration

The DNP curriculum includes Interprofessional Collaboration for Improving Patient and Population Health Outcomes as an essential element for the DNP-prepared leader. Only through reliable evidence-based care delivery will our health care systems realize the quadruple aims throughout the continuum of care. A nurse leader who has obtained a DNP degree is equipped to partner with interprofessional teams to improve care delivery and health care

outcomes.[12] The CNO is involved in interprofessional collaboration constantly throughout each day. Members of the interprofessional team include nurses at all levels and in all settings of the organization, nurse leaders, interdisciplinary team members and leaders, executives, medical staff, universities and schools of nursing, and board members. The focus of these discussions is rarely specific to application of DNP education. The only discussions where it has been significant is with the medical staff when discussing the nurses and advanced practice nurse scope of practice, human resource members when discussing education preparation for specific nursing positions, and with the chief operating officer and chief executive officer in discussing the skills of a DNP-prepared CNO.

Discussing the value of a DNP for the organization should be conducted more frequently. Nurses are almost half of the organizational team members, and close to one-third of the organizational expenses. The practice of nursing is continually changing and the environment in which we practice is complex and high risk. Nursing practice directly impacts patient safety, engagement, length of stay, and outcomes. Nurses and the practice of nursing should be led by doctorate-prepared nurses who have knowledge and experience with performance improvement, implementing evidence into practice, and driving improved outcomes for patients and teams. Nurses who have undergraduate degrees in nursing and graduate degrees in other fields, such as business or health administration, are not as equipped or knowledgeable to evaluate current nursing practice and implement effective change.

# Professionalism

Organizational professionalism was included in the Nursing Strategic Priorities plan with measurable goals for all nursing team members. Key process measures to improve nursing professionalism include goals aligned with 80% of registered nurses obtaining a Bachelor of Science degree in nursing by December 2020; increasing American Nurses Credentialing Center–certified nurses; revision of the Clinical Ladder for nurses, and implementation of a CNA ladder; publishing in peer-reviewed journals or presenting at state or national conferences; and most importantly, exceeding national benchmarks for nursing engagement. In 2019, nurses exceeded the national Nursing Excellence average in all 7 categories including: autonomy; adequacy of resources and staffing; fundamentals of nursing quality care; interprofessional relationships; leadership access and responsiveness; professional development; and registered nurse to registered nurse teamwork and collaboration. This improvement was accomplished through a commitment and dedication to improving work environment using evidence, strategic planning, and collaboration.

Promoting the practice of nursing has been a professional goal of mine since first starting in a bachelor's degree program. This passion has become stronger as I advanced my education and increased the scope of my responsibilities. I have also had many mentors who had this same passion for nursing practice. Since obtaining my DNP degree, I have had the opportunity to expand my professionalism by publishing my capstone DNP project and presenting it at a national conference. I have also taken the opportunity to partner with nurses at all levels and interprofessional team members to publish in peer-reviewed journals and present at state and national conferences.

Certification is a measure of professionalism and although I had nursing administration certification prior to obtaining my DNP degree, I have been successfully sustaining this certification. As part of my DNP clinical hours, I was able to become a certified professional in health care quality and sustained it since that time. I have also served as an officer in a regional professional organization, a board member of a state professional organization, and a member of a national CNO steering committee. Prior to earning my DNP degree, I served on a community hospice board and as the board representative to their Quality Council. Since earning my DNP degree, I was elected to serve on the hospice system board of directors along with the executive and finance committees of the board.

Since obtaining a DNP degree, I have been relentless in encouraging nurses and interprofessional team members to present and publish our many successful practices. One increase in my professionalism since earning my DNP degree has been serving as a preceptor and mentor for bachelor's, master's, and doctorate-prepared nurses and administrative fellows. The DNP education has made advancing my and others' professionalism and advocating for nursing practice a constant topic of discussion.

## Pearls/Takeaways

Nurses at all levels and in all settings should take a risk, get involved, conduct research, and offer to lead or facilitate improvements. Speak up, find your courage, and empower yourself with education. While in a DNP program, use your clinical time to your career advantage by obtaining national nursing and professional certifications such as Lean Six Sigma. Seriously consider using at least some of your clinical time outside of your organization, and branch beyond nursing with other professionals or executives in information technology, finance, or process engineering.

Even after obtaining your doctorate degree, never stop learning and getting involved at your organization, with professional organizations, or serving on boards. Seek additional certifications, attend and present at state and national organizations, publish your results even if they do not reach goals, and/or be active with public policy. Obtain public speaking education and experience through programs such as Toastmasters International, a professional organization committed to improving public speaking skills.

Public speaking and emotional intelligence are critical skills for nursing leaders and not a significant focus in the DNP Health System Leadership curriculum. Nurses with a DNP need to be able to successfully advocate for the practice of nursing, promote advances in nursing practice, and engage nurses, other professionals, executives, and politicians. CNOs and DNPs must be collaborative interprofessional partners, which requires excellent communication and emotional intelligence skills.

In addition to courses in communication, the DNP Health Systems Leadership program should expand on the clinical topics of pharmacology, pathophysiology, and genetics to address pharmacology and care management issues at a system level with implementation of high-risk or high-cost medication or transition of care instead of the intense focus on diagnosis and prescribing. Pharmacology is a high expense and high risk for organizations. The lectures and exams could have focused on both clinical concepts and organizational concepts to make it more applicable to a DNP leadership program.

The DNP Health Systems Leadership program was developed to provide the nurse leader with advanced education to practice in a high-level leadership role and to achieve improved patient outcomes through evaluation and implementation of evidence-based practices. The Master of Business Administration or Master of Health Administration programs can provide comprehensive skills with financial and business practice but cannot exclusively prepare the nurse leader or CNO to address the health care system challenges present in today's organizations.[12]

## Conclusion: Impact of the DNP Degree

As a result of obtaining my DNP degree 2 years into the CNO role, I have improved my skills in the areas of evidence evaluation, data analysis, strategic planning, prioritizing, execution on goals, operational efficiency, and change management. Likewise, I have gained significant respect from my medical partners, executive team peers, and practicing nurses. Evidence evaluation and data analysis are routinely conducted using meta-analysis and evidence tables to guide practice decision making. Progress on the nursing strategic priorities is communicated monthly at the nursing leadership forum. During my tenure, nurse leader competencies have been established and the requirement of a DNP degree has been promoted for nursing executive positions. Change management strategies enabled biomedical device integration with the EMR. Case reviews were enacted as a performance improvement methodology to prevent future patient harm. Measured outcomes from practice change occurred with changes to the nurse manager span of control decreasing nurse turnover below the state benchmark and an initiative to improve care for the vulnerable population with SDPD led to decreases in hospital-acquired pressure injuries, length of stay, and improved communication. Implementation of my DNP project, which utilized video monitoring in place of room sitters, led to a multi–million-dollar cost savings for the organization.

Completing a DNP degree will provide a nurse with methods, tools, and experience to be more effective and efficient. The essence of the DNP program is to implement evidence-based care to improve patient outcomes and the system. As a nurse leader, this is my daily mission. Working on DNP-type projects is how I spend the majority of my time. The DNP program has provided me with additional knowledge and skills to be more effective, efficient, and scientific in my work. The DNP degree is an excellent program for nursing leaders and should be a requirement for CNOs.

## Acknowledgments

My success as the CNO has been made possible by the TGH nursing team members, interprofessional and interdisciplinary partners, my mentors and preceptors, and the organizational leaders who took a chance on me years ago and continue to do so.

## References

1. Falkenberg-Olson, A. Research translation and the evolving PhD and DNP practice roles: A collaborative call for nurse practitioners. *J Am Assoc Nurse Pract*. 2019;31:447-453.

2. Fulton J, Kuit J, Sanders G, Smith P. The role of the professional doctorate in developing professional practice. *J Nurs Manag*. 2012;20:130-139.

3. Hartjes T, Lester D, Arasi-Ruddock L, Bradley S, Munro S, Cowan L. Answering the question: is the doctor of philosophy or doctor of nursing practice right for me? *J Am Assoc Nurse Pract*. 2019;31(8):439-442.

4. Rugs D, Barrett B, Chavez M, et al. Doctoral-prepared nurses in the Veterans Health Administration: a cross sectional survey. *J Prof Nurs*. 2019;36(1):62-68. doi:https://doi.org/10.1016/j.profnurs.2019.06.008

5. Malloch, K. Leading DNP professionals practice competencies for organizational excellence and advancement. *H Nurs Admin*. 2017;41(1):29-38.

6. Altman SH, Butler AS, Shern L. *Assessing Progress on the Institute of Medicine Report The Future of Nursing*. National Academies Press; 2016.

7. Redman R, Pressler S, Furspan P, Potempa K. Nurses in the united states with a practice doctorate: implications for leading in the current context of health care. *Nurs Outlook*. 2015;63:124-129.

8. Tussing T, Brinkman B, Francis D, Hixon B, Labardee R, Chipps E. The impact of the doctorate of nursing practice nurse in a hospital setting. *J Nurs Adm*. 2018;48(12):600-602.

9. Beeber A, Palmer C, Waldrop J, Lynn M, Jones C. The role of doctor of nursing practice-prepared nurses in practice settings. *Nurs Outlook*. 2019;67:354-364.

10. Barry J, Winter J. Health system chief nurse executive is a DNP the degree of choice? *J Nurs Adm*. 2015;45(11):527-528.

11. Morgan D, Somera P. The future shortage of doctoral prepared nurses and the impact of the nursing shortage. *Nursing Admin Q*. 2014;38(1):22-26.

12. Stuart W. Why seek a doctorate-prepared nurse to join your team? *Health Care Manag*. 2018;37(3):220-224.

# CHAPTER 15

# LEADERS, CHANGE AGENTS
## THE UNIQUE CONTRIBUTIONS OF A DNP-PREPARED NURSE EXECUTIVE

*Kelly Hancock, DNP, RN, NE-BC, FAAN*

## INTRODUCTION

As the system chief nursing officer (CNO) of a large academic health system, I have the responsibility to lead the strategic direction for Cleveland Clinic's 28 000-member nursing team, including 15 000 bedside nurses, 1600 advanced practice nurses, 610 nurse leaders, and more. The nursing executive team consists of 9 associate chief nursing officers (ACNOs), 14 CNOs, and 4 nursing administration team members. Spearheading our health system's largest caregiver group (representing nearly half of the health system), I oversee nursing practice, development and education in inpatient, outpatient, rehabilitation, and home care fields throughout the systems' 165-acre main campus, 15 regional hospitals, 150 northern Ohio outpatient locations (including 18 full-service, family health centers and 3 health and wellness centers), and locations in Weston, Florida, Las Vegas, Nevada, Toronto, Canada, Abu Dhabi, United Arab Emirates, and London, England. I am a member of Cleveland Clinic's executive leadership team, reporting directly to the president and chief executive officer of our health system. I continually act to help Cleveland Clinic achieve and exceed established financial, operational, and clinical goals that include reducing care costs, making Cleveland Clinic a best-in-class workplace, developing superior clinical care, research, education and innovation, and improving quality, safety, and care experience. This executive role in nursing leadership has positioned Cleveland Clinic nursing as the world leader in nursing excellence.

In 2010, the Institute of Medicine (IOM) released "The Future of Nursing" report. In this report, nurses were encouraged to step up and prepare for the future. The report included educating leaders at all levels and the authors recommended that nurses receive leadership development at every level in order to transform the health care system. It was recommended that we double the number of nurses holding doctoral degrees to enhance nursing's ability to work collaboratively with physicians and lead change in health care. I assumed my role as executive CNO in 2012. I quickly realized that I wanted to and had an obligation to pursue my Doctor of Nursing Practice (DNP) education. I graduated with my DNP degree in 2015. The decision to pursue my DNP degree was my own. I felt that I was positioning my organization well to meet the IOM's call to action for higher education for all nurses. I also knew that I would have to create a culture

Benson LA, ed. *The DNP Professional: Translating Value From Classroom to Practice* (pp 167-171). © 2021 SLACK Incorporated.

that would fuel creativity, elevate novel solutions, and develop new or improved resources to drive costs down, advance care, improve outcomes, and propel Cleveland Clinic nurses onto the national platform.

The evidence shows that DNP nurse leaders have served as experts for change in health care environments through systems thinking, knowledge of health policy, health economics, and building interprofessional teams.

# DNP Essentials: The Impact of the DNP-Prepared Nurse Executive

The health care environment is experiencing a significant overhaul and organizations must be prepared to respond quickly and effectively to extreme, groundbreaking change. The DNP-prepared nurse executive has positively impacted health care organizations through increasing quality, strengthening patient outcomes, decreasing costs, and influencing health policy.

Recommendations were made by the 2010 IOM report for new health care delivery models to support quality care that favorably impacts clinical outcomes. Due to the increase in medical errors, the report also called for educating health care professionals so they can effectively develop strategies to address those errors.[1] DNP-prepared nurse executives have gained new knowledge on the importance of quality improvement and therefore will promote the engagement in and support of quality initiatives to prevent harm from occurring.[1] DNP Essential V: Interprofessional Collaboration for Improving Patient and Population Health Outcomes provides knowledge and the importance of high-functioning interdisciplinary teams. I have used the knowledge I acquired through my DNP education to enhance the way we think about building a culture of improvement in my organization. It is about creating organization alignment, using visual management, building problem-solving capabilities, and standardizing processes for sustainment of efforts. In partnership with the Department of Continuous Improvement, we co-created and provided education to nursing professionals at the bedside to encourage their engagement and ownership of quality and clinical outcomes. The idea was to create a culture where our nursing caregivers are capable, empowered, and expected to make improvements every day. The implementation of this new approach has allowed for those delivering the care to be directly involved in the improvement efforts; we have seen a decline in hospital-acquired infections, decrease in overall fall rate by 15%, and an increase in both patient and caregiver experience.

As it relates to health care policy, the DNP-prepared nurse executive has an opportunity to act as a change agent to effect health care policy.[2] As the national landscape of the health care environment continues to evolve from volume to value, health care needs leaders who can influence and challenge normative thinking about how the care is being delivered and by whom.[3] The DNP-prepared nurse executive has gained new insight through their education to influence health care policies, regulations, and reimbursement associated with care delivery models.[4] Additionally, DNP Essential V: Health Care Policy For Advocacy in Health Care provides insight on how to critically analyze health policy from the perspective of the stakeholders.[5] This knowledge can assist a nurse executive to create a framework either locally or nationally to influence the delivery of health care services across the continuum of care.

An example of how I utilized that knowledge in my organization was establishing a Cleveland Clinic Nursing Institute Legislative and Health Policy Council. This council focuses on education, analysis, and influence of political and practical issues that impact the nursing profession and the delivery of health care. Caregivers that participate on this council represent a broad range from bedside nurses, to managers, to leaders in regional hospitals, to our family health centers. One of the nurse leaders involved in this council was instrumental in working to pass an Ohio State House bill that allowed advanced practice providers to admit patients to hospitals in our state under certain conditions. Another example would be how a clinical nurse who is a diabetic educator works closely with the American Diabetes Association's National Advocacy Committee on multiple state and federal issues. This work has influenced practice and policy changes that were necessary to better deliver care to patients with diabetes.

DNP Essential VIII: Advanced Nursing Practice is where I gained knowledge on how to better leverage the role of the advanced practice registered nurse (APRN) in my organization. Cleveland Clinic's APRNs provide patient care throughout its numerous hospitals, family health centers, outpatient clinics, and ambulatory care settings. To further train the growing number of nurses in pursuit of advanced practice roles, Cleveland Clinic strategically developed its first-ever APRN fellowship. Additionally, members of this fellowship, which was created in 2014, were actively involved in the promotion of the APRN Modernization Bill. State House Bill 216 officially expanded APRN authority in the state of Ohio. With cost and access as primary drivers of current and projected APRN growth, we identified specific growth areas: expansion of express care clinics and implementation of novel APRN roles, such as the house officers and hospitalist/intensivist role, e-hospital and distance health roles, and expansion of international APRN services. Cleveland Clinic Abu Dhabi is the first Middle Eastern country to utilize APRNs since 2017. The APRN-led house officer program allowed Cleveland Clinic to transition house officers from contracted physician providers to advanced practice providers. In a 1 year, post-implementation survey completed by caregivers at the first 2 community hospitals to implement the program, findings showed improved intensive care unit patient management, global house officer responsiveness, nurse-provider communication, procedural competencies, and a proactive approach to identifying barriers to discharge of patients.

There are many milestones in the advancement of nursing education and in academia. Following Florence Nightingale and the first established appprenticed-based nurse training program in 1860 at St. Thomas Hospital in London, the education of nursing professionals at its core emphasized direct nursing care and how to educate for that care. New York University granted the first PhD in nursing in the 1930s.[6] As a result of allocated federal funding in 1960, an effort was now underway to prepare nurses as scholars and researchers.[6] Over the years, there was an increase in nursing programs granting PhD degrees with an emphasis on academics, science, and research. A gap still existed to earn a doctoral degree that had an emphasis on clinical expertise and scholarship that could be used in a variety of settings including academia.[6] This is where the DNP education was being considered to fill that space.

DNP-prepared educators in academia and in health care organizations make the connection between education and clinical practice.[6] In my health care organization, the senior nurse educators are all DNP-prepared. Our organization has a nurse residency program for new nurse graduates, which is competency-based and supported by simulation. The lead for our residency program is a DNP-prepared nurse educator. The advantage of having her in that role with the knowledge she has garnered through her DNP program is that it has allowed her to bridge the gap between academia and clinical practice. The 2 overarching goals of the residency are to improve practice readiness of novice nurses to ensure a competent workforce and enhance training, skills, and knowledge needed to deliver both safe and effective care.

A professional enrichment experience designed to support and challenge clinical nurses on the frontlines of health care was founded and led by a DNP-prepared clinical nurse specialist. This experience allowed for clinical nurses to examine their profession and reinforce the idea that they are indeed leaders. The content of this course includes readings and discussions on topics essential to clinical leadership to include communicating emphatically, expressing appreciation, and harnessing the science of stamina to remain resilient. The outcomes of this experience include an increased awareness by the participants of their crucial role in health care as well as an increased and renewed sense of purpose.

# SWOT Analysis: Overarching Challenges in the Field

The complexity and evolution of the health care system in the United States has created fragmented care delivery models that are not cost-effective. The United States spends 2.5 to 3.0 times more on health care than any other country.[7]

The challenges facing health care providers today are enormous. Pressure to maintain and improve quality, safety, and patient and caregiver experience in an environment that is resource constrained is concerning for health care leaders. The lack of coordinated care across providers, as well as settings particularly for patients at risk such as those with chronic illness, can be attributed to the increases in costs and decreases in quality that are seen.

Health care environments are at the same time experiencing workplace violence by patients and visitors. This has become a major health and safety issue for health care workers and can lead to a series of adverse consequences.[6] Declining reimbursements, along with rising costs of care, have contributed to lack of resources available to address the challenges that organizations are facing today.

Many organizations are addressing these challenges by seeking DNP-prepared nurse executives who can balance the need to increase quality of care while making it affordable.[8] The education gained through a DNP program allows nurse executives to redesign systems of care and provide cost-saving solutions to patient care challenges.

In my organization, one of our DNP-prepared leaders is leading an interdisciplinary effort to decreasing central line blood stream infections (CLABSI). I lead monthly operating reviews with the leaders that have responsibility for the quality and patient safety indicators. This review allows for recognition of the efforts and discussion on the opportunities. The system intensive care units CLABSI rates have a reduction of 23%, which equates to approximate cost saving of $17 000 per CLABSI. The key elements of the strategies focus on implementing practice changes, evaluating the impact of those changes to include the clinical outcomes for patients, and the cost of care to decreasing the infection rates.

Another example in my organization is that one of the DNP leaders is co-leading a workplace violence committee along with one of our physicians. I am one of the executive sponsors of this committee, and I participate in a quarterly report with the leaders of this committee. The quarterly meetings review work that has been completed and what needs to be done in order to meet the established objectives and key outcomes. The DNP leader has been able to work collaboratively to design an education program that curtails workplace violence incidents and improves the resiliency of caregivers. The best practices that have come out of this interprofessional council include de-escalating training, development of an online system for caregivers to report incidents, and support resources for caregivers affected by workplace violence. We have seen a decrease in workplace violence incidents as measured through our internal event reporting system and an increase in caregiver engagement measured by our recent caregiver engagement survey.

The need for insightful leaders in health care organizations can be addressed through DNP-prepared nurse executives. The broad-reaching impact of these type of leaders can be seen from clinical practice, continuous improvement, and care affordability efforts.

# SWOT Analysis: Current Problems

The nursing shortage of the future involves new driving forces that include global economic and health care reform. In the United States, the nursing shortage has been cyclic over the years. In the next 10 to 15 years, it is expected that close to 1 million nurses will retire due to the fact that 55% of the nursing workforce is more than 50 years old.[9] The complexity of today's health care environment as described in this chapter has led to nurse turnover in organizations, which is also contributing to the shortage. Health care organizations are then faced with paying premium dollars for staff to work additional shifts as well as bringing in agency temporary staff. Among newly licensed registered nurses, the first year turnover rate is on the rise. This comes at a tremendous cost to an organization. According to NSI Solutions, the average cost for turnover for a registered nurse is estimated at \$37 700 to \$58 400.[9] Reasons for this turnover include nurse burnout, the balance of career and family, the threat of workplace violence, and advances in technology.

Nursing is rooted in a holistic approach to caring for patients and their families. Caring and respecting each patient's dignity and integrity is fundamental to that approach. The increasing demands of today's nursing workforce along with diminishing resources has at times compromised the values and beliefs of the professional nurse. This can lead to moral distress. The American Nursing Association's Code of Ethics (2015) requires professional nurses to speak up when we feel something is not right, unjust, and inequitable.[10,11] Education is key. Fitzpatrick speaks about the concept of teaching moral courage to nursing students, so they are empowered early in their career to speak up.[11] The need to educate early on may help mitigate future moral distress and burnout. Conversely, in the acute care setting, the need to have senior-level nurse leaders able to address these concerns is imperative.

DNP-prepared nurse executives can help prepare nurses to deliver that high-quality care they want to give and address their concerns when their values are challenged. These leaders have the knowledge to understand different perspectives of all team members and their professions. They provide strategic operational awareness that supports caregivers at all levels in identifying and addressing barriers. In our recent caregiver experience survey, the nursing caregivers highest scoring questions were (1) my team discusses ways to prevent errors (93rd percentile rank) and (2) caregivers feel they can speak up regarding negative patient care (82nd percentile rank). These leadership skills create a sense of empowerment amongst all team members.[12] Empowerment is essential to the advancement of the profession of nursing.

# Outcomes and Value Added

It is critical for health care systems who employ DNP-prepared nurse executives to evaluate and capture their value and contributions to the organization. This is done by developing a standardized approach to communicating clinical and operational outcomes of DNP nurse executives. The knowledge that a DNP-prepared nurse executive has is beneficial to health care organizations impacting health care decisions at all levels of practice management and executive administration. Their contributions are extraordinary. Sharing exemplars of their impact on the profession itself, providers, partners, and the overall health care system is the first step. This can be done by a variety of mechanisms, the first of which is publishing. The promotion of the value to a health care organization of having a DNP-prepared nurse executive can be done through publications.[13] The publications should include a focus on how the leader is able to facilitate organizational change that is evident by favorable impact to both clinical and business metrics. The DNP-prepared nurse executive is in a prime position to collaborate with partners in academia to ensure that proposed student capstone projects are focused on current issues in health care. In my organization, we mentor many students pursuing a DNP degree. The mentor will often suggest a project that is addressing a strategic priority that can have a measurable impact. Create a forum to ensure all DNP students (whether they are employed at your organization or not) have the ability to share the results of their project to your organization's executive team. This creates an awareness of the education provided in the curriculum, the value of that work, and demonstrates the need to have nurse leaders prepared at that level.

# Professionalism

As the number of DNP students interested in leadership roles continues to grow, we have a professional obligation to ensure we provide more opportunities for mentorship and capstone projects. Inviting and incorporating these students into our organizations will allow for a better understanding of how to utilize the knowledge gained from that experience in the future. I routinely have provided mentorship and preceptorship to a variety of DNP students. I also provide input through my involvement in a variety of advisory councils for nursing programs both locally and nationally. One example of providing an opportunity for a capstone project in my organization is that I have a DNP student working with me and my team on the monthly operating reviews that I have with the nurse leaders. As mentioned earlier, not only do we discuss quality, patient safety, and experience, but we also review established metrics around caregiver growth and development, caregiver engagement, and financial stewardship. This student is actively involved in reviewing the overall data, identifying the opportunities, participating in the monthly reviews, and is actively involved in one of the strategies around quality. This experience will allow the student to reflect on her learning from her DNP program thus far and help her understand how the DNP Essentials are core to being an effective systems-level nurse leader.

# Conclusion: Impact of the DNP Degree

As a result of obtaining my DNP degree, I have been able to create a culture of innovation and transformation within Cleveland Clinic nursing and the health system. This is a culture that fuels creativity, elevates novel solutions, and develops new or improved resources to drive costs down, advance care, and improve outcomes. The impact of this culture directly affects practice, advocacy, clinical research, and innovative thinking, which enhances nurse engagement, clinical outcomes, and professionalism.

Specifically, I have helped foster a culture of improvement that embraces the DNP degree and its associated value. Preparation of DNP professionals has been encouraged and promoted. All nurse educators are DNP-prepared. Other DNP nurse leaders have led successful initiatives for CLABSI reduction, reduction of workplace violence, and professional experience enrichment designed to engage frontline clinical nurses in exploring their role as nurse leaders. I have served as the organizational coordinator for the monthly operating reviews with the leaders that have responsibility for the quality and patient safety indicators. Through this new enculturation there has been a decrease in health care acquired infections and falls and an increase in patient and nurse satisfaction.

Health care systems today need organizational leadership that can drive change effectively. DNP-prepared nurse executives are those change agents. They acquire leadership strategies that allow them to draw from their new competencies to impact patient and organizational outcomes. They have new knowledge on how to best lead interprofessional teams to ignite sparks for change in complex health care delivery systems.

# Acknowledgments

I would like to start by thanking my inspirational mentor, Dr. Nancy Albert. Her example of life-long learning and service to others has always inspired me during my professional nursing career. Thanks to everyone at Cleveland Clinic who has helped shape me as an executive nurse leader. I am honored and humbled to serve with a community of great leaders and I am privileged to follow in the footsteps of those who came before me. Lastly, I would like to thank my wonderful husband, Eric, and our 2 extraordinary children, Eric and Amanda. Your unwavering support of my career has been my foundation of strength and I will always be grateful for your love.

# References

1. Dunbar-Jacob J, Nativio D, Khalil H. Impact of nursing practice education in shaping healthcare systems of the future. *J Nurs Educ.* 2013;52:423-427.

2. Fain J, Asselin M, McCurry M. The DNP. Why now? Several broad-scale healthcare factors influenced nursing policy makers to roll out the doctorate of nursing practice degree in the midst of a national shortage. *Nurs Manage.* 2008;39(7):34-37.

3. Kendall-Gallagher D, Breslin E. Developing DNP students as adaptive leaders: a key strategy in transforming in transforming healthcare. *J Prof Nurs.* 2013;29(5):259-263.

4. Sherrod B, Goda T. DNP-prepared leaders guide healthcare system change. *Nurs Manage.* 2016;49(9):13-16.

5. Hain A, Schlosser S. Using problem-based learning to teach health policy at the DNP level. *Nurse Educ.* 2014;39(3):118-121.

6. Bellini S, McCauley P, Cusson R. The doctorate of nursing practice graduate as faculty member. *Nurs Clin North Am.* 2012;47(4):547-556.

7. Salmond S, Echevarria M. Healthcare transformation and changing roles for nursing. *Orthop Nurs.* 2017;36(1):12-19.

8. Tussing T, Brinkman B, Francis D, Hixon B, Labardee R, Chipps E. The impact of the doctorate of nursing practice nurse in a hospital setting. *J Nurs Adm.* 2018;48(12):600-602.

9. Ackerson K, Stiles K. Value of nurse residency programs in retaining new graduate nurses and their potential effect on the nursing shortage. *J Contin Educ Nurs.* 2018;49(6):282-288.

10. Code of ethics for nurses with interpretive statements. American Nurses Association. https://www.nursingworld.org/practice-policy/nursing-excellence/ethics/code-of-ethics-for-nurses/coe-view-only/

11. Fitzpatrick J. Teaching moral courage: obligation and challenge. *Nurs Educ Perspect.* 2018;39(4):200.

12. Grace P. Enhancing nurse moral agency: the leadership promise of doctor of nursing practice preparation. *Online J Issues Nurs.* 2018;23(1).

13. Malloch K. Leading DNP professionals: practice competencies for organizational excellence and advancement. *Nurs Adm Q.* 2017;41(1):29-38.

14. Us, sunt. Officid estium es nonsentis de aut lacerrum accabo. Nam, quam endit libus a autem aut quiae venes rectat.

# CHAPTER 16

# Aligning DNP Practice With the Mission and Strategic Priorities of the Organization

*Debra A. Burke, RN, DNP, MBA, NEA-BC*

## Introduction

The role of senior vice president for patient care and chief nursing officer (CNO) at a large, academic medical center is complex. Responsibilities include creating an environment that attracts and retains talented individuals and fostering a spirit of innovation and creative problem-solving. The job requires professional advocacy within and outside the organization, fiscal responsibility, and fundraising. But first and foremost, the CNO is responsible for ensuring the delivery of high-quality care throughout the institution. Leading in this ever-growing dynamic health care environment takes both progressive leadership experience and strong educational underpinnings to help navigate and prioritize the daily challenges and develop the longer-term strategic plan.

Our organization's 4-part mission focuses on advancing practice, education, research, and service to the community. As the chief nurse, I must address each of these important areas of the mission within my role. The following is the mission of the Massachusetts General Hospital:

*Guided by the needs of our patients and their families, we aim to deliver the very best health care in a safe, compassionate environment; to advance that care through innovative research and education; and to improve the health and well-being of the diverse communities we serve[1]*

In the following sections, I will discuss these 4 areas of the mission and how incorporating the Doctor of Nursing Practice (DNP) Essentials guides the practice of the CNO. But first, let's discuss why the DNP degree is important for the CNO.

## The DNP Degree and the Role of Chief Nursing Officer

For many years, the terminal degree for nurses was the Doctor of Philosophy (PhD). But as a nurse administrator, the PhD education does not necessarily align well with the required competencies of the practicing nurse executive. As described by the American Association of Colleges of

Benson LA, ed. *The DNP Professional:*
*Translating Value From Classroom to Practice* (pp 173-180).
© 2021 SLACK Incorporated.

Nursing (AACN), a PhD is the "formal education for a career in research and the scholarship of discovery."[2] This is generally not the focus of the CNO role. However, within the DNP program, there is education that addresses leadership skills, system analysis, and critical thinking that are all necessary competencies for the nurse executive.[3]

The Institute of Medicine "The Future of Nursing" report[4] also looked at the issue of how nurses can be fully engaged in addressing the needs of our health care system. This report called for life-long learning, including increasing the percentage of bachelor's-prepared nurses and a challenge to double the number of nurses prepared at the doctoral level of education. The AACN also addressed the need for higher education in their DNP position statement identifying the need for "a transformational change in the education required for professional nurses who will practice at the most advanced level of nursing."[2]

These reports have collectively called on health care system professions to theoretically examine how we educate our clinical disciplines as well as enhance our workforce knowledge and skill level.[5] Berwick describes that we need a health care leadership development strategy amongst health care professions. In order to meet the challenges ahead and the recommendations outlined in these reports, our profession has been called upon to address both the improvements needed in health care and the educational preparation of our nurses. The clinical doctorate has gained renewed invigoration as one way to fundamentally address these challenges.

Finally, working in an academic medical center where life-long learning is expected, continuing my education was not only encouraged but highly recommended. As I thought about my role as a nurse leader, I also viewed the pursuit of my DNP degree similar to the focus that we place on encouraging our clinical nurses to become certified. We know that certification is a way for nurses to demonstrate their knowledge and skill in a particular specialty. Should I not also hold myself to that same standard?

# DNP ESSENTIALS AND THE FOUR-PART MISSION

The DNP Essentials are considered the foundational outcome competencies for graduates of a DNP program (AACN).[2] As a nurse executive, I have integrated these Essentials into the CNO role using them to guide me in enhancing the professional practice environment. Of course, some of these are fundamental to the daily practice of the CNO while others are less prevalent. In the following sections, I will showcase examples of how I integrate the DNP Essentials in my administrative practice to address the 4 areas of my organization's mission statement; practice, education, research, and service to the community.

## *Mission Part I: Patient Care and the Practice Environment*

### DNP Essentials

- Scientific Underpinnings for Practice
- Clinical Scholarship and Analytical Methods for Evidence-Based Practice
- Advanced Nursing Practice
- Information Systems/Technology and Patient Care Technology for the Improvement and Transformation of Health Care

### Creating a Supportive Professional Practice Environment

The CNO is ultimately accountable for patient care delivery so they must create a practice environment that is safe and supportive for the practicing clinician. There is clear evidence that a healthy work environment is critical to ensure safe, quality patient care and serves as an environment where nurses chose to work.

The ability to attract and retain high-quality employees is crucial for ensuring excellence in patient care. In her book *Talent Magnetism*,[6] Matuson describes how creating an environment that is a "talent magnet" will ensure that you have the best employees and that they will come to you vs you needing to recruit. Crucial to creating that environment is constantly connecting with employees, being visible and approachable, and purposely staying close to those who you most value. It is also about meeting the needs and expectations of employees in what they are looking for in a leader. Based on extensive research done by Kouzes and Posner,[7] when asked what employees expect from their leader, they articulate the following 4 traits: (1) honesty, (2) someone who is forward looking, (3) competent, and (4) inspiring. These important traits and others described in the literature inform my own leadership practice.

Some of the ways that I stay connected with staff include attendance at unit staff meetings and hosting a staff nurse advisory committee where clinical nurses from across the organization meet with me and my leadership team every month. I also conduct night rounds so that I can connect with our off-shift staff.

As CNO, I need to continuously use objective data to inform me whether our practice environment is one that health professionals find supportive of their practice and result in high retention rates. In our organization, we utilize the Staff Perceptions of the Professional Practice Environment Survey, which is comprised of a psychometrically sound scale to assess nurses' and other health professions' perceptions of what is working and (as importantly) what is not working in the practice environment. A core component of the survey is the Professional Practice Work Environment Inventory (PPWEI) scale, which measures autonomy and control over practice; communication about patients; cultural sensitivity; handling disagreement and conflict; sufficient staff; time and resources for quality care; staff relations with physicians, staff and hospital groups; supportive leadership; teamwork; and work motivation.[8] Administration of this scale every 2 years provides me and my executive team with key signals about where we should focus. This has been critical in developing our strategic plan as well as addressing existing or emerging problems that staff might identify in a timely manner.

## Cultivating Transformational Leaders

Evaluation and continuous assessment of patient care delivery is the most important role of the CNO. One of the characteristics of an academic medical center are our highly acute patient populations who present with complex disease processes. These patient care needs demand a clinical workforce who are bringing the best art and science to their practice every day. Nurses need the support of leadership to help create an environment that supports their practice and helps them to grow in their profession. Our clinical leadership model of the nurse director (ND) and clinical nurse specialist (CNS)/nursing practice specialist (NPS) leadership team provide the support that meets the needs of the front-line clinician.

## Nurse Director or Nurse Manager

For years, I have known that the role of the ND (frontline nursing leader) is pivotal in creating a positive, professional practice environment. The literature described the ND as the chief retention officer and that nurses do not leave their hospitals, they leave their managers. This was the impetus for my DNP capstone project. I designed my project to explore the positive characteristics of NDs that contribute to high registered nurses' satisfaction. Utilizing units with high satisfaction scores, my study used a qualitative design to explore this question. Nine clinical nurses and 9 NDs met the inclusion criteria and each group identified 4 themes that reflect those positive characteristics of NDs (Table 16-1).[9]

I was struck that 3 of the characteristics that both staff and directors identified as important to staff satisfaction were identified by both groups: empowerment, visibility, and role modeling. Literature in this area often cite a difference in what managers and staff believe affect satisfaction. Clinical nurses also identified 1 unique characteristic, a "passion for excellence," as an important characteristic of NDs that provided them with excitement and inspiration to strive for excellence. NDs also identified a unique theme. Authentic presence was important and a key way for them to get to know and connect with staff in meaningful ways. They described authentic presence as interactions that were both "purposeful and deliberate" on their part. That presence was most often described as creating "meaningful" connections with staff. Those connections that they created with staff were both personal and professional.

These characteristics define transformational leadership. Recognizing what clinical nurses value in their nurse leaders helps to guide our leadership development efforts and the recruitment of effective leaders.

## Role of Clinical Nurse Specialists and Nurse Practice Specialists in Driving Quality Outcomes

Our clinical leadership model also includes the role of the CNS or NPS as part of the unit-based nursing leadership team. Both professionals are master's-prepared registered nurses who have clinical expertise within their specialty. I have set the expectation that pursuing a DNP or PhD degree is highly encouraged as their primary role is to enhance the skills and knowledge of our clinical nurses, utilizing scientific underpinning for practice. They provide leadership and coaching to staff to advance evidence-based practice (EBP) and quality improvement initiatives. The CNS/NPS also provides direct patient care. This affords them the opportunity to role model best practice to both novice and expert clinical nurses. The overarching goal of this role is to continuously improve patient outcomes on their respective units as well as meet organizational priorities such as prevention of pressure injuries, catheter-associated blood stream infections, and other nurse-sensitive quality indicators.

The ND-CNS/NPS dyads collectively address both unit-based needs as well as priorities of the organization. These priorities are based on specific patient outcomes that we seek to improve or the advancement of our performance. The following projects describe interventions to address some of those areas. Multiple units have tackled our "quiet at night" and "staff responsiveness" scores, as measured by the Hospital Consumer Assessment of Healthcare Providers and Systems (HCAHPS). We have struggled with our quiet at night scores in particular, since only 38% of our inpatient beds are private. These units have implemented initiatives found in the literature and also unique strategies based on the specific clinical area and patient populations that they serve. Significant staff input has also been important to ensure engagement in the process of change. These targeted strategies have resulted in improvement in our scores.

The ND-CNS/NPS leadership team is also responsible to ensure that we apply and then sustain changes in practice. This includes best practice for fall prevention and pressure ulcer prevention and other nurse-sensitive patient outcomes of care.

## Translating Evidence to Practice

EBP is a clinical decision-making process that integrates the best research evidence with clinical expertise and patient values and preferences to improve care. At our organization, we use the Johns Hopkins Nursing Evidence-Based Practice Model[10] and utilize their EBP toolkit to guide the process.

Semi-annually, we host an EBP educational program targeted to teams of nurses who want to address an issue

**Table 16-1**

## THEMES REFLECTING POSITIVE CHARACTERISTICS OF NURSE DIRECTORS FROM CLINICAL NURSE AND NURSE DIRECTOR PERSPECTIVES

| CLINICAL NURSE THEMES | NURSE DIRECTOR THEMES |
|---|---|
| • Empowerment: Empowering and reflective practice strategies enhance nurse autonomy<br><br>• Visibility: Visibility promotes interpersonal connections and a safe and caring environment<br><br>• Role modeling: Clinical nurses appreciate and value the high expectations and professional behaviors role modeled by NDs<br><br>• Manager passion and vision for excellence: ND passion and vision fosters the quest for excellence | • Empowerment: NDs empower clinical nurses by balancing autonomy and support/advocacy<br><br>• Visibility: Visibility fosters staff accountability, autonomy, and responsiveness<br><br>• Coaching/role modeling: In role modeling professional behaviors, NDs set clear standards and expectations for all staff<br><br>• Authentic presence: Authentic presence allows nurse directors the ability to come to know staff |

Adapted from Burke D, Flanagan J, Ditomassi M, Hickey P. Characteristics of nurse directors that contribute to registered nurse satisfaction. *J Nurs Adm*. 2017;47(4):219-225.

identified in their practice. These projects are also influenced by our organization's quality and safety data. The program provides the team with a comprehensive overview of the EBP process. Teams develop P-I-C-O questions (Patient/ Problem; Intervention; Comparison; Outcome) and are assigned an EBP mentor to guide them through their project. Those mentors are our CNS/NPS and other EBP experts. But most of the ideas for projects come from our clinical nurses. One recent project questioned why we were still using intravenous dextrose for the management of infant hypoglycemia. The outcome of this project was the evidence-driven shift to glucose gel.

This project, along with many others, have impacted cost of care by reducing patient length of stay, utilizing lower cost interventions, or eliminating unnecessary invasive procedures. I plan to share many of these EBP projects with our board of trustees during my annual address to illustrate the impact that nurse-driven evidence-based initiatives can have on patient outcomes and cost-effectiveness.

### Enabling Practice Through Technology

With the rapid development of enabling technology modalities to enhance practice, it is key that in my role, I create an environment where leveraging technology is embraced. Technology is part of our everyday work environment in health care since we utilize an electronic medical record (EMR).

We also use handheld technology to enhance our communication between providers and plan to exploit this technology further in the coming years to also include direct communication between providers and patients. We see opportunities to utilize this communication device to deliver information directly to clinicians (eg, patient monitoring data) and become a platform for direct linkage with our EMR thus reducing documentation time. We have plans to also utilize handheld devices to deliver just-in-time staff education and assist with staff scheduling.

It is crucial when establishing our technology goals to engage the frontline clinician in all of this work. We know that all of these enhancements are possible, but we need to meet the needs of the practicing clinician and patient as we examine what are the best uses of our technology.

## Mission Part II: Teaching and Education

### DNP Essential

• Interprofessional Collaboration for Improving Patient and Population Health Outcomes

Care delivery is a team sport requiring all clinical disciplines to come together to design the plan of care for each patient by integrating their respective discipline's expertise and domain of practice.

Interdisciplinary dedicated education units provide a structure for such learning and collaboration and allows for synthesis of ideas and the synthesis of characteristics from many disciplines. At the same time, it addresses students' individual differences and helps to develop important, transferable skills that they will bring to their professional practice.

## Interprofessional Dedicated Education Unit

A strategy we have employed to foster interdisciplinary education is a partnership we have launched between our organization and the Massachusetts General Hospital Institute of Health Professions (IHP). The Massachusetts General Hospital IHP is an independent graduate school of health sciences with students in nursing, physical therapy, occupational therapy, speech-language pathology, and physician assistant studies. This collaboration gave rise to the Interprofessional Dedicated Education Unit (IPDEU) at Massachusetts General Hospital. While the dedicated education unit (DEU) model has been around for many years as a means of supporting clinical instruction of nursing students, our team elevated this model to the next level by training our own clinicians to serve as interprofessional practice instructors (IPIs) for students.

Students spend 2 mornings on 1 of 3 IPDEUs at Massachusetts General Hospital. Each student spends time with a nurse IPI and an IPI from another profession. The students accompany their IPIs throughout all direct and indirect patient care activities, being prompted to focus on specific aspects of interprofessional practice (IPP) and engaging in formative huddles and debriefings throughout the morning.

The IPDEU provides real-world exposure to the Essential and often unexpected aspects of working in interprofessional teams, preparing students to apply these principles throughout their professional curriculum, and carry these skills and attitudes with them into their careers.

## Cultivating a Pipeline of Future Nurses

As the CNO, I need to not only focus on the retention of clinical staff, I also need to use data to analyze our ability to recruit health professionals to our organization. Those data are from our own organization, state level data, and also national market data. We then need to develop a plan to address our recruitment goals. DNP-prepared nurse leaders are in a unique position to develop initiatives to create nursing pipelines, evaluate transition into practice initiatives, and assess current educational programs. Two of my associate chief nurses decided to focus their DNP capstone studies on this topic. Both projects are aligned with addressing the priority of recruiting and retaining hard-to-recruit for specialty nurses such as oncology and perioperative nurses. This has resulted in strategies to attract both these specialty nurses as well as a more focused and individualized onboarding strategy.

## *Mission Part III: Research*

### DNP Essentials

- Scientific Underpinnings for Practice
- Clinical Scholarship and Analytical Methods for Evidence-Based Practice
- Organizational and System Leadership for Quality Improvement and Systems Thinking

## Research

With the goal of bringing the best art and science to patient care delivery, a nursing research infrastructure is critical to support nurses who bring clinical questions forward from their practice. As an academic medical center, we also have the responsibility to advance new nursing knowledge. Fostering a nursing research-intensive organization is a priority for our organization. Toward that end, the official dedication of the Yvonne L. Munn Center for Nursing Research was held in 2008. The center provides an infrastructure that promotes innovation and the mobilization of resources to support research initiatives that advance clinical practice and optimize quality patient-centered outcomes.[11] Goals of the center include:

- Accelerate research in core areas of focus
- Design strategies to promote the development, use, and translation of evidence into practice
- Foster innovation through the establishment, implementation, and evaluation of interventions that promote changes in care delivery
- Implement mentoring strategies to support a nursing research agenda
- Enhance visibility of research conducted by nurses through dissemination in high-impact journals and presentation at internal and external scientific meetings

As the CNO, I support this program by generating new partnerships and funding mechanisms within the organization and with external funding sources.

## DNP-PhD Forum

We are fortunate to have approximately 40 PhD-prepared and 40 DNP-prepared nurses in our organization and have recently launched the DNP-PhD Forum. The focus of the forum is to provide an opportunity for DNP- and PhD-prepared nurses to advance knowledge and promote an environment of inquiry and quality within our nursing practice environment. These professionals work independently and collaboratively to develop evidence, knowledge, and science to optimize nursing practice and drive improvements in patient care. During a recent forum, the members reviewed the article "Regenerating Nursing's Disciplinary Perspective".[12] The article analyzes the literature on the focus of the discipline of nursing, synthesizes the themes, and suggest areas of knowledge development for the discipline and strategies for moving forward in claiming, clarifying, and strengthening the discipline. The dialogue that ensued led to a call-to-action to leverage the education and expertise of the members of the forum to foster inquiry through EBP, quality improvement, innovation, and research. To accomplish this, the forum will be tapped to provide coaching and support for strategic initiatives.

## Quality Improvement

The late quality guru W. Edwards Deming[13] said that organizations must have a consistency of purpose and a deep and abiding dedication to constant, ongoing improvement in order to satisfy patients, beat the competition, and retain jobs. Deming's focus was on ensuring that continuous improvement was bred into the culture, not something that was momentary or occasional. He often challenged managers for being short-sighted and focusing on the wrong measures. He encouraged managers to invest in the long-term by focusing on meaningful measures of continuous improvement.

Organizations that excel at continuous improvement incorporate it into their values and reflect it in their hiring and training. They also incorporate it into their employee evaluation and compensation system. Continuous improvement is a way of life, not a passing fad or short-term fix.

In my role as chief nurse, I recognized that we needed to hardwire the performance improvement process into the clinical setting. Toward that end, we entered into a partnership with the American Association of Critical-Care Nurses to launch the Clinical Scene Investigator (CSI) Academy[14] to foster the integration of quality improvement into practice in 2018. The curriculum includes the following components: leadership; teamwork; project identification; social entrepreneurship; business case for quality; project implementation; data-collection and analysis; strategic communication; and scaling and sustaining projects. Over a 12-month period, with on-site and virtual training and coaching, clinical nurses are being empowered to lead change through innovation to drive improvement in patient outcomes and fiscal performance. Projects were selected based on their availability to advance or improve practice, promote change, replicability in other settings, and the ability to impact outcomes. Some of the topics chosen include improved ambulation for patients to reduce deconditioning, improving handoffs between clinicians, and addressing ICU delirium. The impact of this program is immeasurable. The program has provided development for both nursing leaders and clinical nurses and engaged them throughout the process, resulting in demonstrable outcomes and improved efficiency and cost-effectiveness. Because of the success of this program, planning is underway for the next cohort.

## *Mission Part IV: Service to the Community*

### DNP Essentials

- Organizational and System Leadership for Quality Improvement and System Thinking
- Health Care Policy for Advocacy in Health Care
- Clinical Prevention and Population Health for Improving the Nation's Health

The goal for the community service part of our mission is to elevate the health of the populations that we serve, particularly those in our closest geographic communities. Through community assessments, data analysis of patient outcomes, and patient satisfaction data, we were able to look at the health of our communities and assess equity in care amongst different patient populations. This information provides the basis on which we define our service to the community goals and strategies to reduce disparities and enhance the overall health of our communities.

As a member of the executive committee on community health, the CNO's responsibility is to support and develop strategies to advance this part of our mission. The community mission is described during new employee orientation to introduce all employees to this important part of our mission and also build into the strategic goals for each hospital executive, including the CNO.

The following are some of the programs that we have outlined as important to address the identified needs of our communities.

### Patient Assessment of Social Determinants of Health

Many people believe good health is determined by their access to doctors. Although important, about 80% of health status is determined by the social and economic conditions where you live and work. These social determinants of health include the financial and social supports available in our homes, neighborhoods, and communities; the quality of our schooling; the safety of our workplaces; the cleanliness of our water, food, and air; and the nature of our social interactions and relationships. They shape our health and the length and quality of our lives. Our organization is committed to ensuring its employees recognize social determinants of health barriers faced by their patients and the resources available to address them so they can be treated successfully.

### Anchor Institution Strategy

The anchor institution strategy at this academic medical center is intended to utilize hospital resources to benefit our local communities, specifically those who we have determined experience disparities and inequities. One strategy is to employ people from these communities. As CNO, our recruitment and pipeline programs are geared toward identifying those health professionals and non-professionals in our community and designing programs to support their successful transition into the workforce.

### Certified Nursing Assistant Training Grant

A good illustration of this is an initiative where I have partnered with human resources, a local educational institute, and my patient care services' team to remove obstacles to support career advancement for our service workers (eg, nutrition service coordinators, environmental service aides, unit service associates). We were successful in submitting a grant to support service workers who want to pursue training to become certified nursing assistants (CNAs). The program will provide training, career coaching, and CNA test preparation to enrollees while maintaining their regular weekly pay.

This program addresses both race equity and social determinants of health by making opportunities available to our employees to advance their education and careers while maintaining their income. Obtaining CNA certification and moving into the role of patient care associate is a stepping stone to other clinical opportunities in the future. The program aligns with the organization's strategy as an anchor institution to address inequality in communities by providing economic stimulus to under-served communities to combat disparities around health care, education, and employment. The nature of anchor work is that the impact is felt locally. Since this proposal targets the hospital community, the institution's employees are the beneficiaries. So, what is initially an internal effort will impact the community by way of impacting the families of the institution's employees.

### Hausman Fellowship

The Hausman fellowship is designed to promote recruitment of minority nurses and meet the needs of a diverse patient population. The fellowship provides an opportunity for senior nursing students of diverse backgrounds, from local universities, to work in a variety of patient care settings under the mentorship of a minority nurse preceptor. Fellows gain clinical experience and enhanced clinical skills in patient care. The Hausman fellowship advances both our diversity mission and fits well into our anchor institute strategy of employing people from our local communities. The ultimate goal of this fellowship is to expose nursing students to this organization and then hire them as registered nurses upon graduation from their bachelor's degree program.

### Dorothy A. Terrell Diversity Nursing Leadership Fellowship

In reviewing the demographic profile of our leadership and clinical staff, I have identified that we need more focused initiatives to promote the diversity in both groups. I have recently been successful in securing funding for the Dorothy A. Terrell Diversity Nursing Leadership Fellowship designed to create opportunities for clinical nurses of diverse backgrounds to gain exposure to a variety of leadership roles that can help inform and shape their career direction in leadership roles.

With this fellowship, clinical nurses will be provided a mentored experience in 1 of 3 tracks: administrative, practice, or education roles. They are also provided career counseling regarding a particular role to help guide the clinical nurses in next steps, (eg, pursue graduate education). I feel fortunate to have donors who want to invest in the infrastructure to advance this important aspect of our mission.

# Conclusion: Impact of the DNP Degree

Looking back on my education, I am reminded often of the value of the DNP coursework and educational experience and how it has considerably impacted my ability to serve in the CNO role. DNP-prepared nurses hold a variety of influential roles within the health care system. As described in the DNP Essentials, nurses who complete a DNP program are prepared in either an advanced practice nursing role or with a systems/organizational focus.[2] In this chapter, I have shared how in my role as CNO, I have created a culture where nurses with DNP preparation use their skills to ensure that the best evidence reaches the bedside in the most effective and efficient manner. This occurs through transformational leadership, translational research, and effectively using data to drive system improvement and practice. I have also highlighted the importance of PhD- and DNP-prepared nurses collaborating to implement new nursing science and practice innovations.[15]

The DNP degree has greatly influenced my leadership as a CNO and has prepared me well for the challenges of this role. My decision making is more analytical, informed, and strategic. My leadership is more purposeful, tactical, and responsive, and I realize that I must impact the practice of nursing both at the local and national levels if we are to impact the health of the communities that we serve today and into the future.

# Acknowledgments

The importance of life-long learning cannot be overstated. It is the key to excellence in any endeavor and a prerequisite for strong, effective leadership. As you see in my chapter, I have been fortunate to be surrounded by an exceptional team whose unwavering commitment to quality has helped elevate patient care and contributed to the advancement of nursing practice. I am grateful for the support I have received over the years, both from Massachusetts General Hospital and our donors, that has allowed me to pursue advanced degrees and enhance my own life-long learning.

# References

1.  MGH mission. The General Hospital Corporation. https://www.massgeneral.org/assets/MGH/pdf/medicine/HTLInsert020317.pdf

2.  DNP essentials. American Association of Colleges of Nursing. https://www.aacnnursing.org/DNP/DNP-Essentials

3.  Kaplan L, Brown MA. Proud to be a pioneer: perspectives of a first cohort of DNP students. *J Nurse Pract.* 2009;13(3):10-20.

4.  Institute of Medicine. The future of nursing: leading change, advancing health. The National Academies of Sciences. http://books.nap.edu/openbook.php?record_id=12956&page=R1

5.  Berwick D. A user's manual for the IOM's 'quality chasm' report. *Health Aff.* 2002;21(3):80-90.

6.  Matuson, RC. *Talent Magnetism: How to Build a Workplace That Attracts and Keeps the Best.* Nicholas Brealey Publishing; 2013.

7.  Kouzes JM, Pozner BZ. *The Leadership Challenge.* 4th ed. Jossey-Bass; 2002.

8.  Erickson JI, Duffy ME, Ditomassi M, Jones DA. Development and psychometric evaluation of the professional practice work environment inventory. *J Nurs Adm.* 2017;47(5):259-265.

9.  Burke D, Flanagan J, Ditomassi M, Hickey P. Characteristics of nurse directors that contribute to registered nurse satisfaction. *J Nurs Adm.* 2017;47(4):219-225.

10. Dearholt S, Dang D. J*ohns Hopkins Nursing Evidence-Based Practice: Model and Guidelines.* 3rd ed. Sigma Theta Tau International; 2018.

11. Erickson JI, Ditomassi M, Jones DA. *Fostering a Research-Intensive Organization: An Interdisciplinary Approach for Nurses From Massachusetts General Hospital, 2015 AJN Award Recipient.* Sigma Theta Tau International; 2015.

12. Smith MC. Regenerating nursing's disciplinary perspective. *Adv Nurs Sci.* 2019;42(1):3-16.

13. Deming WE. *Out of the Crisis.* MIT Press; 1982.

14. AACN clinical scene investigator (CSI) academy. American Association of Critical-Care Nurses. https://www.aacn.org/nursing-excellence/csi-academy?tab=Nurses%20Leading%20Innovation

15. Trautman DE, Idzik S, Hammersla M, Rosseter R. Advancing scholarship through translational research: the role of PhD and DNP-prepared nurses. *Online J Issues Nurs.* 2018;23(2):manuscript 2.

# SECTION VII

## ACADEMIA EXEMPLARS

# CHAPTER 17

# CULTURAL COMPETENCY THROUGH A STUDY ABROAD EXPERIENCE FOR DNP STUDENTS AND ITS IMPACT ON THE DNP ESSENTIALS

*Mary C. Loughran, DNP, RN, MHA*

## INTRODUCTION

The United States is becoming more culturally diverse with mass immigration and globalization. We are home to more immigrants than any other country, with more than 40 million people living in the United States who were born in a foreign country.[1] The increase in immigrant and refugee populations in the United States is expected to continue. As a result, the nurses of the 21st century are facing global health care issues and will need to provide care for these typically vulnerable minority groups.[2] One measure that has been shown to decrease health disparities is cultural competence in nursing students and professional nurses.[2] Nurses that provide culturally competent nursing care have the ability to increase access to health care, improve quality of care, and improve patient satisfaction, which may lead to better health outcomes for culturally diverse groups.[2,3]

Cultural diversity is a fact of life. There are differences and similarities among people and groups. In 2008, the American Association of Colleges of Nursing (AACN) formally called for cultural competence education to be included in nursing curricula.[4] Their rationale identified the persistent disparities in health that lead to poorer health and shorter lifespans.[4] They challenged nursing educators to develop curricula that would prepare students to be able to provide culturally competent care. This has been embraced at Duquesne University for all levels of nursing education: baccalaureate, master's, Doctor of Nursing Practice (DNP), and Doctor of Philosophy (PhD).

The DNP degree is the terminal degree for advanced practitioners and nursing administrators. DNP graduates are uniquely qualified to lead efforts that provide culturally competent care in their practices and health care organizations. It is up to the DNP programs to provide their students with educational activities to achieve this cultural competence.

Duquesne University has a long-standing commitment to developing cultural competence in all its nursing students. Transcultural and global health content is contained in courses across all programs as early as 1998. Classroom and clinical activities as well as study abroad opportunities have resulted in positive outcomes for the participating students. As the DNP program coordinator, I have had the opportunity to experience firsthand the study abroad experience of the DNP students in their "Transcultural Care and Global Health Perspectives" course that is taken during a 12-week

Benson LA, ed. *The DNP Professional:*
*Translating Value From Classroom to Practice* (pp 183-191).
© 2021 SLACK Incorporated.

summer semester of their first year in our DNP program. The DNP students have a study abroad immersion experience for 2 weeks at Duquesne University's campus in Rome, Italy. According to some of the students who have experienced the study abroad program, they say that it has been life changing. I would like to discuss Duquesne University's rich history of taking students abroad in the context of Campinha-Bacote's cultural theory, and "The Process of Cultural Competence in the Delivery of Healthcare Services," and to reflect on how this supports the achievement of scientific foundations and cultural competence as noted in DNP Essentials I and VII, respectively.

# CULTURAL COMPETENCE

Completion of all 8 DNP Essentials is a mandatory requirement to achieving the DNP degree. DNP Essential I: Scientific Underpinnings for Practice reflects on the complexity of doctoral practice and conceptual foundation of nursing.[5] The scientific foundation of nursing practice not only includes the natural sciences, but it has also made room for psychosocial sciences and the science of complex organizational structure.[5] The objectives of this DNP Essential that need to be met in the DNP program include the following:

- Integrate nursing science with knowledge from ethics, the biophysical, psychosocial, analytical, and organizational sciences as the basis for the highest level of nursing practice.
- Uses science-based theories and concepts to:
  - Determine the nature and significance of health and health care delivery phenomena.
  - Describe the actions and advanced strategies to enhance, alleviate, and ameliorate health and health care delivery phenomena as appropriate.
  - Evaluate outcomes.
- Develop and evaluate new practice approaches based on nursing theories and theories from other disciplines.[5]

During this cultural immersion, the DNP students have the opportunity to experience a variety of cultural practices. The "Transcultural Care and Global Health Perspectives" course will include content on various transcultural theories, practices, and models. The students also compare the impact of cultural, religious, economic, and political influences on the Italian health care system and global health care systems in general. Evidence-based research findings as they apply to global problems and initiatives are discussed, along with strategies for care collaboration with domestic and global stakeholders.[6] Campinha-Bacote's transcultural theory will be reviewed to further explore DNP Essential I and to look at cultural competence and its role in achieving DNP Essential VII: Clinical Prevention and Population Health for Improving the Nation's Health.[5]

Campinha-Bacote defined cultural competence as the "ongoing process in which the health care provider continuously strives to achieve the ability to effectively work within the cultural context of a client (individual, family, or community)."[7] Her model requires that the health care providers see themselves as *becoming* culturally competent vs already being culturally competent.[7] Assumptions of the model include:

- Cultural competence is a process, not an event.
- Cultural competence consists of 5 constructs: cultural awareness, cultural knowledge, cultural skill, cultural encounters, and cultural desire.
- There is more variation within ethnic groups than across ethnic groups (intra-ethnic variation).
- There is a direct relationship between the level of competence of health care providers and their ability to provide culturally responsive health care services.
- Cultural competence is an essential component in rendering effective and culturally responsive services to culturally and ethnically diverse clients.[7]

The 5 constructs act as the pillars of Campinha-Bacote's model. Cultural awareness is the in-depth examination of one's own personal and professional background. The premise is that unless you are aware of the influence on your own culture and professional values, there is the risk of cultural imposition, or imposing your beliefs on the other culture.[7] Cultural knowledge is the process of seeking and obtaining a solid foundation about diverse cultural and ethnic groups in order to understand the health-related beliefs of the client and how illness is interpreted.[7] Cultural skill is the ability to collect relevant cultural information and perform a culturally based physical assessment that takes into consideration the physical, biological, and physiological variations.[7] Cultural encounters encourage the health care provider to directly engage in cross-cultural interactions with clients from different cultures. This allows the health care provider to appreciate that there is intra-ethnic variation in cultures and that the clients seen may or may not represent all the members of that culture.[7] Cultural desire is the motivation of the health care provider to *want* to, rather than *have* to, engage in the previous 4 constructs; it involves the concept of caring and a genuine passion to accept differences and build on similarities.[7] All 5 of these constructs are interdependent and must be experienced by the health care provider in order to become culturally competent.[7] This framework when applied to the study abroad experience provides opportunities for the DNP students to continue the process of developing their cultural competence.

DNP Essential VII specifically states the following: Clinical Prevention and Population Health for Improving the Nation's Health[5] and addresses the issue of being culturally competent for the DNP student. It addresses the need for cultural diversity and sensitivity that guide the practice of DNP graduates. This DNP Essential is concerned with the health promotion and illness prevention for individuals and families. Central to achieving the national goal of improving the health status of the US population is the implementation of clinical prevention and population health activities.[5] The concepts of health promotion and illness prevention, along with the corresponding evidence-based recommendations, must take into consideration the cultural diversity and sensitivity of the populations that are being served.[5] The objectives of this DNP Essential that need to be met in the DNP program include the following:

- Analyze epidemiological, biostatistical, occupational and environmental, and other appropriate scientific data related to individual, aggregate, and population health.
- Synthesize concepts, including psychosocial dimensions and cultural diversity, related to clinical prevention and population health in developing, implementing, and evaluating interventions to address health promotion/disease prevention efforts, improve health status/access patterns, and/or address gaps in care of individuals, aggregates, or populations.
- Evaluate care delivery models and/or strategies using concepts related to community, environmental, and occupational health and cultural and socioeconomic dimensions of health.[5]

Data sets involving epidemiological, biostatistical, occupational, and environmental information need to be analyzed by the DNP to be able to develop, implement, and evaluate care delivery models and strategies involving clinical prevention and population health.[5] At Duquesne University, these skills are obtained in their "Epidemiology and Biostatistics" course. However, if the DNP graduate is not culturally competent, how can they achieve the health promotion and illness prevention outcomes that are envisioned in this DNP Essential? Duquesne University's study abroad program provides those experiences, which will promote and enhance the cultural competency of our DNP graduates.

As the world continues to get smaller with the advent of communication technologies and easier global travel, the need for culturally competent nurses continues to increase. Students in study abroad programs where they are the minority culture develop an enhanced awareness of the many challenges that minorities experience when adjusting to a new location.[8] Students that have international experiences develop personal awareness of social consciousness,[9] increased self-efficacy, and the ability to adapt to new situations, greater sensitivity to other cultures' beliefs and values,[10] and increased self-confidence and self-reliance.[11] A study abroad experience can help bridge that theory-to-practice gap, however, many nursing students, even graduate nursing students, have had little exposure to different cultures and worldviews.[3]

# Study Abroad Program at Duquesne University School of Nursing

Given Duquesne University's history of providing study abroad experiences, our faculty felt strongly that a cultural immersion experience should be included in the DNP program when it began in 2008. This approach fit nicely into the philosophy of the clinical and research agendas of the School of Nursing, which include social justice, cultural competence, health disparities, and wellness within chronic illness.[12] The cultural immersion experience takes place in the "Transcultural Care and Global Health Perspectives" course. DNP students are given the opportunity to think about their own cultural heritage as well as the health and illness in a health care system outside of the US health care system. The study abroad experience is not a mandatory requirement for this course, but it is strongly encouraged. However, I am pleased to note that the overwhelming majority of students choose to study abroad. For students who do not go to Italy, they are required to identify a non-Western medicine setting where they will complete a minimum of 10 hours of observation and participation to complete their field notes assignment. These students are encouraged to investigate possible settings in their local areas, for example, traditional healers such as shaman, midwife, or Eastern medical practices like acupuncture. The students need to have their setting approved by the course faculty. Additionally, these students are encouraged to get out of their comfort zones by eating at an ethnic restaurant, watching any foreign channel television, spending time with a person from a different culture, and/or attending a religious service of another culture.

The first 2 study abroad experiences for DNP students occurred in 2009 and 2010. Two nursing faculty members took these students to Montreal and Toronto where they were placed in non–English-speaking environments. They were required to learn about the Canadian health care system and the role of nursing. Since 2011, the DNP students have been traveling to Italy for a cultural immersion and observation experience of the public and private Italian health care institutions. Duquesne University's Rome campus opened in 2002 and is located in the Sisters of the Holy Family of Nazareth Generalate. Its campus is within the Acquafredda Nature Reserve just 7 miles from Vatican City and St. Peter's Basilica. The walled property encloses lovely gardens and walkways. This is an idyllic location in Rome that contains all of the amenities of a college campus: classrooms, a library, computer labs and wireless internet, dining room, recreational areas, laundry facilities, and each double room has its own private bathroom. Our Italian campus is safe and comfortable making for an enjoyable visit whether studying for just a Maymester or for an entire semester.

Two nursing faculty accompany the students to our campus in Rome and work closely with the director and assistant director of the Italian campus to plan the 10-day immersion experience. This course is offered during the 12-week summer semester, which allows the students to complete some of their course activities prior to and after the study abroad experience. The activities are designed to enable the DNP students to experience a new culture, observe differences in health care and health care disparities, and understand the influences of culture on these health care systems.

The "Transcultural Care and Global Health Perspectives" course that has been mentioned is a required core course in the DNP program at Duquesne University School of Nursing. This course explores the impact of globalization on health care and health care planning, and the need to design health care systems that are responsive to diverse cultural needs. The focus is on select global health problems assessed in a multidisciplinary manner to ensure attention to the under-served and their complex cultural needs and requirements. Attention is directed at increasing the capacity of health care professionals to develop culturally sensitive health care systems.[13] Keeping the objectives outlined in both DNP Essentials I and VII, the course objectives were designed using various cultural care theories to remind the DNP students that theory does reflect and guide practice. The course objectives include the following:

- Identify global health problems and diverse cultural needs across various culture groups.
- Understand the utility of theories, models, and approaches in promoting health from a global perspective.
- Compare health systems across cultures for methods of success to facilitate positive health outcomes within the cultural context.
- Analyze caring practices in the context of comparative health systems through immersion in the cultural context in which it is occurring.
- Analyze evidence for practice to promote culturally congruent care from a global perspective and influence health policy.[13]

Using the theory of Campinha-Bacote, this immersion experience allows the students to see themselves *becoming* culturally competent due to the integration of her constructs (ie, cultural awareness, cultural knowledge, cultural skill, cultural encounters, cultural desire) into course assignments and experiences.[7] Activities that support the course objectives will be discussed using Campinha-Bacote's 5 constructs.

Cultural awareness is the first construct in Campinha-Bacote's theory. It involves student exploration of their own cultural and professional backgrounds through required readings and completion of the "Cultural Icon" assignment. This assignment requires that the students think about their culture inclusive of their values, beliefs, and traditions to discover their cultural self. The students are asked to reflect on their cultural self and select a cultural icon that reflects their cultural beliefs, values, or traditions. The cultural icon

usually has a personal meaning. It may be something that the student wears or carries with them, or a gift passed down to them within their family. The students bring the icon or a picture of it with them and do a 3-minute presentation for the class when they are in Rome. This exercise is a great way for the student to get in touch with their cultural self and assist their colleagues to understand who they are culturally. Students doing this assignment say that it really made them look into their family backgrounds, and they discovered things about themselves and their families that they did not know. They are more than excited to present their cultural icons and really enjoy sharing this part of themselves with their colleagues. The students who do not participate in the study abroad program are required to do this assignment and post a 3-minute "Voice Thread" presentation that is able to be reviewed by the faculty instructors and fellow colleagues. This is the first construct toward achieving cultural competency.

The second construct is cultural knowledge. During their time in Italy, the students have several opportunities to learn about the Italian culture and its health-related beliefs. They attend a special presentation on "Intercultural Sensitivity in Health Care" in Italy by Dr. Ida Castiglioni, professor of sociology and cultural processes in the Department of Sociology and Social Research, University of Milano-Bicocca. This event is held on campus and allows for the students to ask questions and interact with the guest speaker regarding the cultural nuances of health care in Italy. Examples of activities that focus on health care within the Roman culture include visiting the public hospital, Fatebenefratelli Hospital, located on Tiber Island. It is currently run by the Brothers Hospitallers of Saint John of God. This public hospital offers medical and surgical services typically seen in US hospitals. They even have acupuncture and homeopathy clinics. Traveling to Palermo, Sicily, the students have the opportunity to learn about a transplant hospital which is owned and operated by a US organization collaborating with the Italian health care systems. It is important to note that Italy does not allow foreign students to provide hands-on care to their patient populations. Therefore, at both of these hospital visits, a presentation by the director of nursing and/or physicians on the Italian health care system is offered regarding the role of nurses and other health care professionals in their organization, as well as the services provided to their clients. Students have the opportunity to tour the facilities, and talk with nurses, physicians, and other hospital personnel to learn about specialty areas and common practices in public and private hospitals. The students also visit the Community of Sant'Egidio with Dr. Paolo Mancinelli. This is an organization that is completely staffed by volunteers who reach out to the marginalized people in Rome, including the sick, poor, migrants, and others. Duquesne University has a special connection with Sant'Egidio through their work with the DREAM Program (Disease Relief through Excellent and Advanced Means). DREAM addresses the challenges for global health for Africa focusing on HIV/AIDs, malnutrition, and other infective and chronic diseases with access to universal treatment, which is still the ultimate goal for these patients. The students attend a prayer service in the Santa Maria in Trastevere church. The service is led by lay people and will usually focus on current country and global issues. Afterwards, the students meet with Dr. Mancinelli to discuss the community initiatives of the Sant'Egidio community. At the end of the study abroad, the students complete an assignment that compares the Italian health care system to the US health care system and explores how the DNP promotes culturally congruent health systems and health policies when caring for a patient with an acute or chronic health problem that has just come to live in the United States. This assignment will allow the student to articulate the impact and influences of culture on health systems.

Cultural skill involves learning how to conduct a culturally specific physical assessment while also appreciating the physical, biological, and physiological variations of ethnically diverse clients.[13] Since Italy does not allow direct patient interaction, this is a difficult construct to complete during the study abroad experience. The students may observe these interactions as they are happening, and they may also ask questions of the nurses, physicians, and other hospital personnel regarding the assessment of their patients. Otherwise, assigned readings specific to the Italian culture as well as other cultures may be helpful in assisting the students to achieve this construct.

Probably the easiest construct to achieve during a study abroad experience is cultural encounters. With Italy as their classroom, the students were provided with the cultural encounters in the hospital and community organizations noted above, in addition to exploring the historical and contemporary Roman culture in Rome and Palermo. A wide variety of planned activities that immerse the students in the Italian culture and engage them in fieldwork allows them to observe cultural influences on health care. There are many examples of cultural encounters that occur during this study abroad immersion. A few of them will be presented that showcase the range of experiences arranged for the students.

To help the DNP students understand the religious and faith expressions of the culture, they attend a papal audience at St. Peter's Square on Wednesday mornings during the summer when the Pope is at his Vatican home. Short readings and prayers are said in several languages. Visitor groups from various countries are announced. Our group is announced as "pilgrims from Duquesne University in Pennsylvania." Students may tour St. Peter's Basilica on their own, and a tour of the Vatican Museum and Sistine Chapel is provided by a noted Vatican art historian. Prior to this evening tour, the students attend an aperitivo (happy hour buffet) and a concert in the Vatican courtyard.

One of the most interesting experiences is attending an Italian cooking class. The students prepare the meal: homemade pasta, marinara sauce and, for dessert, tiramisu. The chefs of the restaurant will cook the homemade pasta and sauce for the students to eat, followed by the dessert. It is a wonderful opportunity to see the importance of fresh food in the Italian culture. A similar experience is the farm-to-table Sunday lunch that the students eat while in Palermo. This meal is sacred to the Italian people as it is a time to gather with family and friends. Another encounter while in Palermo is the walking tour of the local markets that are a hybrid of European and North African markets. The importance of diet, food, and popular medicine in the Sicilian culture is discussed. The students also get to experience the Segestan thermal baths where the thermal waters are provided by the 2 active volcanoes that are located on Sicily. These waters are full of minerals that are thought to promote healthy circulation, muscles, and healing for respiratory problems. These combined experiences reveal the importance of food and family in the Italian culture and the belief in the healing power of water.

From a different perspective, the students become familiar with the everyday routines of the Italian people. For example, they experience the public transportation systems by using the bus or underground metro to travel throughout the city. Duquesne University's campus is just outside of Rome, so it requires the use of public transportation. Each encounter that has been described presents a different facet of the Italian culture that enables the students to become immersed in their day-to-day living. Instruction on how to do research-oriented fieldwork inclusive of observation and interpretation are taught through readings and assignments prior to the study abroad. The students reflect on and maintain their field notes about the various experiences which they must synthesize and summarize the overarching themes in a written assignment to enable them to better understand the unique Roman/Italian culture in the contexts of their health care and daily living.

The final construct in Campinha-Bacote's cultural care model is cultural desire. This construct involves the health care providers desire to "want to" engage in the process of cultural competence[13] by seeking cross-cultural encounters and becoming more culturally knowledgeable, aware, and skillful.[14] This is in contrast to the feeling of "have to" participate in these cross-cultural encounters. Genuine caring is an intrinsic quality that cannot be measured in health care providers. The goal of health care providers is to offer words from the heart that reflect true caring. It is important for their clients to feel valued and to see that their providers' actions and words are congruent.[13] It is often said that people do not care how much you know, until they first know how much you care. The DNP students engaged in this travel abroad immersion showed their cultural desire to want to engage in the cross-cultural experiences among the Italian people. Assuming the students desire to "want to" interact with the various ethnics in this culture, their pathway to cultural competency has been enhanced. Through the various interactions and experiences with and among the Italian people, the outcome for the students is to approach others that are culturally different with a genuine passion to treat others like they would like to be treated.

The travel abroad experience provides opportunities for the DNP students to learn, observe, and ask questions about the interprofessional health care team in Italy. During their stay, they visit the Center of Excellence for Nursing Scholarship–IPASVI where they meet with the associate director for nursing and health policy to discuss the roles of nurses in Italy's health care system and the interprofessional health care team. DNP Essential V: Health Care Policy for Advocacy in Health Care[5] also needs to be briefly mentioned. During this immersion trip to Rome, the DNP students get to observe the Italian health care systems, and to make comparisons with the health care systems in the United States. They will take focused courses on health policy and social justice; however, this experience will support a global perspective of health care and health policy providing support for the DNP students' appreciation of their leadership roles in health care policy and advocacy. They visit public and private health care organizations, which allow them to appreciate their roles as advocates for ethical and equitable health policies regardless of the health care settings.

Additionally, the DNP students may experience their study abroad with non-nursing Duquesne students that may be there for the Maymester, which is a 1-month immersion in Italy for those students. For example, in 2018, students from Duquesne's Mary Pappert School of Music were also staying at the Rome campus. The Mary Pappert School of Music challenges its students to connect historical and current music practices, therefore, a study abroad to Italy fits nicely into these goals. This made for interesting experiences and dining conversations with the music students on their perceptions of the Italian culture in the context of art and music. The music students were also genuinely interested in the Italian health care systems and the explorations of the DNP students. Duquesne University's School of Nursing also supports a joint faculty appointment with the Mary Pappert School of Music. Collaboration on how music therapy is used in health care is a clinical as well as a mutual research agenda item. On the last day of our study abroad the music students performed for us. This was their final exam. It was amazing to see and hear the talent of these musicians, as well as a wonderful and collaborative way to end our stay in Rome.

During the summer semester when the study abroad occurs, the DNP students are also taking the "Social Justice and Vulnerable Populations" course. This course dovetails nicely with the "Transcultural Care and Global Health Perspectives" course. The instructor from this course may be one of our faculty members who has a joint faculty appointment in the School of Nursing and the Ethics department. The objectives of this course are to:

- Discuss the relationships between social justice, determinants of health, and vulnerability.
- Analyze selected policies and protocols for their impact on vulnerable populations and their fidelity to social justice principles.

- Integrate evidence about vulnerable populations, determinants of health, and social justice teachings into research, practice, and education.
- Develop interventions that liberate and empower.[15]

These objectives complement the cultural competency study broad experiences with a focus on vulnerable populations that are examined through the lens of "social justice theory, the Catholic social justice tradition, and determinants of health."[15] Having the course taught by an ethicist also brings another perspective for the DNP students to consider, and provides opportunities to engage in conversations where they can reflect their cultural and global experiences in Italy.

## OUTCOMES

An integrative review by Kelleher[16] suggests that nursing students who participate in study abroad experiences receive many benefits: personal and professional growth, cultural sensitivity and competence, and cognitive development. This has been the experience of Duquesne's nursing students at undergraduate and graduate levels. Student learning outcomes from studying abroad have been "life changing" experiences according to Dr. Richard Zoucha, Joseph A. Lauritis, CSSp Endowed Chair for Teaching and Technology, and professor and chair of advanced role and PhD programs.[17] He has been the initiator and visionary of the study abroad programs for both the DNP and PhD programs at Duquesne University since they began in 2009. According to Dr. Zoucha, the main purpose of the study abroad programs is to get the students "out of their comfort zones."[17] The study abroad immersion allows the students to learn how to relate to a population where you do not speak their language, and reflect back to patients in the United States that do not speak English, ultimately, leading the student to identify how they will change their practice.[17] Students are challenged to think about their experiences and observations when working with patients, families, and communities who may come from a different culture but are here in the United States using our health care system. One of the students that traveled to Rome in 2018 stated, "I did feel uncomfortable when I spoke English to someone in Italy and they did not speak English. It made me feel somewhat anxious, so then I tried to speak with my limited knowledge of Italian and somehow we connected … it made me realize how uncomfortable it must feel when people travel to the United States and we get impatient with them." Students also state that the study abroad experience has helped them feel part of the global nature of nursing with a new respect for those who care for the vulnerable. As one student noted, "The professors were helpful because of their experience, but the learning came from the interaction with the people who came to us or who we visited with." The DNP students who have engaged in this study abroad immersion in Italy have stated that they were able to recognize the impact of one's culture on their perspectives of health and wellness. Their cultural competence journey has begun. The study abroad experience enables the DNP students to appreciate the complexities of culture, and that it is necessary to consider whenever looking to develop, implement, and evaluate interventions that they may be designing to address the health care needs of populations in support of DNP Essential VII.

# PROFESSIONALISM

Currently, I am the program coordinator for the DNP program at Duquesne University School of Nursing. The faculty of our DNP program consists of both DNPs and PhDs. We collaborate to ensure that the DNP program is up-to-date with rigorous and creative courses that prepare a DNP graduate who is ready to contribute and make an impact in 3 areas: clinical and administrative health care, academia, and health policy. The fact that our DNP program has both DNPs and PhDs teaching these courses provides the DNP student with examples of the collaborative efforts between DNPs and PhDs.

The DNP degree was not meant to supply the nursing education workforce, but that is what is happening and will continue to happen.[18] You may be asking what has led to this influx of DNPs into the academic arena. A reason for this trend can be seen in AACN's report, "Special Survey on Vacant Faculty Positions" in October 2016. A total of 1567 vacancies were identified in 821 nursing baccalaureate and/or graduate programs in the United States (85% response rate). These data show a faculty vacancy rate of 7.9% with 92.8% of the vacant positions requiring or preferring a doctoral degree.[19] The AACN's report "2016-2017 Enrollment and Graduations in Baccalaureate and Graduate Programs" states that 64 067 qualified applicants were turned away from nursing programs due to faculty shortages.[19] In order to handle this demand for nursing schools, these nursing programs stated that they would need to fill the current vacancies plus an additional 133 faculty positions.[19] Additionally, with the impending retirements of a large number of faculty and academic administrators, efforts need to be made to encourage more nurses and nursing students to pursue academic careers.[18] These factors have led to the recruitment of DNPs to fill these vacancies. It has been suggested that DNPs do not receive the educational preparation for the role of a nurse educator and, therefore, are not qualified to be in academia. My reply to that question is, neither does the nursing research doctorate receive the educational preparation to teach, and no one is challenging their preparation to teach in academic settings. When it comes to DNPs or PhDs assuming academic administrative positions, the best preparation, until formal graduate programs that prepare academic administrators become available, may be on-the-job training that is supported by mentoring programs and specific coursework that adds to the new administrator's background and experiences.[18]

It is important to note that the National Organization of Nurse Practitioner Faculties (NONPF), the National League for Nursing (NLN), and the AACN support advanced practice nurses with clinical doctorates to work in academia.[18] They believe that the "DNP degree is the answer to getting our most talented clinicians, executive leaders, managers, and educators the advanced practice experiences, which will deepen their critical thinking and analytic skills and widen their network of colleagues in leadership roles."[18] The nurse educator with a terminal DNP degree is able to prepare a future generation of nurses that will be able to lead and collaborate with interprofessional teams, understand organizational systems, and use data to improve patient outcomes and influence health policy.

# PEARLS/TAKEAWAYS

The impact of immigration and globalization in the United States has increased the cultural diversity of patient populations using our health care systems. This has ushered in the imperative that all nurses, especially DNPs, be culturally competent. DNP Essentials I and VII provide the context for our transcultural course that uses the study abroad immersion experiences in Italy to support our students' development and continuing growth of cultural competence that will guide the practice of our DNP graduates. We have found that our immersion experiences change our students and broaden their worldviews when they realize that the rest of the world does not live like them.[8] I would strongly encourage DNP programs to look into adding a cultural immersion experience into their programs, making sure that the DNP curricula emboldens the DNP students' growth in cultural competence.

Campinha-Bacote's cultural care theory and the 5 constructs—cultural awareness, cultural knowledge, cultural skill, cultural encounters, and cultural desire[7]—are relevant to this study abroad experiential learning. Using these constructs as the framework provides the DNP students with opportunities to understand the Italian culture and the social, political, and religious values and beliefs that impact their views on health care. It is hoped that the DNP students will reflect on these unique experiences and identify ways that they will change their practice when caring for clients from diverse backgrounds in the United States.

The DNP education should prepare DNP students to be confident in their ability to practice and be leaders in transcultural care.[20] Health care leaders are responsible for managing diversity and maintaining a healthy and productive work environment.[20] For example, DNPs can support an organization at all levels: clinical, system, and organizational. At a clinical level, they can be involved in ensuring that nurses and other health care providers are knowledgeable on the cultures of the patients that they care for in their organizations. With the creation of health care systems throughout the United States, DNPs can become involved in evaluating these systems to make sure that they are culturally appropriate for their patient populations. DNPs, especially nurse executives, can get involved at the organizational level to ensure that hiring practices aimed at diversity are in place, and create positive work environments.

Nursing faculty play a critical role in educating DNP students. They need to be culturally competent and model culturally sensitive behaviors. Their role is critical in designing and assessing curricula to support the achievement of cultural competency. By following the DNP Essentials and the objectives that are noted under each one, nursing educators will be able to design DNP courses where theory and cultural competency are threaded throughout the curricula. The DNP Essentials serve as the template to achieve this goal in DNP programs.

More rigorous research is needed on cultural competence, especially in the DNP and other graduate nursing programs. The effectiveness of teaching methods and how this translates to the student or graduate student when they care for culturally diverse patients needs to be researched.[10,17] Some of the methods that we have highlighted included use of reflection in assignments, study abroad immersion, and a dedicated "Transcultural Care and Global Health Perspectives" course and our "Social Justice and Vulnerable Populations" course.

DNPs need to understand the relationships between culture, health values, and behaviors in order to support care for diverse populations.[21] Regardless of their professional work settings, it has become necessary for DNP students to be culturally competent in order to achieve the DNP Essentials and to be effective in their future roles as transformational leaders.

# Conclusion: Impact of the DNP Degree

As a result of obtaining my DNP degree, I was able to assume the role of DNP program coordinator at Duquesne University in 2015. My first-hand experience as a DNP and former chief nursing officer allows me to strategically implement what is needed in our DNP curricula. In addition to the courses on transcultural nursing care and vulnerable populations that have been mentioned, our coursework focuses on leadership while exploring ethical management and change theories, project management and evaluation, health policy, evidence-based practice, and biostatistics and epidemiology that coincide with the AACN's DNP Essentials. This past academic year, as chair of the DNP committee, we successfully completed a review and alignment of our DNP course objectives and outcomes anticipating the announcement from AACN on the new DNP Essentials.

When I assumed the role of DNP program coordinator, our DNP program was not accredited. Working collaboratively with Duquesne University faculty and staff, I am pleased to report that we received accreditation from the Commission on Collegiate Nursing Education in 2016. We are currently preparing for our 5-year accreditation review in 2021.

I have the privilege of working with faculty, DNP- and PhD-prepared, who are committed to the DNP program and its students. We continuously improve our DNP program, which focuses on clinical leadership, and have just launched a post-master's and post-baccalaureate Executive Nurse Leadership and Health Care Management DNP programs.

Having earned the DNP degree, I have been able to contribute to the education of graduate students on the roles that nursing, especially a DNP-prepared nurse, can play in health care organizations, academia, and health policy in creating change. I am looking forward to continuing the success of our current DNP programs where we teach our students to identify problems, propose evidence-based solutions, and implement changes that will improve patient outcomes as advanced practice nurses and nursing and health care executives.

# Acknowledgments

To the nursing faculty at Duquesne University who enthusiastically foster the practice of transcultural and holistic nursing among our students by using the best of their nursing education, practice, and research. To my family, especially my husband, Joe, who has always been a trusted source of encouragement regarding my professional practice.

# References

1.  Radford, J. Key findings about US immigrants. Pew Research. Accessed September 4, 2019. https://www.pewresearch.org/fact-tank/2019/06/17/key-findings-about-u-s-immigrants/

2.  Gallagher RW, Polanin JR. A meta-analysis of educational interventions designed to enhance cultural competence in professional nurses and nursing students. *Nurse Educ Today.* 2015;35:333-340. doi:10.1016/j.nedt.2014.10.021

3.  Kokko R. Future nurses' cultural competencies: what are their learning experiences during exchange and studies abroad? A systematic review. *J Nurs Manag.* 2011;19:673-682. doi:10.1111/j.1365-2834.201.01221.x

4.  Lonneman W. Teaching strategies to increase cultural awareness in nursing students. *Nurse Educ.* 2015;40(6):285-288. doi:10.1097/NNE.0000000000000175

5.  The essentials of doctoral education for advanced nursing practice. American Association of Colleges of Nursing. Accessed August 26, 2019. https://www.aacnnursing.org/Portals/42/Publications/DNPEssentials.pdf

6.  Transcultural care and global health perspectives. Duquesne University School of Nursing. Syllabus; 2019.

7.  Campinha-Bacote J. The process of cultural competence in the delivery of healthcare services: a model of care. *J Transcult Nurs.* 2002;13(3):181-184.

8.  Levine M. Transforming experiences: nursing education and international immersion programs. *J Prof Nurs.* 2009;25(3):156-169. doi:10.1016/j.profnurs.2009.01.001

9. Kirkham SR, Hofwegen LV, Pankratz D. Keeping the vision: sustaining social consciousness with nursing students following international learning experiences. *Int J Nurs Educ Scholarsh.* 2009;6(1):article 3. doi:10.2202/1548-923x.1635

10. Edmonds, M. An integrative literature review of study abroad programs for nursing students. *Nurs Educ Perspect.* 2012;33:30-34.

11. Green BF, Johansson I, Rosser M, Tengrnah C, Segrott J. Studying abroad: a multiple case study of nursing students' international experiences. *Nurse Educ Today.* 2008;28:981-992.

12. Zoucha R, Turk M. Using the culture care theory as a guide to develop and implement a transcultural course or doctor of nursing practice students for study in Italy. In: Mcfarland MR, Wehbe-Alamah HB. *Culture Care Diversity and Universality.* 3rd ed. Jones & Bartlett Learning; 2015:521-534.

13. Campinha-Bacote J. A model and instrument for addressing cultural competence in health care. *J Nurs Educ.* 1999;38(5):203-207.

14. Schim SM, Doorenbos A, Benkert R, Miller J. Culturally congruent care: putting the puzzle together. *J Transcult Nurs.* 2007;18(2):103-110. doi:10.1177/1043659606298613

15. Social justice and vulnerable populations. Duquesne University School of Nursing. Syllabus; 2018.

16. Kelleher S. Perceived benefits of study abroad programs for nursing students: an integrative review. *J Nurs Educ.* 2013;52(12):690-695. doi:10.39/01484834-20131118-01

17. Zoucha R. Interview conducted by Mary C. Loughran. May 2019.

18. DeNisco S, Bellini S. When the DNP chair is a DNP graduate: the DNP in the academic role. In: Dreher M, Glasgow MES. *DNP Role Development for Doctoral Advanced Nursing Practice.* 2nd ed. Springer; 2017:505-524.

19. Nursing faculty shortage fact sheet. American Association of Colleges of Nursing. Accessed September 3, 2019. http://www.aacnnursing.org/portals/42/news/factsheets/faculty-shortage-fact-sheet-2017.pdf

20. Bjarnason D, Mick J, Thompson JA, Cloyd E. Perspectives on transcultural care. *Nurs Clin North Am.* 2009;44:495-503. doi.10.1016/j.cnur.2009.07.009

21. Hunter J. Applying constructivism to nursing education in cultural competence. *J Transcult Nurs.* 2008;19(4):354-362. doi:10.1177/1043659608322421

# CHAPTER 18

# Transforming DNP Systems Leadership Education

*Melinda Earle, DNP, RN, NEA-BC, FACHE*

## Introduction

The Rush University College of Nursing (RUCON) established one of the first clinical practice doctorates in the country, the Nursing Doctorate (ND), in 1990. As the American Association of Colleges of Nursing (AACN) endorsed the Doctor of Nursing Practice (DNP) degree in 2004, the RUCON ND transitioned to the DNP. The first specialty track to transition to the DNP was the leadership track in 2007, followed by all specialty advanced practice programs in 2012. Currently, more than 1200 graduate nursing students are enrolled in the master's entry in nursing for non-nurses, the post-licensure clinical nurse leader master's program, 15 DNP advanced practice nursing specialty tracks, and the Doctor of Philosophy (PhD) in nursing.

The RUCON transformative systems leadership (TSL) DNP has 2 tracks: systems leadership and population health leadership. The TSL DNP is focused on preparing nurse leaders to lead interprofessional teams in developing and implementing system- and organization-level evidence-based change to improve patient outcomes. As defined by AACN, the TSL DNP is an appropriate degree for applicants providing "indirect care such as nursing administration, executive leadership, health policy, informatics, and population health."[1]

In this chapter, I will discuss my evolution as an educator and program director, revisions to the TSL DNP program to maintain competitive advantage in the marketplace, my personal growth as an interprofessional leader, and my activities to advance the nursing profession.

## Expansion of DNP Education

Although I had 5 years of part-time teaching experience, the learning curve from full-time health care executive to full-time teacher is steeper than one would imagine. The AACN's *Essentials for Doctoral Education for Advanced Nursing Practice* clearly state the DNP education does not prepare graduates for "a role as an educator."[1]

Not planning a faculty career, I did not avail myself of the elective teaching course offered through the RUCON during my DNP studies. Anecdotally, I have found this is

Benson LA, ed. *The DNP Professional: Translating Value From Classroom to Practice* (pp 193-204).
© 2021 SLACK Incorporated.

often the case. A quick scan of TSL DNP graduates reveals students from a variety of settings: clinical practice, administrative practice, community health, public health, consulting, school nursing, and informatics. Most students, during the time they are students, do not picture themselves becoming full-time faculty. As long as teaching courses and teaching certificate programs are electives within DNP programs, they will be sought out by more than a handful of students. DNP faculty should encourage students to take a more long-term view of their career and the potential to become faculty in the future.

During my first year as faculty, I immersed myself in learning how to teach and develop curriculum. I audited the teaching course I had eschewed previously, attended a university-based teaching excellence series, and studied for the National League for Nursing's certified nurse educator examination. Since most courses are taught online, I also earned an online teaching certification from the Online Learning Consortium. One year into my faculty role, I was asked to take on the position of program director for the TSL DNP program. As a graduate of the RUCON TSL DNP program, I hoped to bring my nurse executive leadership experience, my formal RUCON DNP education, and my new-found teaching experience together to lead the program.

# INCORPORATION OF DNP ESSENTIALS

As the new program director, my first priority was to fully comprehend the AACN DNP Essentials[1] as the foundational document for DNP education. Obviously as a DNP graduate, I was familiar with the Essentials and had demonstrated the requisite outcomes in my education. Living the Essentials as a DNP program director required a higher level of understanding. I immersed myself in the DNP Essentials as the "foundational outcome competencies" for DNP education.[1]

Fortunately I found the RUCON DNP terminal objectives for all DNP education are congruent with the DNP Essentials. The DNP Curriculum Committee had recently completed a review of all course objectives for alignment with the terminal objectives. I was pleased to note alignment between terminal objectives and course objectives with few exceptions. Major and minor focus on the DNP Essentials is determined at the time every course is approved by the DNP Curriculum Committee. I reviewed all the course approval forms to assess which DNP Essentials are emphasized in the courses. As I expected, all DNP Essentials were represented in the 15 courses in the program of study. I found a major emphasis on DNP Essential II: Organizational and Systems Leadership for Quality Improvement and Systems Thinking in 12 of the 15 courses followed by DNP Essential III: Clinical Scholarship and Analytical Methods for Evidence-Based Practice in 10 of 15 courses.[1] This is consistent with the RUCON TSL DNP program goal of preparing DNP

graduates to implement evidence-based changes in health care systems. DNP Essentials with the least attention were Essential VI: Interprofessional Collaboration for Improving Patient and Population Outcomes[1] (2 of 15 courses), and DNP Essential VIII: Advanced Nursing Practice[1] (3 of 15 courses). After much discussion of these results at DNP Curriculum Committee, it was determined having 2 courses in outcome management was appropriate. The discussion also determined a need to apply an advanced nurse specialty competency-based model to a formal advanced nurse leadership practicum. For example, RUCON DNP nurse practitioner (NP) programs offer 252 clinical practice clock hours in addition to the 252 clock hours the students use to design, implement, and evaluate their scholarly project. The NP programs use the National Organization of Nurse Practitioner Faculties (NONPF) and the specific NP specialty certification competencies to design their curriculum. These competencies were not a good fit for a leadership DNP program. The American Organization for Nursing Leadership (AONL), formerly American Organization of Nurse Executives (AONE), is the specialty nursing professional organization representing more than 9800 nurse leaders. AONL publishes competencies for executive nurses, system chief nursing executives, post-acute care nurse leaders, and nurse managers. As DNP education prepares nurses as advanced practice nurse leaders, the AONL Nurse Executive Competencies[2] were chosen to guide the TSL DNP curriculum. Five areas of competency are identified by AONL: communication and relationship building, knowledge of the health care environment, leadership, professionalism, and business skills. Each of the 5 competency areas are broken down into 28 sub-areas such as governance, patient safety, performance improvement, and change management.

# SWOT ANALYSIS: REGAINING STUDENT ENROLLMENT

As I began my tenure as program director, the TSL DNP program was experiencing declining enrollment. Prior to 2015, the program admissions were averaging 33 students per year. In 2017, admissions dropped to 11 annual students. This drop in admissions was rationalized by the exponential growth in DNP programs across the country. In 2007, only a handful of DNP programs existed. By 2017, more than 300 DNP programs had opened with many more in development.[3] RUCON administration believed that with the competitive DNP program market, we could anticipate an average of 12 students a year. I was determined to recruit an annual enrollment of 24 students.

Obviously, a program environmental assessment was needed. I evaluated the current program using a SWOT (Strengths, Weaknesses, Opportunities, Threats) analysis (Table 18-1). A major strength of the TSL DNP program is its

**Table 18-1**

## RUSH UNIVERSITY COLLEGE OF NURSING TRANSFORMATIVE SYSTEMS LEADERSHIP DNP SWOT ANALYSIS

| STRENGTHS | WEAKNESSES |
|---|---|
| • One of the oldest leadership DNP programs in the country<br><br>• NursingCAS application process<br><br>• Top ranked DNP program by *US News and World Report*<br><br>• Experienced core faculty<br><br>• Experienced advisors and second readers<br><br>• Online format with only three 2-day on-site visits<br><br>• Many faculty are fellows in the American Academy of Nurses<br><br>• Several faculty are graduates of the program<br><br>• Program director is lead faculty for IONL fellowship program | • Course content developed by primarily PhD faculty<br><br>• Few core faculty with nurse executive experience<br><br>• No core faculty with nurse executive certification<br><br>• No core faculty are fellows in ACHE<br><br>• Core faculty do not attend state or national nurse leader conferences<br><br>• Clinical practicum hours are limited to scholarly project development, implementation, and evaluation<br><br>• Only 1 leadership course in program of study |
| **OPPORTUNITIES** | **THREATS** |
| • Rush Health Systems employees have a pre-paid 90% tuition plan<br><br>• Partnering with IONL to offer reduced tuition<br><br>• Creating an advisory committee of former graduates<br><br>• Attracting early nurse leader careerists | • 300% increase in DNP programs since 2007<br><br>• Turning away applicants with non-nursing master's degrees<br><br>• Turning away applicants that do not have 500 clinical practicum clock hours from their master's degree<br><br>• More master's-prepared APRN applicants accepted than experienced executive nurse leaders<br><br>• Confusion between Population Health and Systems Leadership DNP programs |

longevity. As one of the oldest clinical practice doctorates in the country graduating more than 300 leadership DNP students, the program has more than 2 decades of experience and reputation to build on. The reputation of the program is validated by US News and World Report (USNWR)[4] graduate nursing school rankings. In 2020, the RUCON DNP programs in their entirety were ranked second and the TSL DNP specialty program ranked seventh in the country.[4]

Other strengths of the TSL DNP program include: experienced faculty, online format with only three, 2-day on-site visits, and more than a decade of experience in developing and delivering online curriculum.

Weaknesses of the program in 2018 were: having only 1 leadership-focused course in the curriculum, few course faculty with nurse executive work experience, only 1 faculty member with advanced executive nurse certification and a member of AONL, and, as previously identified, no formal leadership practicum.

Leveraging my strengths as the program director (as an experienced, certified nurse executive), the program could create opportunities within the nursing leadership community. For example, the program could recruit students, faculty, and advisory council members from my network, established through decades of involvement in national, regional, and local leadership professional organizations. Additionally, using my experience to create a contemporary, attractive program for experienced nurse executives as well as advanced practice registered nurses (APRN) seeking leadership development and early nurse leader careerist.

The biggest threat to the TSL DNP program is the growing shortage of nursing faculty due to faculty retirements, growth in nursing education programs, and competitive salaries offered by practice sites. In 2018, AACN reported 1715 national nurse faculty vacancies (a 7.9% national nurse faculty vacancy rate).[5] This threat is compounded within leadership DNP programs by the salary discrepancies between nursing faculty and nurse leaders, especially in executive nurse leader positions. I, personally, took a 55% salary cut to become full-time nursing faculty.

The exponential growth of DNP programs is a threat to the program. However, this can be mitigated by thoughtful attention to the student experience: (1) admission processes and requirements; (2) contemporary plans of study with engaging courses; and (3) relevant experienced faculty.

# IMPLEMENTING EVIDENCE INTO PRACTICE

## Admission Processes and Requirements

Several weaknesses in the admission requirements were identified. Master's of Science in Nursing Administration (MSN-NA) degrees do not have a standardized number of clinical practice clock hours. The DNP degree requires 1000 post-baccalaureate clinical practice clock hours. TSL DNP applicants with less than 500 clinical practice clock hours in their MSN-NA program were denied admission to RUCON as the TSL DNP curriculum only provided 500 clinical practice clock hours. A review of applicants verified clinical practice clock hours from their MSN-NA programs noted 120 to 500 clinical practice clock hours with 350 clinical practice clock hours most common. As an MSN-NA graduate myself, it appeared that we were excluding the students that would benefit most from the TSL DNP program. Shouldn't current executive nurse leaders have the opportunity to earn the leadership practice doctorate?

The solution was to add availability of clinical practice courses for these applicants or acknowledge leadership experience through executive nurse leader certifications. In 2015, AACN clarified that schools could credit practice hours for national certifications.[6] We selected the American Nurse Credentialing Center's (ANCC's) Advanced Nurse Executive Board Certification (NEA-BC) and the AONL Certified in Executive Nursing Practice (CENP) certifications for awarding 500 clinical practice clock hours.

Another solution was needed for those applicants that could not qualify for a national executive nurse certification. Review of our applicant pool indicated several candidates willing to add 2 to 4 credit hours of clinical practicum courses to make up the deficit between their master's programs verified clinical practice clock hours and the required 1000 post-baccalaureate clinical practice clock hours. An existing clinical practicum course was revised to add more structure, clinical supervision, and variable course hours.

Nurse leaders with baccalaureate nursing preparation pursuing graduate degrees have made choices based on regional availability of graduate programs and perceptions of the value of particular graduate degrees by non-nursing colleagues or superiors. When confronted with a nationally recognized health care system chief nursing officer applicant with a Master's of Business Administration Degree, I had to explore a path for applicants with non-nursing master's degrees. It is clear from the AACN DNP Essentials[1] that the practice doctorate education builds on the AACN's *Essentials of Master's Education in Nursing* (MSN Essentials).[7] How do you build on the MSN Essentials without a master's degree in nursing? Putting my DNP education into practice, it was clear I needed to gather evidence.

During the fall of 2018, I conducted telephone interviews with 13 program directors from the USNWR top-ranked DNP programs.[4] Two of the top-ranked DNP programs were excluded as they did not offer a leadership specialty program. Of the 11 remaining programs, 10 offered admission to applicants with a baccalaureate degree in nursing and a non-nursing master's degree. The non-nursing master's degrees most commonly accepted for admission were a master's in business administration, health administration, public administration, and public health. Most program directors referred to the 2015 AACN "White Paper"[6] as their rationale for admitting non-nursing master's graduates. AACN states, that "to provide some additional clarity and flexibility, schools may credit practice hours to a post-master's DNP student who holds current national certification: (1) in an area of advanced nursing practice, as defined in the DNP Essentials; and (2) requires a minimum of a graduate degree."[6] Two further rationales were frequently cited, the program directors believed experienced nurse executives with non-nursing master's degrees met the definition of advanced nursing practice provided by AACN as they were in the business of "administration of nursing and health care organizations."[1] A few program directors also cited the IOM "Assessing Progress on the Institute of Medicine Report The Future of Nursing" stating that DNP-prepared leaders are needed "for leadership roles in academics, health care delivery, health care planning and policy, and other arenas."[8]

All leadership DNP programs surveyed required non-nursing master's degree applicants to currently practice in an area of advanced nursing practice such as health services leadership management, nursing informatics, or community and public health. Programs varied in the years of experience required in these roles with some programs requiring as little as 1 year and others as much as 5 to 10 years.

Program directors were also queried as to how their programs ensured the MSN Essentials were met. The most common response was that the DNP Essentials were a higher standard than the MSN Essentials, so achievement of the DNP Essentials through the DNP program coursework ensured the MSN Essentials were met. Many program directors noted similarities between a Master's of Science in Nursing (MSN) coursework and non-nursing master's coursework when reviewing student's master's transcripts. One program director had devised challenge examinations for master's in nursing courses for non-nursing masters' applicants. Two of the 11 program directors provided courses to bridge the gap between non-nursing master's degrees and required MSN courses determined by review of transcript, usually requiring graduate nursing theory, biostatistics, nursing research, and epidemiology courses. However, the majority of program directors (7 out of 11) did not require additional coursework.

The third area of inquiry in the program director survey was the methodology for meeting the 1000 post-baccalaureate clinical practice clock hours. All programs awarded clinical practice clock hours for national nursing certification. The range of hours awarded was 250 hours to 500 hours with 500 hours being the most common response. An array of nursing certifications are accepted: certified nurse leader, nursing informatics, nurse executive-board certified (NE-BC), nurse executive advanced-board certified (NEA-BC), nurse executive advanced certification, certified nurse manager and leader, CENP, and Lean Six Sigma green belts and black belts.

While many program directors accepted leadership experience as evidence for mastery of the MSN Essentials, RUCON leadership was clear that experience would not be considered a substitute for formal education. It did seem to me that national nurse executive certification examinations could assess attainment of MSN Essentials gained through nursing leadership practice. As a certified advanced nursing executive with decades of nursing executive practice, as I reviewed the MSN Essentials I realized I could not lead a nursing workforce without familiarity with the MSN Essentials. I compared the MSN Essentials outcomes with the nurse executive outcomes assessed by the CENP and NEA-BC certification examinations (Table 18-2). The congruencies were evident. I verified the crosswalk with other faculty in the program.

Armed with the evidence from the program director survey and the crosswalk, I was prepared to share my findings with the RUCON DNP Curriculum Committee and Admissions and Progressions Committee. Based on the findings from the program director survey, admission of non-nursing master's-prepared nurses was approved under the following conditions:

- All admission requirements are met.
- Evidence of national nurse executive certification.
- Review of transcripts for graduate nursing research, biostatistics/epidemiology, and population health courses. Missing courses will be added to the plan of study.
- At least 2 years of documented executive nursing practice.

## Contemporary Plans of Study With Engaging Courses

The TSL DNP curriculum is designed to develop nurse leaders from a variety of employment backgrounds. Nearly 50% of each cohort is comprised of APRNs either in clinical practice or faculty practice. The other 50% are nurse leaders in formal leadership roles in a variety of settings (acute care hospitals, provider practices, community health clinics, home health, public health, and skilled nursing facilities). Length of experience with formal and informal leadership roles can vary from 2 years to more than 30 years. The challenge is to meet the curricular demands outlined in the DNP Essentials with engaging courses for all experiential levels. In review of the courses, many were meeting the needs of APRNs leading change in clinical practice environments but did not adequately advance the knowledge of seasoned nurse executives.

Murphy, Warshawsky, and Mills emphasize the importance of alignment between the DNP Essentials and the specialty-focused AONL Nurse Executive Competencies in graduate nursing leadership education.[9] I used the crosswalks provided in the article and identified tenets from their work to review courses in the current RUCON TSL DNP program. My analysis formed the structure for a RUCON TSL DNP program faculty retreat. In advance of the retreat, I prepared a 1-page course summary that included the course title, hours, description, objectives, and learning assessments for each course in the curriculum. The course summaries were displayed on classroom tables and participants were asked to review for alignment with the DNP Essentials and AONL Nurse Executive Competencies. Overall, faculty felt the program was aligned with the dual competencies, but a few gaps were identified. All of the gaps identified came from the AONL Nurse Executive Competencies. The least-represented competency areas identified by faculty participants were communication and relationship building (influencing behaviors, diversity, community involvement, medical/staff relationships, academic relationships); knowledge of the health care environment (delivery models/work redesign, governance, patient safety, performance improvement/metrics, risk management); leadership (personal journey disciplines, systems thinking, succession planning); and business skills (strategic management). Since the retreat, the findings have been shared with the DNP Curriculum Committee. The Committee members added the importance of threading diversity and global leadership throughout coursework. I spoke with lead course faculty for each course to identify opportunities for inclusion. Courses have been revised or newly developed incorporating many of the topics identified in the gap analysis.

In addition to the AONL Nurse Executive Competencies, retreat faculty reviewed the results of a website survey of the published programs of study of 12 top leadership DNP programs across the country. Within the limitations of course titles rather than full course descriptions or syllabi, the

**Table 18-2**

## AMERICAN ASSOCIATION OF COLLEGES OF NURSING MASTER'S ESSENTIALS AND EXECUTIVE NURSE COMPETENCIES CROSSWALK

| MASTER'S ESSENTIALS | NURSE EXECUTIVE BOARD CERTIFICATION | AMERICAN ORGANIZATION FOR NURSING LEADERSHIP CERTIFIED IN EXECUTIVE NURSING PRACTICE |
|---|---|---|
| Essential I: Background for Practice from Sciences and Humanities | II. Exemplary Professional Practice<br>IV. New Knowledge and Practice Applications | 2. Knowledge of Health Care Environment<br>4. Professionalism |
| Essential II: Organization and Systems Leadership | I. Structures and Processes<br>II. Exemplary Professional Practice<br>III. Transformational Leadership<br>IV. New Knowledge and Practice Applications | 1. Communication and Relationship Building<br>2. Knowledge of Health Care Environment<br>3. Leadership<br>4. Professionalism<br>5. Business Skills |
| Essential III: Quality Improvement and Safety | I. Structures and Processes<br>II. Exemplary Professional Practice<br>III. Transformational Leadership | 1. Communication and Relationship Building<br>2. Knowledge of Health Care Environment |
| Essential IV: Translating and Integrating Scholarship into Practice | IV. New Knowledge and Practice Applications | 2. Knowledge of Health Care Environment |
| Essential V: Informatics and Healthcare Technologies | I. Structures and Processes | 4. Professionalism<br>5. Business Skills |
| Essential VI: Health Policy and Advocacy | I. Structures and Processes<br>II. Exemplary Professional Practice<br>III. Transformational Leadership | 1. Communication and Relationship Building<br>2. Knowledge of Health Care Environment |
| Essential VII: Interprofessional Collaboration for Improving Patient and Population Health Outcomes | I. Structures and Processes<br>II. Exemplary Professional Practice<br>III. Transformational Leadership | 1. Communication and Relationship Building<br>2. Knowledge of Health Care Environment<br>4. Professionalism |
| Essential VIII: Clinical Prevention and Population Health for Improving Health | I. Structures and Processes<br>IV. New Knowledge and Practice Applications | 1. Communication and Relationship Building<br>2. Knowledge of Health Care Environment<br>4. Professionalism |
| Essential IX: Master's-Level Nursing Practice | Master's or higher degree in nursing or bachelor of science in nursing and non-nursing master's; 4160 hours of executive nursing practice | Master's or higher degree in nursing or bachelor of science in nursing and non-nursing master's and 4160 hours of executive nursing practice or bachelor of science in nursing plus 8320 hours of executive nursing practice |

courses were analyzed for consistency with DNP Essentials. Developing evidence-based practice as recommended in DNP Essentials I and III was evident in course titles at all schools. Similarly, all schools had multiple courses aligned with the successful completion of a scholarly project. In alignment with DNP Essentials II, IV, and V, most programs had leadership, informatics, and policy courses. Courses focused on DNP Essential VII with quality and safety in the course title was evident in 8 of the 12 programs. The DNP Essential VI focus on interprofessional collaboration was less evident in course titles but could be incorporated in any number of courses including leading the scholarly project.

Comparing RUCON TSL DNP coursework to the other 12 leadership DNP programs, there were more similarities than differences. Opportunities for expanded content included communication and relationship building, informatics, and quality and safety.

The DNP Essentials clearly prepare leaders to implement change at the macrosystem level rather than the microsystem level.[1] However, according to Murphy et al, specific skills needed to lead macrosystem change are systems thinking, strategic management, and health policy.[9] Of the 12 leadership DNP programs reviewed, only 1 program referred to systems thinking in a course title, with half of the programs referring to systems in their course titles, none of the programs had strategic management in their course titles, and all but 2 programs had specifically titled policy courses. Additional course content in systems thinking and strategic management was recommended for the RUCON TSL DNP program.

Total credit hours for leadership DNP programs varied from 34 to 41 credit hours with 35 credit hours the most common. The RUCON TSL DNP programs of study is 35 hours.

# COURSE REVISIONS AND NEW COURSE DEVELOPMENT

Based on the environmental analysis, many minor course revisions were completed. Three major course revisions and the development of an entirely new course became my responsibility: DNP Specialty Practicum, DNP Specialty Immersion Residency, Finance and Business Concepts, and the creation of an Advanced Leadership Course.

## DNP Leadership Specialty Practicums

Historically, 3 separate clinical specialty practicum courses focused on completing the scholarly project. During a RUCON review of all DNP specialty programs, an inconsistency was identified in the RUCON TSL DNP program. While all the other DNP specialty tracks awarded 252

practicum clock hours related to the scholarly project, the TSL DNP program awarded 500 practicum clock hours for completion of the scholarly project. For uniformity across programs, practicum courses for completion of 252 non-project related practicum clock hours needed to be developed. Additionally, in order to admit students with less than 500 clinical practicum clock hours from their master's education, additional terms with variable course hours would need to be folded into this course. In other specialty DNP programs at RUCON, students completed 2 types of non-related specialty practicums: specialty practicums and a residency immersion.

The college had no history of creating leadership-focused practicums. This is where my particular skill set as a TSL DNP graduate, work experience, and certification as an advanced executive nurse leader were essential. In the other specialty DNP programs, advisors certified in the student's clinical specialty provide clinical supervision while site facilitators or preceptors oversee the day-to-day experiences. As the only certified advanced executive nurse leader in the college, I provide the supervision for all students while an on-site facilitator oversees the day-to-day experiences. I designed the course to provide leadership practice for the student in individually focused identified development areas for the student. Students can choose leadership in clinical practice, health care administration, education administration, informatics leadership, or policy development. Many students choose a variety of practice areas.

At the start of the course, students are encouraged to complete leadership assessments to identify opportunities for leadership development. The DNP Essentials and AONL Nurse Executive Competencies provide the framework for creating learning objectives, learning activities, and measurable outcomes from their practicum experiences. During the 15-week course, students submit a practicum proposal, a practicum form with learning objectives, learning activities, and expected outcomes, and 3 practicum clock hour tracking forms with narrative reflective journals. Students are encouraged to seek out experiences with leaders from a variety of settings and backgrounds. However, they select 1 facilitator to monitor their overall practicum experience. At the end of the term, a practicum evaluation form is completed by the student and their facilitator.

Although a pass/fail course, the assignments are graded and returned to students with comments by me as the course director. The course consistently receives student evaluation ratings of 3.6 and above on a 4-point scale.

## DNP Leadership Residency Immersion

Like the specialty practicum course, the residency immersion was focused on completion of the scholarly project. Now, the specialty immersion course needed to follow a similar path as the other specialty DNP immersion courses: practicum clock hours tracking and reflective journals.

However, in nurse practitioner, clinical nurse specialist, and certified nurse anesthetist practicums, the students are developing and presenting patient cases. I needed to develop a comparable format for leadership students to demonstrate the application and synthesis of the knowledge gained through the program to real-life scenarios. Again, the DNP Essentials and AONL Nurse Executive Competencies provided the framework for creating course learning activities. Each student presents an exemplar pulled from their practicum experiences in an interactive web-based class session.

## Finance and Business Concepts

The Finance and Business Concepts course focused on using Excel worksheets to prepare a 5-year project budget and writing a financial position paper requesting funding for the student's project. A change in project course sequencing required a change in the assignments from direct application of budgeting principles to the student's project to theoretical application through case studies. Opportunities for course development also included:

- Skills in interpreting financial statements
- Billing and coding compliance skills
- Basic health care economic principles with financial benchmarks
- Developing metrics for monitoring financial performance
- Legal, ethical, and policy issues in health care financing
- Global health care financing.

The new 15-week course addressed all these topics using a less acute care hospital–focused textbook and adding videos, asynchronous class sessions, and more engaging assignments for students in all practice settings. More emphasis was placed on critical thinking exercises where students applied financial concepts to real-life situations from their practice setting.

## Advanced Leadership Course

As an experienced health care executive, from my experience as a DNP student and DNP-prepared organizational leader, I discovered several key areas for contemporary leadership development not present in the current curriculum including:

- Evidence-based advanced leadership skills such as systems thinking
- Developing emotional intelligence: self-awareness, self-regulation, motivation, empathy, and social skills
- Board governance and shared governance leadership competencies
- Interprofessional team leadership skills (communication, collaboration, conflict management, negotiation, and shared leadership)
- Competencies for leading innovation, diversity, change, and global health initiatives

I designed an advanced leadership course with the following objectives: (1) adapt advanced evidence-based leadership skills for the role of executive nurse leader; (2) maximize evidence-based communication and relationship building skills to lead organizational system changes; and (3) leverage executive leadership skills to lead interprofessional teams. Students view YouTube videos by national leaders and participate in interactive webinars with faculty. Assignments include self-reflections, self-assessments, discussion postings, creating an ethical leadership plan, negotiation strategy paper, strategic communication plan, and a paper focused on analyzing the student's leadership of a high profile initiative.

Technology, Entertainment, and Design (TED) Talk videos have become a popular addition to the course. TED, a nonprofit, recruits internationally recognized thought leaders to distill their wisdom into short (ie, less than 18 minutes), impactful, videotaped presentations. In one assignment, students are required to create a video of their leadership wisdom using a TED Talk approach.

## Relevant Experienced Faculty

Former program directors asked faculty from all departments to conduct applicant interviews. Although a standardized interview form was used, faculty differed in their assessment of applicant potential, particularly in evaluating leadership potential and assessing the feasibility of the student's project idea. To provide consistency in applicant interviews, I began conducting all applicant interviews. This was a learning curve. Initially, I accepted all applicants. Over time, based on degree completion rates, I was able to develop several key questions gleaned from successful student characteristics. For example, students with no formal or informal leadership experience struggled with courses. Students with a range of formal leadership roles coupled with volunteer leadership roles had higher degree completion rates. Also, students unprepared for the rigor of 12 to 18 hours of coursework a week often left the program within the first 2 terms. Most students continue their full-time employment during their education. I learned to ask the applicants for their plan for balancing work and school and how they were preparing their family and friends for their unavailability.

Another reason for interviewing all the candidates was the need to match the student to the appropriate advisor. I found assigning an advisor to a student difficult if I had not interacted with the applicant. I found the interpersonal match as important as the advisor's expertise. The advisor is the student's main contact with all aspects of the educational process. Advisors meet monthly with students, assisting them with the transition to school; developing, implementing, and evaluating their scholarly project; supervising their clinical practicums; and coaching the student through the DNP program and often beyond toward new career options. Student complaints about advisors or request for advisor changes decreased dramatically with this simple change.

To fully prepare RUCON TSL DNP students for advanced leadership roles, I believe faculty should have experience as a nurse executive. It has taken years of speaking openly about the mission of preparing future nurse leaders to convince a few colleagues to transition to faculty roles. A successful, but rare, strategy has been a shared position with a hospital. One experienced chief nursing officer gave half of her position to a designated successor and took a half-time position with the RUCON. Another colleague needed a half-time faculty position due to family caregiving needs. I have to stay active in the nurse leader community to identify potential faculty recruits.

## OUTCOMES

The many changes implemented in the years I have been program director have resulted in a consistent applicant pool of 40, recommending 28 applicants for admission per year, and 22 graduates per cohort. On average, student satisfaction for courses range from 3.5 to 4.0 on a 4-point rating scale and student satisfaction with course faculty ranges from 3.5 to 4.0 on a 4.0-rating scale. End of program student satisfaction surveys between 2017 and 2018 demonstrated improved student satisfaction with curriculum and meeting students' expectations and an increase from 88% of students' likelihood to recommend program to a prospective student to 100%.

# INTERPROFESSIONAL COLLABORATION AND POPULATION HEALTH

Early in my tenure as an academic, I was asked to lead an interprofessional and multi-organization team to answer a call for proposals from the Robert Wood Johnson Foundation (RWJF) to establish a National Leadership Program Center for the Multisector Health Leaders program. RWJF's stated purpose for creating this program was to "develop, train, and network leaders who will drive action toward building a culture of health."[9] RWJF further defines a culture of health as "individuals, businesses, and governments working collectively to foster healthy communities."[10]

The National Leadership Program Center for the Multisector Health Leaders program was charged with structuring a 3-year program to "develop, harness, and leverage a diverse group of leaders representing key sectors, who as a result of this program, will take their leadership and influence to the next level to lead communities, organizations, and the nation to a Culture of Health."[10]

The funding request to accomplish this goal was more than $10 million and required the coordinated efforts of the National Center for Healthcare Leadership (NCHL), Rush University (RU), DePaul University Center for Community Health Equity, the Illinois Institute of Technology Lewis College of Health Sciences, the University of North Carolina Gillings School of Global Public Health, and Rippel Foundation ReThink Health. The proposal recommended the creation of the RWJF Multisector of Health Leadership (MLH) Center comprised of all the named entities. Developing the proposal took 1 month and the concerted effort of more than 25 team members.

I drew on much of my DNP education to facilitate this team, first, turning to published literature to understand the problem RWJF was hoping to solve with their culture of health leadership development programs and then finding the evidence-based leadership practices needed to lead these changes. When bringing together multi-sector leaders to improve the culture of health in communities, determining the best practices and the best people in the country to teach these skills was needed.

Secondly, it took all the team leadership skills I learned in my DNP education to meet the application deadline. Assembling the correct team of leaders was the first charge. I had to use my networks to unearth their networks to create the diverse team necessary to meet the demands of the proposal. The design principles and operating model were agreed upon at the first meeting. Five work groups were created: (1) program design and approach; (2) applicant recruitment and selection; (3) cross-program collaboration and synergies; (4) organizational capacity and staffing; and (5) application deliverables, outcomes, and budget. Two lead individuals took responsibility for each work group. Timely distribution of meeting minutes with follow-up accountabilities and deadlines were critical. My communication with work group leaders between meetings kept work moving at the necessary pace. A grant writer was hired to ensure the document read with 1 cohesive voice.

Thirdly, although DNP education does not focus on curriculum development and alignment between course objectives, learning activities, and student outcomes, my recent educational experiences prepared me to lead the team creating an innovative curriculum for multisector leaders. The team fashioned a contemporary approach to leadership development using collaborative (action-based inquiry intensives), independent (leadership portfolios and online learning), action (regional networks), and experiential (business simulation) learning. Networks of thought leaders, innovative practitioners, and renowned university scholars from within and outside health care were formed to guide participant development during group learning sessions and individual coaching sessions.

Finally, without my DNP education I would not have understood the impact of the social determinants of health on the overall health of individuals and communities. It was through my DNP studies that I learned to value the work of non-health care sectors on health. For most of my nursing career I was focused on acute care rather than primary prevention. The concept that unsafe neighborhoods or a lack of walking paths contributed to obesity was learned in my DNP studies.

Unfortunately, despite our best efforts, our proposal was not accepted for funding. However, many valuable lessons were learned from the project. Preparing a $10 million project in 1 month improved my project management skills. Leading a team with such diverse backgrounds taught me the value of listening to everyone's ideas. Meeting thought leaders from across the country greatly enhanced my professional network and refocused me on the need for teaching and leading colleagues from all areas within health care and the surrounding community leaders.

Throughout my career I have valued the contributions of my non-nursing colleagues. I have been a member of the American College of Healthcare Executives (ACHE) for more than a decade, attending their annual Congress and local Chicago Healthcare Executives Forum meetings regularly. I became a Fellow in ACHE after joining the RUCON faculty. Although I value nursing and nursing leadership, I believe it is through the relationships developed outside of nursing that we can maximize the breadth and depth of our leadership abilities. This is also my reasoning for maintaining an appointment within the RU College of Health Sciences (CHS) Health Systems Management (HSM) master's program. Working with non-clinical master's students challenges my traditional thinking of how health care should function. To maintain my faculty rank within RU CHS, I chair students' project committees and assist them in publishing their work.

# PROFESSIONALISM

I wish I could say that I advanced the nursing profession by publishing my DNP scholarly project. I will always regret not submitting a manuscript as soon as I completed my doctoral work. I took the more comfortable option of presenting my work at multiple national conferences. For a time I was definitely seen as a national expert on patient throughput (the subject of my DNP project work). I submitted abstracts for 7 international and national meetings during the last term as a student and was accepted for podium presentations at all of them: ACHE Congress, Academy of Management international meeting, several World Research Group national conferences, American Organization for Nursing Leadership national meeting, annual Magnet conference, and several Teletracking User Group meetings.

One dramatic impact my DNP education had on me was reviving my interest in health care policy and advocacy. While still a student, I worked with RU's nursing shared governance organization to initiate a legislative and patient advocacy (LPA) standing committee. The goals of the LPA committee are to: (1) communicate, educate, and provide information to the professional nursing staff about Illinois and federal legislation and patient advocacy issues; (2) act as liaisons with Illinois representatives and lobbyists; and (3) comply with RU policies and procedures regarding dissemination of information and political activities. Since its inception, the LPA committee has hosted multiple policy educational forums, an environmental health and justice summit, voter registration drives, provided an advocacy toolkit for nurses, and facilitated state legislator visits.

Individually, I have attended professional organization lobby days in Illinois and Washington, DC. Through my DNP education, I learned the National Collaborating Centre for Healthy Public Policy's "Framework for Analyzing Public Policy."[11] This tool prepared me for an informed discussion with legislators that could add to their knowledge of the impact of proposed bills on complex health care systems. I was able to speak directly to the impact of the plethora of nurse staffing laws in the State of Illinois.

Given my interest in policy, I jumped at the chance to teach one of the DNP policy courses when I joined the RUCON faculty. Teaching this course keeps me current on proposed federal and state legislation. All of the 21 students I teach each term use the framework described in the previous section to compare and contrast 2 proposed policy solutions to a high-cost health care issue. I learn as much about health care policy as the students do.

I have a strong commitment to advancing nursing leadership locally, regionally, and internationally. In the state of Illinois, I am an active member of the Illinois Organization of Nurse Leaders (IONL). I've been a board of directors member, a regional director, elected president of the organization, founding chair of the Past-Presidents Council, and lead faculty of IONL Nurse Leaders Fellowship Program. Recently, I was recognized for my work with the Most Valuable Member Award.

By far the greatest honor in my career was being selected from among 130 national applicants for the RWJF Executive Nurse Fellows (ENF) program in 2013. The 3-year fellowship prepares you to lead and advance the profession of nursing. Learning activities ranged from traditional lectures at the Center for Creative Leadership to action learning team projects, learning teamwork through working with horses, developing your executive presence with a drama coach, fine-tuning your interview skills with a live television interview, executive coaching, and developing an individual leadership project. Throughout the program, national thought leaders were embedded in learning activities and discussions.

My action learning team convened a national health care summit in Washington, DC. Fifty individuals including payers, health systems/providers, advocacy groups, consumers, and technology experts focused on using technology to improve transitions in patient care. Key themes of the summit included the importance of:

- Human/patient/consumer centeredness
- Inter-operability within and across organizations and sectors
- Communication

The summit outcome was a collection of project ideas and prototypes that were shared at national meetings and in 1 publication.[12] The goal was for all participants to continue working on prototypes that improve communication, focus on patients, and utilize technology to improve care transitions.

My individual leadership development project took me out of my comfort zone. When choosing an individual leadership project that would have impact on the health outcomes of our nation, I worked with a federally qualified health care center (FQHC) that provides health care to the homeless in Chicago. The project I led for the organization was creating a Health Neighborhood (HN) within several transitional housing complexes. The HN aims were to improve the health outcomes for this population through increasing access to health services and education, support for adopting healthy behaviors, and self-management of chronic health conditions. The Kellogg Foundation's Logic Model learned in my DNP program became the organizing framework for the multiple activities needed to create the HN.

The fellowship was a once-in-a-lifetime, life-changing experience that truly prepared me for a more expansive role in leading my profession. It was during the RWJF ENF program that I made the decision to move from practice leadership to academia. Through the fellowship, I discerned my personal impact on the profession would be greater by teaching, coaching, and mentoring current and future nurse leaders. The fellowship provided the safe space and new insight needed for that discernment to occur.

Unfortunately, the RWJF ENF program ended in 2018. Alumni from the fellowship created NurseTRUST, an organization to continue the work of the fellowship. Professional organizations can provide leadership development programming, but they do not have the capacity to create the safe space, trust, and depth of relationships created within RWJF ENF programming. The mission of NurseTRUST is "to engage nurses in life-changing leadership, with a vision to transform health through optimizing nursing … to intentionally disrupt health care to improve health, add unparalleled value through trusted and collaborative relationships, and inspire and equip nurses to lead courageously."[13]

I am a program committee member for NurseTRUST. We are developing programming and products to deliver on the mission. I like to refer to the work of NurseTRUST as paying it forward. In the RWJF ENF program, we developed the competencies to disseminate throughout the nurse leadership community. One example is how NurseTRUST members serve as mentors, bringing nurse leaders that will never have the formal RWJF ENF experience into our programs and leadership circles through mentor/mentee relationships.

Another area of contribution to the profession is board leadership. Based on the project I completed with the FQHC for the homeless, I was asked to join their board of directors. I was recently elected vice chairperson of the board of directors and also chair the Quality Management Committee. I have learned just how many of my acute care executive leadership skills are transferable to the organization. It continues to be a growing experience for me.

# Pearls/Takeaways

**Step out of your comfort zone.** The greatest growth experiences in my professional career came from taking on projects that were a stretch for me. I took on projects that I did not have specific skills or knowledge about. In each case, I used the approach learned from my DNP project to successfully meet the challenge. You do not have to be an expert to succeed, and you can become an expert through doing. I have seen many leadership careers stall because of the fear of taking risks and stepping out of your comfort zone. Often, I learned more from the mistakes I made than the successes. The secret is to learn from the missteps and reframe your thinking to see failure as motion forward rather than a step back.

**Leadership is a journey not a destination.** A successful leader commits to life-long learning. In 4 decades of leadership, I have seen leadership best practices come and go. Remaining vigilant in the quest for new leadership evidence-based practices is as important in leadership as in any clinical practice. It was difficult at times to surrender old leadership practices for the new evidence, but it was always worthwhile.

# Conclusion: Impact of the DNP Degree

As a result of obtaining my DNP degree, I was well-prepared to transition into an academic leadership role and implement a substantive quality improvement project in an academic setting. Through my formal DNP education, I learned to clearly define the problem using data and systems thinking, enlist a group of stakeholders, scan the environment, explore the published literature for best practices and strategies, manage change, and improve measurable educational outcomes that ultimately will improve the health of individual patients and populations. The revised TSL curriculum has seen improvements in program enrollment, student satisfaction, and national reputation. The student applicant pool has grown to 40 and the number of students entering the program remains steady at 28 students, more than double the number admitted at the beginning of the project. Student satisfaction, measured by the end of program student survey, has increased from 88% of students likely to recommend the program to a prospective student to 100%. In the 2021 USNWR rankings, the TSL DNP program climbed from seventh to fourth in the country.

# Acknowledgments

I attribute my successful transition to a faculty role to the unwavering support I received from the faculty and leadership of RUCON. You were patient and kind as I found myself a novice after many years of being an expert. A special thanks to Dr. Beth Bolick, Dr. Janet Engstrom, and my husband, Dr. Jason Earle, for teaching me how to be a teacher, scholar, and program director.

# REFERENCES

1. The essentials of doctoral education for advanced nursing practice. American Association of Colleges of Nursing. Accessed May 7, 2019. https://www.aacnnursing.org/Portals/42/Publications/DNPEssentials.pdf

2. Nurse executive competencies. American Organization for Nursing Leadership. Accessed May 7, 2019. https://www.aonl.org/nurse-executive-competencies

3. DNP fact sheet. American Association of Colleges of Nursing. March 2019. Accessed May 7, 2019. https://www.aacnnursing.org/News-Information/Fact-Sheets/DNP-Fact-Sheet

4. Find the best nursing schools. U.S. News & World Report. Accessed May 7, 2019. https://www.usnews.com/best-graduate-schools/top-nursing-schools

5. Nursing faculty shortage. American Association of Colleges of Nursing. Accessed August 25, 2019. https://www.aacnnursing.org/News-Information/Fact-Sheets/Nursing-Faculty-Shortage

6. The doctor of nursing practice: current issues and clarifying recommendations. American Association of Colleges of Nursing. Accessed May 7, 2019. https://www.aacnnursing.org/Portals/42/News/White-Papers/DNP-Implementation-TF-Report-8-15.pdf

7. The essentials of master's education in nursing. American Association of Colleges of Nursing. Accessed May 7, 2019. https://www.aacnnursing.org/Portals/42/Publications/MastersEssentials11.pdf

8. Altman SH, Butler AS, Shern L. *Assessing Progress on the Institute of Medicine Report The Future of Nursing*. National Academies Press; 2016.

9. Murphy LS, Warshawsky NE, Mill ME. An assessment of the alignment between graduate nursing leadership education and established standards. *J Nurs Adm*. 2014;44(10):502-506.

10. 2015 national leadership program centers call for proposals. Robert Wood Johnson Foundation. Accessed June 23, 2015. https://anr.rwjf.org/templates/external/LPG_Applicant_Web_Conference.pdf

11. A framework for analyzing public policy: practical guide. National Collaborating Centre for Healthy Public Policy. http://www.ncchpp.ca/docs/Guide_framework_analyzing_policies_En.pdf

12. Maughan SE, Green A, Henderson K, et al. Nursing summit: Improving transitions in care through collaboration and technology. *Comput Inform Nurs*. 2016;34(3):105-107.

13. Mission. NurseTRUST. Accessed May 13, 2019. https://www.nursetrust.org/

# CHAPTER 19

# Integration of Telehealth Into DNP Curriculum and Clinical Practice

*Pamela Paplham, DNP, AOCNP, FNP-BC, FAANP;*
*Tammy Austin-Ketch, PhD, FNP-BC, FAANP; and*
*Mallory Andrzejak, DNP, FNP-BC*

## Introduction

To generate an expanded and cutting-edge advanced practice nursing workforce, Doctor of Nursing Practice (DNP) program leadership needs to develop a strong appreciation for the historical perspective of health care. Additionally, DNP leadership should continually scan the landscape for novel approaches to not only curricula, but also further a vigilant appreciation for new horizons in the technology sector. Developing additional practice opportunities for DNP students and health care practitioners serves as a platform to increase access to health care for patients, particularly in underserved areas. Integrating telehealth technology into DNP programming to educate advanced practice nurses in utilization of an innovative modality that has the potential to ultimately increase patient access to primary health care is a challenge that is before us in these turbulent health care times. Not only does the use of telehealth provide expansion of potential clinical sites for students, it also provides faculty with use of a powerful tool to provide oversight and consultation to students in remote, rural, or distant clinical sites.

Introducing telehealth into the DNP curricula requires new didactic content, skill development, and hands-on practice with the telehealth medium. Academic faculty or field-based mentors who have practical experience with telehealth technology is helpful; however, it is not an absolute requirement to guide the acquisition of appropriate technology, development of didactic and experiential components of the curricula, or initiating and monitoring best practices in telehealth utilization. Integrating telehealth into the curriculum requires development of knowledge and competence in the use of technologies, as well as the legal issues around Health Insurance Portability and Accountability Act (HIPAA) requirements, insurance reimbursements, and licensing. Students, faculty, and members of the institutional information and instructional technology teams need practice in utilizing the technologies, management of potential technical problems to maximize time for patient care, and understanding the systems that are needed to provide optimal care.

Another key element in the introduction of telehealth into DNP programming is the development of strategic clinical partnerships where telehealth technology can be implemented to provide maximal benefit to a community-based

Benson LA, ed. *The DNP Professional:*
*Translating Value From Classroom to Practice* (pp 205-214).
© 2021 SLACK Incorporated.

partner, the DNP learner, and the academic institution. This requires a significant amount of pre-implementation effort to glean the required comfort level with use of telehealth technology, providing directions to the student, patient, and/or community partner who may be located at a distant site, as well as knowledge of the type of clinical documentation that is required for utilization of telehealth in order to garner appropriate reimbursement for services provided.

# HISTORICAL PERSPECTIVES AND CREATION OF REMOTE MONITORING TECHNOLOGIES

Entrenched in the daily fabric of our lives are mechanisms propagating the invention and use of remote communication methodologies. Historically, the foundations of primordial distance communication were necessitated mainly by the demand for military logistics and preparedness for battle by increasing knowledge regarding the proximity of the enemy. Ancient distance medical communication used by Greeks, Romans, and Native Americans mainly consisted of smoke signals and light reflection, which conveyed not only births and deaths, but also health catastrophes such as the plague.[1]

With the invention of the telegraph, the rapidity at which military personnel could transmit valuable information about casualties, deaths, supplies, and medicinal consultation was significantly enriched. The telegraph led the armed forces to embrace this distance communication technology. However, the utility of this mechanism for the general population was meager due to lack of a network of telegraph receivers and the specialty skill set required to operate this form of technology.[1]

In 1875, the origination of the telephone laid the foundation for distance communication as we know it today. Unlike telegraph technology, telephones became widely available to the general population, especially those living in metropolitan areas, and did not require a highly specific skill for effective use.[1] It was this type of communication media that *The Lancet* (1879) medical journal reported would diminish unnecessary health appointments through distance consultation and/or informational exchange.[2] The first electrocardiogram (EKG) was transmitted over the telephone in the early 1900s by Dr. Willem Einthoven.[3] This idea was ingenious, but it was not until 1924 when *Radio News* magazine portrayed "radio doctors" by using the technology of a microphone and television to engage in distance communication including the use of heartbeat and temperature indicators. Since most Americans had only started to embrace in-home radio and television, this technology was in its infancy and was considered a futurist vision.[1]

As a visionary, Dr. Hugo Gernsback in 1925 predicted that radio and television would be used for patient-physician communication.[4] Dr. Gernsback would also pioneer the idea of teledactyl, where radio signals were used to generate a patient video image and operate a robotic hand remotely to perform physical examination. This foresight is now thought to be the ancestor of robotic surgery.[5] By 1948, the first radiologic images where sent via telephone across 24 miles in Pennsylvania.[6]

By 1959, Nebraska established a closed-circuit television link between a hospital and psychiatric center in need of consultation services.[7] Nebraska also pioneered the first real-time video telemedicine consultation with interactive neurological examinations.[8] In the early 1960s, NASA began testing transmission of data to scientists on Earth from medical monitoring systems attached to animals on test flights.[9] Later that decade, in a collaborative effort to apply equivalent technology intended for manned space exploration with a Native American reservation, NASA, Lockheed Martin, and the Indian Health Service joined together for the Space Technology Applied to Rural Papago Advanced Health Care (STARPAHC) Project.[10] By the 1970s, the STARPAHC program linked Indian Health Service hospitals by transportable support units to the rural Tohono O'odham reservation in Arizona.[9]

From a practical perspective, business and political facets that led to solidifying distance technology for health care utilization occurred between 1999 and 2016. Augmentation of the use of distance technology in health care reported by the Pew Research Center[11] indicated 65% of the US population utilized the internet and two-thirds utilized social networking sites.[11] As use of the internet and advancing technology merged, key aspects of expanding distance technology in health care included reimbursement for telemedicine by the Centers for Medicare & Medicaid Services (CMS) to rural, underserved areas.[5] Additional expansion of telemedicine and telehealth included the American Recovery and Reimbursement and Health Information Technology for Economic and Clinical Health Acts driving technology advances in medicine[12]; CMS dissemination of "Meaningful Use by Electronic Health Record" conception[5]; the Patient Protection and Affordable Care Act[12]; establishment of Accountable Care Organizations[12]; and the National Defense Authorization Act, which provided telemedicine services to transitioning personnel from military to civilian existence.[13] Federal funding from the Federal Office of Rural Health Policy (FORHP) within the Health Resources and Services Administration (HRSA) resulted in $16 million awarded to focus on expanding distance health technology and access to quality care in rural and underserved communities.[14]

*Telehealth* and *telemedicine* are terms that are often used interchangeably. Telemedicine is simply the delivery of health care services through technology, whereas telehealth also includes patient education, provider education, and mobile health applications.[15] Employing telehealth, which is an efficient way to deliver individualized services, is a means to expand health care access, improve patient outcomes, and patient satisfaction. The US Department of Health and Human Services (DHHS) has included greater use of technology as one of its Healthy People 2020 objectives for improving the health of all Americans.[16] Health communication and health information technology (HIT) can have a positive impact on health, health care, and health equity. A key factor in successfully improving population health outcomes, health care quality, and decreasing health disparities will be in the areas of internet and mobile access through education of tomorrow's health care professionals about new modalities for health care delivery.

In concert with the interprofessional models in health care advocated by the Institute of Medicine (IOM),[17] Healthy People 2020, and major health care educational accreditation organizations, patient-centered care necessitates that educational and practice silos be eliminated or minimized. Employment of telehealth in the academic and health care settings can facilitate interactions of health care professionals from many disciplines. Telehealth is an innovative way to address the health care needs for vulnerable and rural populations whereby providers and patients can connect remotely to a team of providers who can assess and address complex health care needs.

The 2010 Affordable Care Act increased the number of individuals seeking care delivery in the health care marketplace where a finite number of health care providers existed. Health care providers were having difficulties keeping pace with patient needs before enactment of the Affordable Care Act. Identified in 2010 by the IOM,[18] health care provider shortages needed to be addressed in order to meet the increasing demands of individuals who were accessing health care insurance. "The Future of Nursing"[18] report advocated for states to remove legal barriers to allow advanced practice nurses to practice at the fullest scope of their licensure in order to keep pace with intentions of the Affordable Care Act. Advanced practice registered nurses (APRNs) are often frontline providers whose ultimate goal is to provide the fullest spectrum of individualized care possible to their patients and are well positioned to respond to issues of providing health care to diverse populations.

As the DNP developed in nursing education, evolution of the curricula, competencies, and the response to our communities of interest required movement with the technology-driven times to keep clinical academic programs current. In order to maintain technological currency, nursing programs needed to closely examine nurse practitioner core curricula and competencies to determine gaps that exist related to telehealth. The gap analysis could include an interview of students, community stakeholders, and careful review of evidence-based literature landscape relating to clinical care of patients.

Considerations must be given to the expenses associated with initiating an academic clinical program utilizing telehealth, sources of funding needed to continue procurement of telehealth equipment, and trainers for both software and hardware related to the telehealth experience. Incorporation of telehealth as a modality, along with the associated legal, ethical, and billing implications, requires development around the guiding principles of the DNP Essentials, in addition to supporting evidence from evidence-based practice (EBP) literature. In addition to the DNP Essentials as a guide for curricular development, the National Organization of Nurse Practitioner Faculty (NONPF) issued a supportive statement for the incorporation of telehealth in nurse practitioner education.[19] NONPF further recommended that programs should integrate key competencies into the curricular model to include didactic content, simulations and/or standardized patient experiences, hands-on use of telehealth technology, and use in clinical encounters based upon the work of Rutledge and colleagues.[20] The competencies outlined in the NONPF[19] document include Core Competencies that are required during face-to-face student interactions with patients such as utilizing appropriate telehealth etiquette and professionalism during a telehealth encounter, skills in utilizing telehealth and all requisite peripheral equipment, a clear understanding of when telehealth should and should not be utilized, an understanding of privacy and protected information (PHI) regulations, proficient use of the technology, knowledge of documentation and billing requirements for telehealth, a keen ability to collaborate via the telehealth medium, and proficiency in accomplishing all required elements of an appropriate history and physical utilizing telehealth. NONPF[19] supports the use of telehealth as a mechanism to complete observation of students (site visits) to minimize the expense of faculty traveling to remote or distant areas.

As health care has evolved, so too has the technology that drives care in general. From the early years of the Greeks and Romans, to NASA in the 20th century, to computer technology that can remotely monitor patients from the palm of your hand, the use of telehealth in academic and health care environments is here to stay. Academic DNP programs will need to embrace the entrance of this modality into curricular, simulation, and clinical practice models to provide the cutting-edge approach to health care that is required in the 21st century.

# TELEHEALTH AND DNP ESSENTIALS

With an interest in expanding DNP curricula, faculty are tasked with reviewing all germane information related to telehealth, costs of implementation of telehealth into the curricula, as well as identifying faculty champions and facilitators for telehealth utilization in the simulation and clinical practice environments. Review of the American Association of Colleges of Nursing DNP Essentials[21] demonstrates a suitable fit for telehealth in several of the standards. Foundational Essentials were established to guide nursing curriculum, however, they can be considered expectations for the advanced practice profession, making the argument that telehealth education is essential for both students and practicing providers. The acquisition of telehealth knowledge and skills meets criteria within each of the 8 DNP Essential outcomes.

DNP Essential I requires utilization of nursing knowledge and foundation at the highest advanced practice level to improve health outcomes, while Essential III requires the DNPs to provide leadership, translate new science, and improve practice. Telehealth has a growing body of research demonstrating at least on-par effectiveness as traditional face-to-face visits.[22,23] It is a viable delivery method for health care and a DNP should be adequately prepared to provide such care. Telehealth is a change in both product and process creating additional human factor barriers related to resistance to change, use of information technology, and lack of knowledge and/or confidence.[24] In order for telehealth to increase in its use and acceptance, it is imperative for DNPs to be equipped to provide the dynamic leadership that will be needed to prepare health care providers to be ready, willing, and able to provide telehealth care. Despite its potential, only 15% of family physicians utilize telehealth.[25] There is an opening in our health care system for providers who are willing to champion this novel delivery model, and the champion can and should be DNPs.

DNP Essential II requires the advanced practice provider to address social disparities and conceptualize new care delivery models, which dovetails with Essential V, requiring the DNP to participate in policy development and political advocacy for health care practices that work to improve population health, access to care, and social disparities. Telehealth is an effective means of providing chronic care education and monitoring to patients. Further, it can provide efficient primary care to the population as a whole but possibly even more so for vulnerable rural and disabled patient populations who disproportionately lack access to physical and mental health care services.[22,26] Therefore, telehealth as a care delivery modality is an effective means of improving care for vulnerable populations.

Telehealth provides a means of addressing the core tenets of nursing practice. To fully realize the benefits of telehealth, all stakeholders have to perceive the usefulness of such technology. The DNP is an ideal advocate for telehealth due to the evidence of efficacy in the engagement, treatment, and monitoring of patients with chronic conditions.[23] As these chronic conditions are often managed by DNPs, there is a responsibility to create and support policy that advocates for the use of telehealth.

Essential IV requires the DNP to be well versed and accepting of information systems and technology, and to use that technology to promote the efficient and efficacious care of individual patients as well as populations. Though

telehealth is efficacious and cost-effective, its implementation remains low in practice and scarce in nursing school curricula. Due to changes in care required for telehealth involving both products and processes, there are significant human elements that hinder growth, most notably provider acceptance.[24]

It is imperative for DNPs to be able to overcome the human factors that impede telehealth implementation. In order to achieve this, it is essential for nursing curricula to incorporate telehealth education and practice early and often into doctoral (and arguably undergraduate) nursing programs. NONPF[19] recommends increased focus on inclusion of telehealth education into nursing curriculum. The focus should be not only on education of telehealth's efficacy and benefits, but most importantly on the hands-on simulation and clinical practice with telehealth equipment and patient care. DNPs are unlikely to overcome the well-documented human factor barriers related to telehealth use if they are not exposed to telehealth use as students. Creating future DNPs who feel ready and capable to utilize this technology places them at an advantage, and patients will have increased access to cost-effective and efficacious care.

Essential VI calls for the DNP to participate in interprofessional collaboration. Telehealth promotes increased interprofessional collaboration in that multiple providers or providers in different locations are able to meet and communicate in real time. Further, telehealth provides access to specialized care and consultation that may not otherwise be available in certain areas due to shortages of professionals. The use of telehealth can involve any variety of health care professionals and is not limited to occupational and physical therapy, psychotherapy, social work, and specialized medical care such as dermatology, rheumatology, pain management, and teleoncology.

DNP Essential VII seeks to improve population health by advocating for prevention and health promotional activities. DNP Essential VIII requires the DNP to acquire and utilize refined assessment skills and techniques across health and social determinants that can be addressed via telehealth and telehealth student education. Evidence of efficacy and cost-effectiveness exists for telehealth regarding remote monitoring or communication and counseling with improvements found in mortality and quality of life in addition to decreased hospital admissions.[23] Telehealth provides a means to provide care to populations that otherwise would not have access to a variety of specialties. The use of telehealth technology requires an advanced level of nursing practice in that it requires specialized assessment skills and use of different technology and equipment. Additionally, telehealth requires the DNP to engage the patient, create a therapeutic and trusting environment, and demonstrate active listening from a distance. This inherently requires specialized skills and training.

# Telehealth Logic Model to Advance Nursing Practice

Utilizing a logic model approach can help to set the framework for incorporation of telehealth into academic curricula or into clinical practice. Identifying key variables and outcome determinations that will define success can be utilized to assist in setting the stage for engagement in telehealth practice. Historically, there is a paucity of exposure to telehealth in advanced practice academic nursing curricula. However, the health care landscape has evolved in such a way that academic nursing must learn to adapt in order to remain relevant and focus on value-based care while developing a new access point. Insufficiency of this type of technologic innovation for faculty, preceptor, and students accentuates the need for telehealth education in primary care and reflects the 2010 IOM directives to endorse quality care and improve access. To illustrate the use of the logic model for telehealth, Figure 19-1 serves as a template for use in primary care and academic settings.

The key inputs in the logic model include determining partnerships and clinical protocols for practice, establishing a consultative team, and creative ways to engage community stakeholders to promote telehealth use in the community. Each of these inputs will be discussed briefly.

## Inputs

To set up partnership and clinical protocol practices, as well as initiation of access to care with telehealth that will allow for the establishment of new academic-clinical partnership(s) in rural and/or underserved communities, several strategic issues need to be considered. Current health care delivery systems in most rural and underserved communities are unable to be supported by traditional health care models, thus the telehealth model of care would assist on breaking down access to care barriers while potentially enhancing quality of and access to health care.

From an academic-faculty perspective, starting a telehealth program for clinical experiences would allow students to use state-of-the-art mobile telehealth technology while also supporting faculty oversight of students in distant settings. Accepting students that will engage with the latest telehealth technology, the remote preceptor has the potential to expand their own knowledge base while exploring an opportunity for a clinical teaching role in addition to the telehealth clinical practice role.

Establishing an interprofessional consultative team is important to ensure oversight of assessment and plan of care, nurse practitioner student engagement, and effective use of interprofessional collaborative competencies. Effectively engaging the student, faculty, and community partners in interprofessional collaboration with other providers such as physicians, dentists, specialty APRNs, social workers, and community outreach personnel serves to enhance patient care. Utilizing the interprofessional collaborative practice (IPCP) team approach allows for comprehensive care needs to be addressed through use of an EBP approach within a patient-centered care model.

Engaging key community stakeholders to promote telehealth through education of primary care providers on the use and benefits of telehealth is imperative to successful implementation. Enlightening the communities of interest on the availability and use of telehealth for primary care is also imperative for effective execution of this care modality. All key stakeholders having their needs recognized and addressed is vital to the success of telehealth in community settings. Through meaningful information exchange working with stakeholders to identify gaps in services related to rural and underserved populations that could be addressed by telehealth can be undertaken by DNP students as their culminating doctoral project.

## Outputs

Activities and participation are output considerations in the logic model. For faculty, preceptors, and stakeholders, formative evaluation baselines need to be established in order to set the stage to measure success. For DNP programming needs, maximum student capacity at the clinical sites needs to be established to allow for the optimal clinical experience as it relates to the trainee, preceptor, and patient care. In addition to determining maximum capacity, DNP didactic and clinical curricula augmentation must be undertaken to reflect the novel care modality. Knowledge, skills, and attitudes training regarding IPCP and cultural sensitivity should be embedded into the preparatory coursework for clinical experiences.

## Practice and Academic Outcomes

Both short- and long-term outcomes need to be considered when employing telehealth in advanced practice education or in clinical practice situations. Short-term outcomes including telehealth knowledge, skills, and attitudes could be measured through utilization of simulated standardized patients. In the clinical setting, demonstrated use of telehealth in clinical settings by trainees, faculty, and preceptors and evaluation of patient satisfaction with the telehealth modality could serve as practice outcomes. Long-term outcomes could include but are not limited to an increase in either culturally sensitive technology use in primary care, supply of nurse practitioners, clinical faculty, and preceptors, and utilization of IPCP.

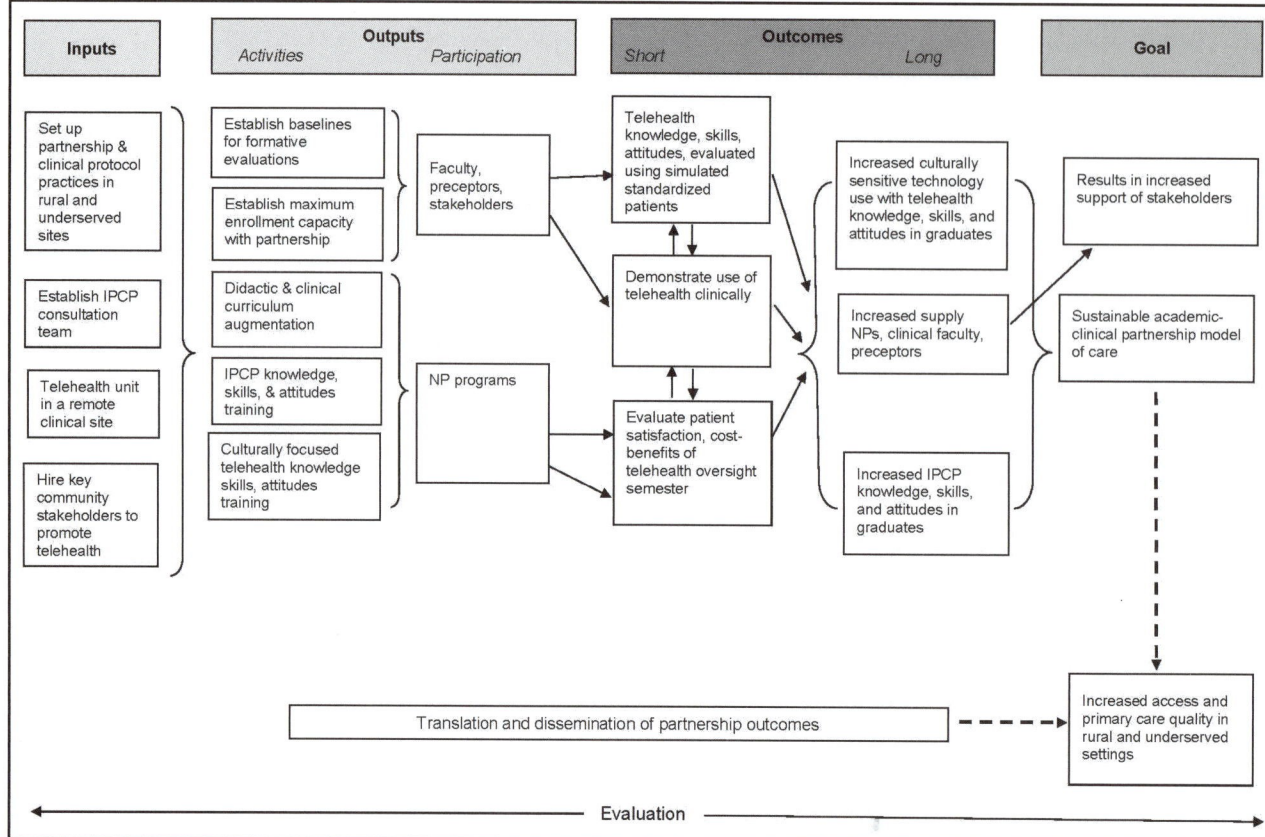

**Figure 19-1.** Partnering to educate nurse practitioners for telehealth practice in rural and underserved settings logic model.

Telehealth is interspersed throughout family nurse practitioner (FNP) coursework that requires primary care clinical experiences. Programmatic quantifiable results are derived from the DNP Essentials, school of nursing outcomes, and measures from the specialty track. From a curriculum standpoint, didactic and experiential exposure to telehealth occurred in advanced physical assessment, FNP specialty track coursework, and the DNP project.

## TELEHEALTH PROGRAM GOALS

The overarching goal of utilizing telehealth in academic programs and primary care practice is to increase the stakeholder support as well as development of a sustainable academic-community clinical partnership model of care. Attaining these goals will increase access and primary care quality in rural and underserved settings. In addition to access and quality, another goal is to include translation and dissemination of the partnership outcomes, which should include successes as well as failures to assist others in undertaking informed decisions as to whether or not telehealth is feasible within their organizations or practices. Table 19-1 illustrates the inclusion of telehealth into DNP academic programming as well as student clinical experience.

## TELEHEALTH VALUE PROPOSITION

In order to build a business plan for the use of telehealth, a long-term financial plan and definitions of the measurements to achieve effectiveness and efficacy need to be key planning goals. The business plan should contain management milestones that are based on reasonable expectations for the stakeholders. The return on investment and patient value of telehealth can be seen across a continuum from academics to clinical practice. From the patient perspective, the value is a reduction in missed medical appointments due to lack of transportation, an increase in patient accountability related to actual participation in their care, and an increase in access to a specialist regardless of the location of both the patient and care provider. From the patient value perspective, incorporating or addressing the aforementioned concepts results in improved coordination of care related efficacy and effectiveness as well as patient outcomes. From an academic perspective, the addition of telehealth to nurse practitioner education increases the reach and breadth of the advanced practice providers upon graduation. It will enhance their ability to increase revenue generation through extended clinical reach. Additionally, telehealth modalities can be used to broaden the oversight of direct and indirect observation of students who are practicing in rural and remote clinical locations. It has increased the pool of potential applicants to access foundational coursework, such as advanced physical assessment, who may live at a distance from the academic center but are seeking to enhance their education. From a clinical practice perspective, patient and provider satisfaction can be increased by ready access to specialty and expert care in real-time. Operationally, there is a potential reduction of wait times for appointments resulting in an open access system.

# INCLUSIONS OF EVIDENCE-BASED PRACTICE

From an academic perspective, there is limited research directly examining the use of EBP protocols delivered via telehealth. Expanded research protocols need to be built into the business plan to make a case for the use of telehealth in clinical practice. As a goal, faculty needs to teach APRNs how to respond if there is an acute change in a patient's condition while using the technology. This may include critical thinking from a technology perspective with the urgency of caring for the patient from a distance while incorporating evidence-based standards.

The implementation of telehealth involves many changes to current health care practices, but it does not reduce the ability to utilize evidence-based care practices. Telehealth has the potential to increase the patient's voice in clinical decision making, a hallmark of both patient-centric and evidence-based care. During student clinical experiences with telehealth, the patient is present throughout the student's clinical presentation to the provider thus allowing that patient to become a more active participant in their care. There is evidence demonstrating that telehealth is efficacious and cost-effective for a wide variety of health care concerns. Telehealth technology allows for the patient to be present and active in all aspects of decision making and provides a means for patients to advocate to multiple members of their health care team simultaneously. In summary, telehealth has the potential to elevate the patient's role, while providing evidence-based accessible care.

# PROFESSIONALISM

Schinasi and Lo[27] suggest that the goal of telehealth professionalism is to convey a level of authenticity, empathy, and presence. In addition to the current curricular model of training, reinforcing, and professional bedside manner for those that deliver health care, the medical virtualist must also develop "web-side-manner," which is an entirely new skill set due to the fact that web visits are more than just conveying data or facts.

# PEARLS/TAKEAWAYS

Telehealth is a change in both product and process. This creates additional human factor barriers related to resistance to change and use of information technology, lack of knowledge, and/or confidence.[24] Providing exposure to the concept of telehealth without creating an opportunity to practice providing care through such a modality is likely not enough to make a student feel comfortable with utilizing equipment as a professional practitioner. Nor are they likely to remember and embrace the utility of unpracticed skills and mindsets.[20,24] APRNs who are not exposed to and comfortable with the use of telehealth may not be able to adjust to these health care changes. It is vital for nursing curriculum to involve not only education on the use of telehealth but also hands-on experience via simulation and clinical settings.[19,20]

# CONCLUSION: IMPACT OF THE DNP DEGREE

As a result of obtaining a DNP degree at an institution that includes telehealth in the curriculum, the utilization of both IOM recommendations and DNP Essentials will enhance patient care by continuing to evolve the role of virtual bedside APRNs. DNP students that understand the worth and breadth of telehealth will become professionals capable to implement such care, advocate for its use, and allow more patients the access to needed health care.

From a faculty perspective, the expansion of knowledge and skills to the student body vs an add-on to the current curriculum adds to the cache of available patient care modalities appropriate to engage in post-graduation practice. Additionally, the use of telehealth has increased our stakeholder pool and built new partnerships with a variety of teams that expands computer, technology, and health care delivery while further breaking down social and structural determinants of health that have traditionally introduced barriers to patient care.

DNPs, those currently practicing and those of the future, need to be ready and able to adopt the most advanced evidence-based patient care as it emerges. It is imperative that DNP graduates are early adopters and champions of this health care delivery modality. The potential impact expanded telehealth care could have on the population's access to needed services, as well as the trajectory for health care services to continue to become more technologically based, create the necessity for the profession to be well versed in telehealth.

**Table 19-1**

## EXEMPLAR OF UNIVERSITY AT BUFFALO TELEHEALTH-RELATED DNP PROJECTS

| DNP PROJECT TITLE/DNP ESSENTIALS ADDRESSED | DNP PROJECT PURPOSE/QUESTION | |
|---|---|---|
| Expanding borders: Implementing mobile telehealth technology to facilitate nurse practitioner clinical education<br>Addresses DNP Essentials IV, VII, and VIII | • Does use of telehealth technology facilitate and/or impeded delivery of efficacious primary care clinical education for patients of a rural health clinic who utilize GlobalMed telehealth technology (ie, bachelor of science-DNP, FNP students and DNP, FNP clinical faculty)? | |
| Implementing telehealth competencies into primary care to enhance clinician education while monitoring patient experience<br>Addresses DNP Essentials I, III, IV, and VIII | • Can identified FNP DNP competencies delivered through telehealth meet the current standards of primary care in a rural health clinic?<br>• Will the telehealth experience (technological, clinical, and interpersonal aspects, the learning experience, and patient care delivery value) provide value to a larger population at a rural health clinic? | |
| Improving education for advanced practice nurses: Developing competencies for telehealth education<br>Addresses DNP Essentials IV, VII, and VIII | • How can academic centers maximize utilization of telehealth equipment available for use in a culturally sensitive manner while minimizing opposition from students?<br>• How will cultural and telehealth competencies influence future DNP programing and the use of telehealth equipment use? | |
| Creation of an evidence-based telehealth training module for primary care provider preceptors servicing vulnerable populations<br>Addresses DNP Essentials II, IV, and VIII | • Creation an evidence-based telehealth training module educating current providers on telehealth, equipment use and the need for telehealth preceptorship.<br>• Determine telehealth components that are necessary to educate and engage potential telehealth preceptors.<br>• Determine effective mechanisms to communicate telehealth education in a short, accessible format. | |

## EXEMPLAR OF UNIVERSITY AT BUFFALO TELEHEALTH-RELATED DNP PROJECTS

| SELECTED RECOMMENDATIONS | SELECTED FUTURE IMPLICATIONS |
|---|---|
| • Major project thematic findings include:<br>  ○ Strengthening the technological-support services foundation<br>  ○ Enhancing the clinical-academic partnership<br>  ○ Optimizing student preparedness | • Continue to examine patient satisfaction and the use of telehealth technology<br>• Develop a mechanism to identify and establish baseline evaluation of telehealth programming<br>• Identification of provider and patient issues that warrant further attention |
| • Value and satisfaction were up as "high" when expanding telehealth competencies, cultural satisfaction, and access to care to a larger population of rural health participants. | • The project revealed students have an interest in incorporating telehealth education into the DNP curriculum for use in clinical practice.<br>• Telehealth integration into academic settings should include simulation experience, physical examination course, and including telehealth in the informatics course. |
| • Collaboration skills and proficiency in telehealth communication technologies are essential competencies for nurse practitioners.<br>• Developing a better working knowledge of telehealth and new communication technologies can enable nurse practitioners in clinical settings to conveniently consult other health care professionals for improved patient care and outcomes | • Incorporating telehealth education into DNP curriculum in regard to which method of education would best prepare students to utilize culturally sensitive telehealth in clinical practice.<br>• Propagating other academic centers to utilize culturally sensitive telehealth training in curriculum |
| • Telehealth training modules should be supplemented with hands-on training and practice.<br>• Training materials should be utilized to exposure all nursing students to telehealth, increasing retention and confidence.<br>• Nursing faculty need to be knowledgeable regarding telehealth, as well as competent and confident in its use. | • Exposing current and potential preceptors to telehealth training materials can lead to increased interest in becoming a telehealth preceptor, filling a needed gap.<br>• Training module can be supplemented as needed over time to various audiences and allows for survey tracking of user feedback |

# REFERENCES

1. Bashshur RL, Shannon GW. History of telemedicine: evolution, context, and transformation. *Health Inform.* 2010;16:65-66.

2. Nesbitt TS. The evolution of telehealth: where have we been and where are we going. In: *The National Academies The Role of Telehealth in an Evolving Health Care Environment: Workshop Summary.* National Academies Press; 2012:11-15.

3. Farris T. A brief history of telehealth. SecureVideo. March 17, 2013. https://www.securevideo.com/blog/2013/03/26/a-brief-history-of-telehealth

4. Novak M. Telemedicine predicted in 1925. Smithsonian. March 25, 2012. https://www.smithsonianmag.com/history/telemedicine-predicted-in-1925-124140942/

5. Lafolla T. History of telemedicine infographic. eVisit. Accessed November 11, 2019. https://blog.evisit.com/history-telemedicine-infographic

6. What is telemedicine? VSee. Accessed November 11, 2019. https://vsee.com/what-is-telemedicine/

7. History of telemedicine. MD Portal. Accessed November 11, 2019. http://mdportal.com/education/history-of-telemedicine/

8. Grigsby J, Kaehny MM, Sandberg EJ, Schlenker RE, Shaughnessy PW. Effects and effectiveness of telemedicine. *Health Care Financ Rev.* 1995;17:115-131.

9. A brief history of NASA's contribution to telemedicine. NASA. August 15, 2013. Accessed June 19, 2019. https://www.nasa.gov/content/a-brief-history-of-nasa-s-contributions-to-telemedicine/

10. Field MJ. *Telemedicine: A Guide to Assessing Telecommunications in Health Care.* National Academy; 1996.

11. Perrin A. Social media usage: 2005-2015. Pew Research Center. October 8, 2015. http://www.pewinternet.org/2015/10/08/social-networking-usage-2005-2015/

12. Gruessner V. The history of remote monitoring, telemedicine technology. Xtelligent Healthcare Media. November 9, 2015. https://mhealthintelligence.com/news/the-history-of-remote-monitoring-telemedicine-technology

13. Wicklund E. Defense bill expands telehealth services in TRICARE. Xtelligent Healthcare Media. December 14, 2016. https://mhealthintelligence.com/news/defense-bill-expands-telehealth-services-in-tricare

14. Davis J. HRSA awards $16 million to expand telehealth, other rural healthcare services. Healthcare IT News. August 12, 2016. https://www.healthcareitnews.com/news/hrsa-awards-16-million-expand-telehealth-other-rural-healthcare-services

15. What is telehealth? How is telehealth different from telemedicine? HealthIT. https://www.healthit.gov/faq/what-telehealth-how-telehealth-different-telemedicine

16. Healthy people 2020 framework. US Department of Health and Human Services. https://www.healthypeople.gov/sites/default/files/HP2020Framework.pdf

17. Institute of Medicine Committee on Quality of Health Care in America. *Crossing the Quality Chasm: A New Health System for the 21st Century.* National Academies Press; 2001.

18. Institute of Medicine. *The Future of Nursing: Leading Change, Advancing Health.* National Academies Press; 2011.

19. NONPF statement in support of telehealth in NP education. National Organization of Nurse Practitioner Faculties. February 27, 2018. https://www.nonpf.org/news/388719/NONPF-Statement-in-Support-of-Telehealth-in-NP-Education.htm

20. The essentials of doctoral education for advanced nursing practice. American Association of Colleges of Nursing. October 2006. https://www.aacnnursing.org/Portals/42/Publications/DNPEssentials.pdf

21. Fraser S, Mackean T, Grant J, Hunter K, Towers K, Ivers R. Use of telehealth for health care of Indigenous peoples with chronic conditions: a systematic review. *Rural Remote Health.* 2017;17(3):1-26.

22. Totten AM, Womack DM, Eden KB, et al. *Telehealth: Mapping the Evidence for Patient Outcomes From Systematic Reviews.* Agency for Healthcare Research and Quality; 2016.

23. Standing C, Standing S, McDermott M, Gururajan R, Mavi RK. The paradoxes of telehealth: a review of the literature 2000-2015. *Syst Res Behav Sci.* 2018;35(1):90-101.

24. Coffman M, Moore M, Jetty A, Klink K, Bazemore A. Who is using telehealth in primary care? Safety net clinics and health maintenance organizations (HMO). *J Am Board Fam Pract.* 2016;29:432-433.

25. Rush KL, Hatt L, Janke R, Burton L, Ferrier M, Tetrault M. The efficacy of telehealth delivered educational approaches for patients with chronic diseases: a systematic review. *Patient Educ Couns.* 2018;101(8):1310-1321.

26. Schinasi D, Lo M. The growing importance of telehealth creates a need for standards. HealthTech. July 23, 2019. https://healthtechmagazine.net/article/2019/07/growing-importance-telehealth-creates-need-standards

27. Rutledge CM, Kott K, Schweickert PA, Poston R, Fowler C, Haney TS. Telehealth and ehealth in nurse practitioner training: current perspectives. *Adv Med Educ Pract.* 2017;8:399-409.

# SECTION VIII

## POPULATION HEALTH EXEMPLARS

# CHAPTER 20

# BUILDING BRIDGES, NOT WALLS
## USING THE DNP TOOLBOX TO ESTABLISH MEDICAL RESPITE FOR THE HOMELESS POPULATION

*Courtney Pladsen, DNP, FNP-BC, RN*

## INTRODUCTION

Nearly 1400 federally qualified health centers (FQHCs) provide comprehensive culturally competent primary care to under-resourced communities across the United States.[1] FQHCs provide care regardless of one's ability to pay. They utilize an integrated care model with a combination of primary care, oral health, mental health, substance use treatment, and a variety of specialty health care. There are specialized FQHCs including Health Care for the Homeless (HCH) organizations that tailor treatment to people experiencing homelessness who are marginalized and live in largely underserved populations. For the past 7 years, I have worked in FQHCs with an HCH program. My energy has focused on improving health care delivery for people experiencing homelessness at the intersection of health care and housing.

In order to meet the needs of individuals who are experiencing homelessness, a system change is essential. When a person who is homeless is diagnosed with cancer, they have to wait to have housing before they are able to initiate treatment like chemotherapy or radiation. When a patient with diabetes with a foot ulcer walks all day to get basic needs met and sleeps in a suboptimal healing environment like a shelter, this often leads to poor wound healing. Both situations lead to delays in care resulting in poor outcomes that could have been avoided if the person has safe and sanitary housing.

Individuals who are in crisis require help immediately, but system-level change is necessary to prevent those crises from occurring in the first place. This work can occur simultaneously. System-level transformation requires centering the community. The change occurs by partnering alongside community members, diverse disciplines, and organizations in order to advocate for more equitable policies at both the state and federal level. This duality is realized for me by providing direct patient care for people experiencing homelessness, while advocating to end chronic homelessness. This practice of meeting the immediate need, while leading efforts to change the system, can be replicated all throughout population health. Our collective efforts are maximized when we advocate and develop a health system that is based on equity for all.

Doctor of Nursing Practice (DNP) nurses are in a unique position to bring the expertise of nursing to make system-level change that will improve the health of our communities.

Benson LA, ed. *The DNP Professional:*
*Translating Value From Classroom to Practice* (pp 217-229).
© 2021 SLACK Incorporated.

This change requires nurses to break down the comfort zone of our silos and build bridges with multidisciplinary teams to foster healthier communities.

# CREATION OF MY ROLE WITHIN THE PRACTICE SETTING

## History of Community Health Centers

In the 1960s, President Lyndon B. Johnson's "War on Poverty" ushered in a new era in health care. During this time, health care pioneers like Dr. Jack Geiger, a civil rights activist and young medical student, witnessed firsthand how a community-based health care model brought health benefits to the most oppressed citizens of apartheid South Africa.[2] Dr. Geiger and other health care pioneers submitted proposals to the Office of Economic Opportunity and subsequently the first proposal for the US version of a community health center was developed. Congress also helped cultivate this new direction in health care by passing several key pieces of important legislation. First, the Social Security Act was amended with the passage of Kerr-Mills legislation (1960), which provided states with grant money for the medically underserved.[3]

The subsequent passage of the landmark Economic Opportunity Act of 1964 marked the birth of US community health centers. The resultant health center model targeted the roots of poverty by combining local community resources with federal funds to establish neighborhood clinics in both rural and urban areas around the United States. This formula not only empowered communities, but also generated compelling evidence that affordable and accessible health care produced compounding positive benefits.[4-6]

## Health Care for the Homeless

The HCH movement was born out of social justice organizing that occurred throughout the 60s and 70s. It has been set apart as a movement through providing compassionate high-quality health care while simultaneously advocating for the end of chronic homelessness through research, policy, and consumer engagement. In 1983, the Robert Wood Johnson Foundation and the Pew Charitable Trusts announced a $25 million, 5-year program to fund the new HCH initiative.[7] There were 19 initial demonstration projects across the United States that were funded. The care team included physicians, nurses, and social workers. The multidisciplinary care model was revolutionary at the time and laid the foundation for patient-centered medical homes.

Barbara Conanan was the nurse pioneer and national leader at the center of the HCH movement from the beginning.[8] In partnership with Dr. Phillip Brickner, the St. Vincent

Hospital team were the directors of the national HCH program.[9] She started in 1981 at the Department of Community Medicine of St. Vincent's Hospital in New York and in 1983 became the manager of the outreach men's shelter. Conanan helped to develop the multidisciplinary approach that distinguishes HCH organizations. In 1987, federal funding expanded to cover HCH organizations, thereby aligning the community health center model with the HCH model. The Health Centers Consolidation Act of 1996 combined these programs under Section 330 of the Public Health Service Act and the programs received the designation of Federally Qualified Health Centers.[10]

Currently, there are more than 1400 community health centers in the United States, with more than 9000 service sites in every state and US territory. These health centers serve nearly 30 million people, 71% of whom live below the poverty line.[11] Half of health center patients live in rural areas, while the other half are located in under-resourced inner-city communities.[11] Health centers serve communities that would otherwise confront economic, geographic, language, cultural, and other barriers to care, making these centers different from hospitals and most private physicians' offices. Health centers are located in high-need areas identified by the federal government as having elevated poverty, higher than average infant mortality, and fewer practicing medical providers.[11]

FQHCs provide access to care to all residents, regardless of insurance status, and provide free or reduced cost care based on ability to pay[12]. With a team-based approach, the care model integrates health care providers such as registered nurses, physicians, dentists, nurse practitioners, midwives, and physician assistants with a variety of other professionals like social workers, mental health clinicians, and community health workers.[11,12] Nearly a quarter of all health center patients are best served in languages other than English, and nearly all patients report that their clinician speaks the same language as them.[11] The services are tailored to fit the special needs and priorities of their communities, and to provide services in a linguistically and culturally appropriate setting.

## Personal Experience

After completing graduate school in 2011, I accepted a position at a large urban FQHC. As a family nurse practitioner, my time was divided between 2 different settings within the organization: a community health center and homeless outreach. The community health center was a large practice with more than 25 000 patients, 6 multidisciplinary primary care teams, and a dental department. The physician providers included pediatric, family, internal medicine, infectious disease, and obstetricians/gynecologists. Advanced practice registered nurse providers included certified nurse-midwives and family, adult gerontology, and psychiatric nurse practitioners. The teams included the integration of behavioral health. More than 75% of the patients were non-English speakers from Central America and Ethiopia. The nurse practitioners had their own patient panels and practiced to the highest extent of their education.

Homeless outreach services included providing primary care, mental health, and substance use treatment to people experiencing homelessness. This occurred in a variety of settings including soup kitchens, shelters, and street outreach. Outreach was done in teams of advanced practice registered nurses/medical doctors/physician assistants, social workers, and peer support workers.

## Impact of Homelessness on Health

However humble, everyone should have a place to call home—stable, safe, and sanitary living conditions greatly impact a person's quality and length of life. The mean age of death for individuals experiencing homelessness is 51 years old, an astounding 28 years less than the 79 years expected for the general population.[13] More than 564 700 people were homeless across the nation in 2015. Sixty-nine percent were in shelters and 31% were on the street.[2] Chronic illnesses, both medical and psychiatric, are disproportionately common in homeless populations and heavily influence these mortality rates.[14] Individuals experiencing homelessness lack the general necessities (ie, housing, financial means, nutrition, consistent and reliable transportation, safety) to manage ongoing illnesses and are more likely to experience exacerbations secondary to lack of resources and inconsistent treatment.[2] These exacerbations correlate with an increase in emergency department visits, inpatient hospitalizations, and increased mortality.[2]

The prevalence of traumatic stress in the lives of people experiencing homelessness is extraordinarily high.[15] Often, these individuals have experienced on-going trauma throughout their lives in the form of childhood abuse and neglect, domestic violence, community violence, and the trauma associated with poverty and the loss of a home, safety, and sense of security.[4] These experiences have a significant impact on how people think, feel, behave, relate to others, and cope with future experiences.[4]

## Starting the DNP Journey

After years of practicing primary care, I realized that providing medical care is not an end in and of itself. I have had countless medical visits overtaken by social emergencies: evictions, domestic violence, deportation threats, racist acts of violence, and the list goes on. In these moments, reviewing their diabetes labs is not the most pressing concern. I became increasingly interested in understanding upstream effects of poor health outcomes. Understanding the barriers to care was not sufficient, I wanted to address health and social inequities. This drove me to pursue a DNP degree. To make broader system-level change, I wanted to expand my quality improvement skills, better understand health care

economics, advance my health care policy knowledge, and focus on translational research to improve health outcomes.

During my doctoral program, my understanding and passion for addressing social determinants of health (SDH) grew. The team-based, community-oriented, and culturally sensitive care provided at FQHCs creates the ideal setting to collect and address SDH information. As my scholarly project was taking shape around screening and addressing SDH, the FQHC where I worked acknowledged that drive and supported my scholarship and quality improvement efforts even prior to completing my degree. Expanding my role started while I was a DNP student, which lead to quality improvement and leadership opportunities.

Out of the scholarly project I developed a multidisciplinary SDH quality improvement working group. This group sought to integrate SDH screening into the primary care visit, as well as infusing SDH into all clinical outcome measures. There were existing quality improvement working groups for outcome measures like vaccination rates, diabetes control, and colon cancer screening. We were able to work with these other groups by aiding in the integration of SDH to all driver diagrams across all of the clinical quality measures. For example, in the diabetes group, access to healthy foods was an SDH. For the vaccination rates, a language barrier was one SDH identified as a potential barrier. Appendix A is an example of a diabetes driver diagram with an integrated SDH approach. By adding the SDH lens to these quality measures, our working group helped to start a cultural shift within the organization. It paved the way for SDH education while taking more upstream approaches to health outcomes.

Leaning into non-clinical roles was challenging. Imposter syndrome is something I certainly experienced throughout my DNP education. Mentors were essential for helping me navigate uncharted territory and affirmed my decisions and skills along the way. These mentors came from various backgrounds including academia as my DNP advisor, a physician who was the vice president of Innovation and Transformation at the FQHC, and nurse leaders. Great mentors distinguish themselves by caring for you as an entire person and not only as a professional. *Harvard Business Review* recommends that professionals focus less on having one mentor and more on have a "personal board of directors,"[16] A singular mentor can be limiting but having multiple informal mentors can help fill multiple professional gaps like time management, personnel management, or networking.

While working in the DNP program I became the medical access director. Responsibilities included providing leadership and supervision of evening and weekend clinic staff, organizing the schedule of more than 50 providers, expanding primary care access, and evaluating staffing models and cost efficacy. This was an incredible learning opportunity. I was part of a multidisciplinary leadership team that supported the largest health center in the city. This opportunity gave me the ability to elevate the role of registered nurses and advanced practice registered nurses in community health. It led to advanced practice registered nurses moving into more leadership positions within the organization and registered nurses taking a more independent role including starting billable visits and triaging patients. These efforts promoted nurses practicing to the fullest extent of their education, which improved staff and patient satisfaction.

With leadership and quality improvement experience under my belt as a practicing advanced practice registered nurse and DNP student, I was chosen to lead the development of a new program within the organization. Medical respite care is acute and post-acute medical care for persons who are homeless and who are too ill or frail to recover from a physical illness or injury on the streets but are not ill enough to require hospital level care.[17] Unlike respite for caregivers, medical respite is short-term residential care that allows individuals experiencing homelessness the opportunity to recover in a safe environment while accessing medical care and other supportive services. Medical respite care is offered in a variety of settings including freestanding facilities, homeless shelters, nursing homes, and transitional housing. The National Health Care for the Homeless Council created the standards for recuperative care and have been leading this model of health care delivery for more than 30 years.[18]

Many patients fall through this gap in our current health care system. For example, a person is admitted to the hospital for diabetic ketoacidosis and with a diabetic foot ulcer. They are inpatient for a week, receive intensive care, and then discharged back to the street with an open wound. This could lead to a cycle of hospital recidivism and poor health outcomes for the patient. Medical respite provides a healthy and safe environment for the person to heal while receiving comprehensive services including medical, mental health, and social services. This patient with diabetes could be admitted to a respite program, have the proper nutrition, a clean place to change the wound, and support to address the SDH-like housing. The FQHC had an existing free-standing, 30-bed men's medical respite program for more than 30 years. Despite the fact that on any given night, 882 unaccompanied (single) women are experiencing homelessness in Washington, DC, there was not a single medical respite bed for women in the entire city.[19] I sought out to fix this.

The FQHC partnered with a women's shelter provider to develop a 12-bed, shelter-based medical respite program. I designed the program by leveraging resources including the Standards for Medical Respite[18] program from the National Health Care for the Homeless Council. I networked with established programs across the country to learn from their expertise. My responsibilities included the design of the staffing model, delineation of the scope of services, development of the policies and procedures, and interdisciplinary care coordination across the 2 partnering organizations.

The development of the medical respite program was my first opportunity to build a program from the ground up. The energy of a new program is infectious when you are able to see a vision come to life with the promise of improving patients' lives. This role sparked something in me that I had not previously experienced and helped to shape a new career path. While I was completing my DNP, I successfully developed and led the program for a year. The quality improvement, leadership, SDH, and program development experiences added many new tools to my toolbox. I was then recruited by a hospital in Maine to move to the state and help them address a length of stay challenge for people experiencing homelessness through the development of the state's first medical respite program. This led to my first experience as a consultant.

## INCORPORATING THE DNP ESSENTIALS

FQHCs provide great opportunity for the incorporation of the DNP Essentials. In a single week, I have provided high quality patient care (DNP Essential VIII), attended a quality improvement meeting about Health Resources & Services Administration's Uniform Data System measures (DNP Essentials II, IV, and VII), provided care coordination with an interdisciplinary team (DNP Essential VI), presented to nursing/medical students (DNP Essentials I, III), and testified at the state house for an upcoming housing bill (DNP Essential V).[20] With the honor of having a terminal degree comes the professional responsibility to contribute to the field and improve our health care system. By taking a system view, one is able to visualize where there is opportunity to create impact at all levels incorporating the DNP Essentials.

## UTILIZING THE DNP ESSENTIALS

Harnessing the academic and professional expertise I obtained through the DNP degree gave me the tools and confidence I needed to become a subject matter expert (SME). I solidified this designation by applying to be a SME through the National Health Care for the Homeless Council.[21] The SME application was a 2-step process. The first entailed submitting a resume, obtaining a letter of recommendation, and having an interview with the National Health Care for the Homeless Council. If you advance through this stage, the second step is to enter into a trial period until you have been favorably evaluated following your first engagement as an SME. Having the title of an SME launched me onto a national platform. This platform opened many professional doors and has enabled me to utilize the DNP Essentials on a regular basis.

Moving beyond professional nursing organizations has been the key to new opportunities and broader impact. In September 2018, I was chosen for the Robert Wood Johnson Culture of Health Leaders Program. It is a 3-year leadership development fellowship that focuses on the promotion of

## Table 20-1

### MEDICAL UTILIZATION OF INDIVIDUALS EXPERIENCING HOMELESSNESS

| TYPE OF UTILIZATION | HOMELESS | CONTROL |
|---|---|---|
| Single men emergency department visits | 9 times higher | - |
| Single women emergency department visits | 12 times higher | - |
| Single men hospitalization rates | 8.5 times higher | - |
| Single women hospitalization rates | 4.6 times higher | - |
| Average emergency department cost per year per patient | $1436 | $175 |
| Average hospital cost per year per patient | $2448 | $517 |
| Maximum emergency department visits per year | 108 | 14 |
| Maximum hospital admissions per year | 14.9 | 2.5 |

1165 insured homeless vs controls. Matched for age, sex, low-income, data over 4.3 years.
Adapted from Hwang SW, Henderson MJ. Health care utilization in homeless people: translating research into policy and practice. Agency for Healthcare Research and Quality. October 2010. https://meps.ahrq.gov/data_files/publications/workingpapers/wp_10002.pdf

health equity in your own community. It is an incredible opportunity for people from diverse professional backgrounds who want to use their position to advance health by promotion of equity, diversity, and inclusion. Of the existing 120 people in the program there are only 2 nurses, which I find appalling. How can we create a culture of health without the largest medical profession in the country? When I asked this question to the program leadership, their answer was simple: nurses do great work in their silos, but when the goal is building cross-sector system change, we are looking for leaders who foster multidisciplinary solutions. If this is the perspective of national organizations, let this serve as motivation for nurses to get outside our comfort zones and break down those silos.

DNP Essential VI is Interprofessional Collaboration for Improving Patient and Population Health Outcomes. As DNP leaders, we have the opportunity, and frankly a mandate per the DNP Essentials, to help our profession develop interprofessional collaboration. An example of this cross-sector partnerships are FQHCs partnering with local farmers markets to increase access to health food through a fruit and vegetable prescription program (FVRx).[22] The FQHC leads a group wellness program focusing on nutrition and exercise while helping the patients, many of whom are first-generation immigrants, to learn how to cook the food from the market. Another example is in rural settings where transportation can be a significant barrier to accessing health care. The FQHC West County Health Centers partnered with a software company, Hitch Health, to address their clients' transportation challenges.[23] When a patient makes an appointment, they receive a text message offering a ride to the clinic on the date of their appointment. If the patient accepts the ride, they receive reminders and are picked up and taken to their appointment. When the appointment finishes, the patient texts again, and a driver comes to take them home. This process is automated and does not involve active management by health center staff. These 2 upstream models can be replicated by nurse leaders across many fields and sectors. To improve population health upstream solutions is complicated, but necessary, and DNPs have the skill set to be at the forefront of these innovations.

# BUSINESS PLAN SUPPORTING THE DNP ROLE

After completing my DNP, I moved to Maine where I worked part-time at a HCH clinic providing primary, mental health, and substance use treatment. Additionally, I worked part-time at an academic medical center hospital as an in-house consultant leading the development of a medical respite program. Prior to being hired as a consultant, I provided some background research on the cost of medical utilization of people experiencing homelessness. The research displayed in Table 20-1 reveals a study done of nearly 1200 individuals. Homeless participants of the study were matched 1:1 to low income controls from the general population based on year of birth and sex. The results are staggering. Emergency room utilization, number of hospitalizations, and length of stay were all significantly higher than the control group.

Utilizing research data paired with the hospital's own analysis of patients who had abnormally long length of inpatient admission, I was able to effectively communicate the scope of the problem, present medical respite as a solution, and provide my consultation as an SME who can deliver this program. The hospital's analysis conservatively estimated there were 1481 avoidable hospital days in 2015. This estimate represents 47 people experiencing homelessness. With the implementation of a 16-bed medical respite program with an average of 22 avoidable days per patient (total of 5840 total days by year 3) yielded a $795 per day cost avoidance. When we utilized backfill economics with an opportunity cost of avoidable days, increasing the revenue of compensated care, an estimated 1000 additional cases could be seen at the hospital. The financial analysis revealed that the revenue from additional cases minus the cost of running the respite program would save the hospital an estimated $12 million per year.

Based off the cost savings to the hospital and the SME consultation fee set by the National Health Care for the Homeless Council, I set a consultation fee of $75 per hour. After negotiating the rate, we signed a 1-year contract with deliverable outcomes for my role. After a year into the project, I developed a business plan that included staffing models, financial analysis, and summary of supporting research. I successfully led 3 partnering organizations on the project, and now in year 2, we renewed the contract for an additional year and the respite program opened in the Fall of 2020.

# Data Mining: Leveraging Data and Creating Impact From DNP Scholarly Projects

## Scholarly Project Background

Social factors such as low level of education, racial segregation, low social support, poverty, and income inequality can lead to premature death.[25,26] There is mounting evidence demonstrating how racism, violence, poverty, and lack of education continue to perpetuate health care disparities across the United States.[27-31] Racial minorities and those living below the poverty level are at a disproportionate risk of being uninsured, lacking access to care, receiving poorer quality of care, and experiencing worse health outcomes.[32] With pervasive health care disparities, a great deal of research is needed to improve the way the health care system understands and addresses social determinants of health.

As health care in the United States has evolved to focus on patient-centered care, care coordination, and quality-based reimbursement, a great deal of interest has emerged surrounding SDH and their significant impact on health outcomes. The World Health Organization defines SDH as the social and environmental conditions in which people are born, live, work, and play.[33] SDH account for approximately 80% of a person's health status, and the current health care system is responsible for the remaining 20%.[34] Over the past 30 years, there has been an evolution in the contextual framework of SDH. Whitehead and Dahlgren developed one of the most widely cited models, which presents a social model of health (Appendix B). The model contextualized an individual's choice and behavior with socioeconomic and environmental factors and the combined impact on health. It is difficult to ascertain how much each specific SDH factor impacts a person's health status, but it is clear that one's zip code can be a predictor of life expectancy.[35]

A growing body of evidence revealing the impact of social determinants on health outcomes, in combination with implementation of the Affordable Care Act in 2010, helped to usher in a new focus on primary care.[36-38] Historically, public health and health care delivery systems functioned in their individual silos. SDH data collection was part of the role of public health and was not viewed as an integral part of primary care. In 1988, the Institute of Medicine (IOM) published "The Future of Public Health", which defined the role of public health in 3 key areas: assessment, policy development, and assurance. Assessment included the collection, assembly, and analysis of the health status of communities, health needs, and epidemiology. More than 20 years later, in 2012, the IOM convened a working group to create a report developed by both the Centers for Disease Control and Prevention (CDC) and Health Resources and Service Administration (HRSA) to help address chronic illnesses by integrating public health with primary care. In the report, one of the areas identified as a space of synergy between public health and primary care was the ability to use clinical practice to identify and address community health problems.

## Information Technology

Many health care providers are not systematically aware of patients' barriers to care, which can greatly impact the effectiveness of treatment plans. The Patient Protection and Affordable Care Act[39] and the Health Information Technology for Economic and Clinical Health Act[40] have been drivers of widespread implementation and utilization of meaningful use within the electronic health record (EHR). The goal of meaningful use is to improve quality, safety, and efficiency with the aim of reducing disparities and improving outcomes.[41] SDH data have traditionally been part of community or aggregate data and have been largely outside the health care setting.[42] Integrating SDH information into the EHR nationwide could lead to an improved understanding about the relationship between SDH and health outcomes and is a natural progression of the technological advances made in the past 20 years.[43]

Current approaches to addressing SDH focus on population-based interventions, which overlook the potential benefit of collecting and addressing SDH in a clinical setting. Integrating SDH information within the EHR provides clinicians with the ability to address and track the impact of SDH on long-term health outcomes.[44] On an individual level, providing this information to a clinician allows treatment plans to be tailored to a patient's needs while also understanding their barriers to care. Additionally, incorporating this information into the EHR could provide insight into how specific determinants impact health outcomes, which could help to fill in current gaps in research and knowledge. On a clinical level, this information would allow organizations to better utilize resources to meet the population's needs.

The purpose of my scholarly project was as follows: (1) assess an education intervention regarding SDH on clinical staff, (2) integrate and evaluate an SDH screening tool called PRAPARE (Protocol for Responding to and Assessing Patients' Assets, Risks, and Experiences) into clinical practice, and (3) describe the findings of patients who were screened. SDH are social and environmental conditions in which people are born, live, work, and play.

The PRAPARE screening tool was embedded within the EHR. An education intervention regarding SDH and the PRAPARE tool was provided to clinic staff. One survey was sent to clinical staff after training, and a second survey was sent 12 weeks later. In addition, a convenience sample of adults in a primary care setting was screened over a 12-week period using PRAPARE. A descriptive analysis was used to illustrate the results of both patient and staff responses.

Of the clinical staff trained, 15 completed both the post-education survey and the second survey evaluating the implementation of PRAPARE. Participants rated the training highly. Nonetheless, participants expressed concern with their comfort in being able to integrate PRAPARE into practice, comfort in utilizing the tool, and identified lack of time as the biggest barrier. Of 222 patients screened, the mean age was 53.4 years, 73.9% were Black, 18% Spanish speaking, 78.8% were living below the poverty line, 40% were unemployed and seeking work, 35% did not have housing, 37% were socially isolated, and 22% lacked access to food. There was no statistically significant correlation between the PRAPARE score and either hemoglobin A1c or blood pressure.

## PRAPARE Results

The demographic data including race and poverty levels were consistent with data reported annually through HRSA.[45] Housing data for HRSA reporting is traditionally collected during registration and 10% of these health center patients in the 2016 report were homeless. PRAPARE data revealed a much higher rate, even when the clinic at the homeless shelter was excluded. The community health center had a low rate of responses to this question on the PRAPARE tool, but of the 13 patients screened, 16.9% reported that they did not have housing.

It is unclear where the discrepancy lies, but the directness and further explanation of the question in the PRAPARE tool may reveal higher percentage of respondents experiencing homelessness. The question asks, "What is your housing situation today?" Choices include "I have housing" or "I do not have housing" (eg, staying with others, in a shelter, hotel, or outside). When patients are being registered, they are asked for an address, rather than asking if they have housing, and this difference may be where the discrepancy arises. Having accurate representation of the number of people experiencing homelessness is not only important in connecting them to social services, but also in grant funding as a HCH organization.

There was a statistically significant difference between each category of education attainment, primary language, and employment status in patients from Clinic A vs Clinic B. Clinic B had the higher percentage of patients who had less than a high school degree, spoke Spanish as their preferred language, but had a higher rate of full-time employment. In Washington, DC, the highest unemployment rate in January 2017 was in Ward 8 at 12.9%.[46] This was only a fraction of what was screened using the PRAPARE tool. Both rates of unemployment (Clinic A at 53.7% and Clinic B at 27.3%) represented a much higher rate of unemployment compared to the city or national averages even when controlled by education level. In January 2017, unemployment rates for those with less than a high school degree were 7.7%, and the rates for those with a high school diploma or GED were 5.3%.[47] Nationally, in 2016, the unemployment rate for Black people was 14.1%, more than double the unemployment rate for White people at 6.5% for those with less than a high school degree. The PRAPARE data revealed that the patients have a disproportionate share of unemployment compared to national averages (Figure 20-1).

Having this type of clinic-level data has the potential to influence allocation of resources within organizations to meet the specific needs identified. When comparing Clinic A and Clinic B, the overall PRAPARE scores had no statistically significant difference, meaning that they both had high levels of SDH barriers to care, but those barriers differed at each site. Clinic A had statistically significant higher rates of homelessness, unemployment, and social isolation, whereas Clinic B had higher rates of low education attainment, non-English speakers, and refugees. This supports tailoring services to each site's unique needs.

## Survey Findings

Survey results revealed that the clinical staff rated the training highly, and felt comfortable addressing SDH, but lacked confidence in the ability to integrate the tool into clinical practice. Eighty percent of respondents felt comfortable addressing SDH with their patients, which is the opposite of the national study conducted by the Robert Wood Johnson Foundation[48] where 80% of physicians did not feel comfortable addressing SDH. The Robert Wood Johnson Foundation survey was a national study evaluating physicians in a variety of settings, thus, location of practice may be a contributing factor to comfort levels (eg, primary care vs intensive care).

Lack of time was expected to be a barrier for the project, and participant responses affirmed this challenge. As the health care system evolves to outcomes-based

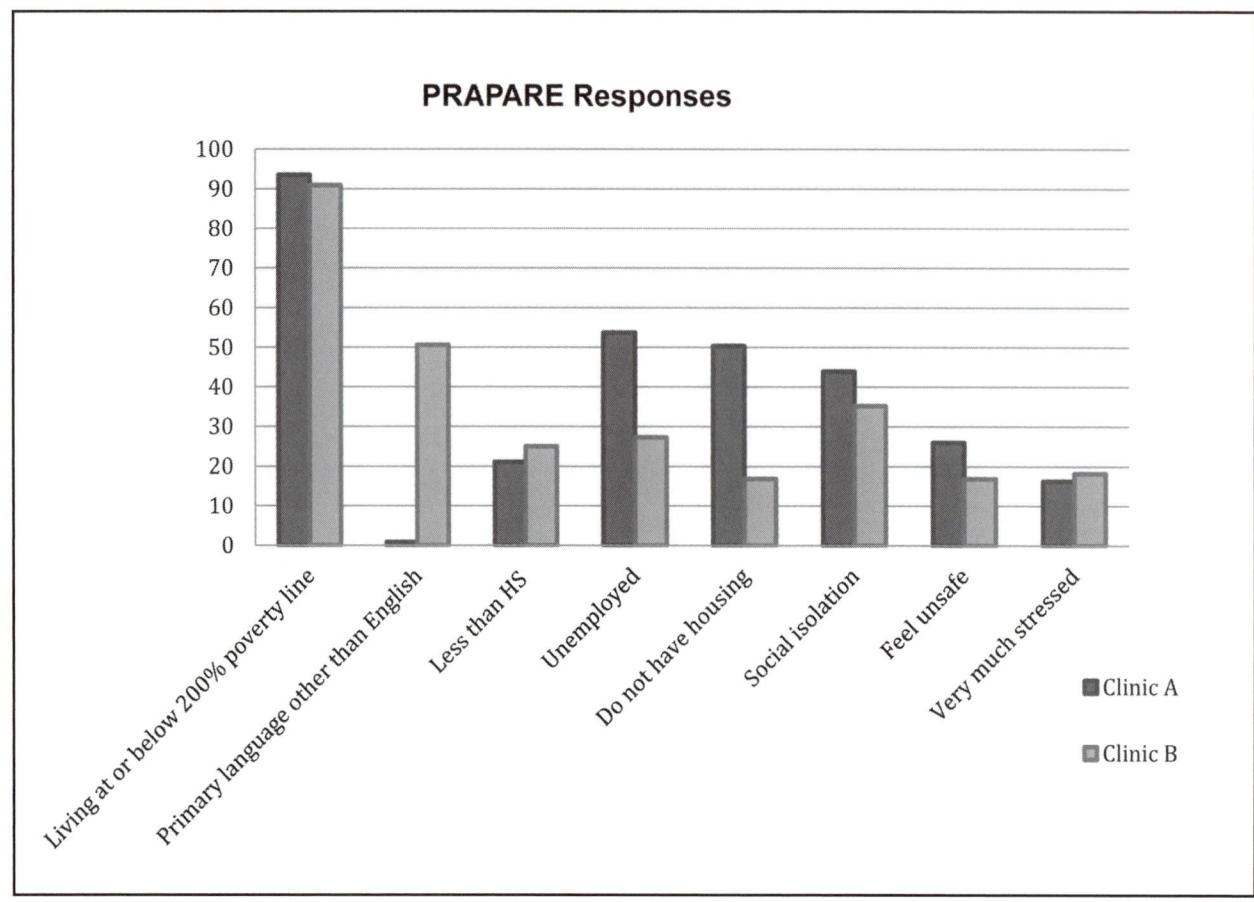

**Figure 20-1.** Abbreviation: HS = high school. Bar graph comparing Clinic A and Clinic B PRAPARE responses.

reimbursement, one consideration for acquiring better patient data is increasing the length of time allotted to the provider with each patient seen. The current reimbursement fee-for-service model incentivizes providers seeing high volumes of patients, which has led to shrinking the length of primary care visits.[49] Medicaid policy change proposals incentivizing health outcomes could help to increase visit times by paying for performance rather than volume, which could in turn provide more time to screen and address social issues.

More than 70% of survey respondents indicated that they were more likely to refer patients to social services after utilizing the PRAPARE tool with the patient, which was an unexpected finding in the project. Further evaluation through longitudinal study could be helpful to evaluate if patients followed through and connected with a social worker, because simply referring a patient does not always translate into a connection to that resource.[50] Despite a variety of clinical staff responding, there was no social service staff represented in the surveys. With social service providers being a key element in addressing SDH, it was unfortunate to not have their voice included.

Despite the knowledge that 90% of a person's health status is shaped by SDH, the relationship between SDH and health outcomes is poorly understood. By educating clinical staff and implementing the SDH screening tool PRAPARE,

222 patients were screened and a significant amount of information was learned about our staff and patients. This information led to better awareness of the patients' barriers to care and also increased referrals to social services. There was no correlation between the PRAPARE score and blood pressure or hemoglobin A1c. Further longitudinal research is needed to explore this relationship with specific determinants. Health inequities continue to be bleak in the United States and with a dearth of research in the area of SDH, there is still a great deal of work to be done.

# INTERPROFESSIONAL COLLABORATION

Whether it has been working with multidisciplinary teams for the scholarly project or with community partners where I provide medical care to patients, my work is constantly collaborative. The HCH model is inherently collaborative, and when working to end chronic homelessness, our partnerships extend beyond the clinic walls to include politicians, activists, housing developers, social service providers, and the list goes on. Of all the partners with whom I collaborate, they know that I am a clinician working directly with patients, and that I have an additional DNP skill set that enables me to look at our system-level challenges and help create solutions.

One example of interprofessional collaboration is a partnership between the HCH clinic and the social service agency that provides residential case management support within Housing First programs. Housing First is a homeless assistance approach that prioritizes providing permanent supportive housing to people experiencing homelessness.[51] It serves as a platform from which they can pursue personal goals and improve their quality of life. This approach is guided by the belief that people need basic necessities like food and a shelter before attending to anything less critical, such as employment, budgeting properly, or addressing substance use disorders.

There are 3 Housing First programs in our city and once weekly I rotate to each of them and have an on-site outreach clinic. After experiencing chronic homelessness, it can be very difficult for people to transition into housing. A study done evaluating mortality of people in Housing First programs revealed a higher rate of mortality than the general homeless population.[52] This partnership helps to decrease barriers and improve care coordination. For those with severe mental illness or with significant mobility challenges I am able to see them in their own apartments. In addition to providing medical support to the clients, I am able to provide education to the case managers about the clients' conditions and how to best support them.

Additionally, through this partnership, we are a part of state-wide effort supporting the application of a Medicaid waiver in support of using Medicaid dollars to finance supportive housing services. Supportive housing services and Medicaid serve many of the same individuals, yet there has been very limited collaboration between these 2 sectors in the past. As states are focusing more attention on addressing SDH, Medicaid programs are increasingly collaborating with state and local housing authorities to assist beneficiaries in their housing needs.[53] This example of an interprofessional collaboration can be replicated across many other fields, and DNPs have a unique skill set to lead these efforts.

# Conclusion: Impact of the DNP Degree

Nurses often self-select to remain siloed as a profession, yet for broader impact on improving the health of our communities we need to break down these silos. The late Congresswoman Shirley Chisholm once said, "If they don't give you a seat at the table, bring a folding chair." Rather than waiting for someone to ask you to be a part of a project, start a new project, lead a study, join a board, or run for office. The 2011 IOM "The Future of Nursing" report recommends that "private and public funders, health care organizations, nursing education programs, and nursing associations should expand opportunities for nurses to lead and manage collaborative efforts with physicians and other members of the health care team to conduct research and to redesign and improve practice environments and health systems."[54] DNPs have been both encouraged by the IOM and directed by the DNP Essentials to step into leadership roles. Interprofessional and cross-sector collaboration is the key to cultivating health equity in communities across the country and DNPs have a unique skill set to lead this effort. It is time that we lean into these opportunities and demonstrate the value of our profession.

As a result of obtaining my DNP degree, I have grown beyond the traditional nursing siloes and have elevated the role of the DNP by becoming an SME with the National Health Care for the Homeless Council, being chosen for the Robert Wood Johnson Foundation Culture of Health Leaders Program, and leading the development of innovative medical respite programs in Washington, DC and Maine. These accomplishments have given me a platform to highlight marginalized populations and promote health equity. Though more research and analysis are necessary, medical respite as a health care delivery model shows great promise of improved health outcomes and several million-dollar cost savings for a significant high-need, high-cost population. My work will continue to support the development of medical respite programs nationally as the clinical director for the National Health Care for the Homeless Council. This new appointment will allow me to promote medical respite programs for the homeless on a national level and improve the continuum of care for people experiencing homelessness. Homelessness should be rare, brief, and nonrecurring, and I will continue to advocate toward this end. I hope that you will join me in utilizing your DNP to create a more equitable health system.

# Acknowledgments

First and foremost I want to thank my patients who have let me into their lives and taught me more about strength, resilience, and joy than I ever thought possible. I have immense gratitude for my mentors and colleagues who have supported and held me up along the way. None if this would have been possible without the endless love and support of my husband, Matt. For him I am eternally grateful. To Thora, for all the joy and laughter you bring to my life. Finally, thank you to my son, Ole, who inspires me to work for a more just and equitable society for future generations.

# References

1. Health center program fact sheet. US Department of Health and Human Services. Accessed May 18, 2019. https://bphc.hrsa.gov/sites/default/files/bphc/about/healthcenterfactsheet.pdf

2. About health centers. National Association of Community Health Centers. Accessed October 13, 2017. http://www.nachc.org/about-our-health-centers/history-americas-health-centers/

3. Peters R. The social security amendments of 1960: completing the foundation for medicare and medicaid. *J Health Hum Serv Adm.* 2004;26(4):438-469.

4. National health center data. Health Resources & Services Administration. Accessed September 16, 2019. https://bphc.hrsa.gov/uds/datacenter.aspx

5. State of healthcare quality report. National Committee for Quality Assurance. Accessed September 16, 2019. http://www.ncqa.org/report-cards/health-plans/state-of-health-care-quality/2016-table-of-contents

6. Yoon SS, Carroll MD, Fryar CD. Hypertension prevalence and control among adults: United States, 2011-2014. *NCHS Data Brief.* 2015; 220,1-8.

7. Zlotnick C, Zerger S, Wolfe PB. Health care for the homeless: what we have learned in the past 30 years and what's next. *Am J Public Health.* 2013;103(suppl 2):S199-S205. doi:10.2105/AJPH.2013.301586

8. Philip W. Brickner National Leadership Award. National Health Care for the Homeless Council. Accessed September 16, 2019. https://nhchc.org/membership/brickner-award/#:~:text=Barbara%20Conanan%2C%20RN%2C%20MS%2C,winner%20of%20the%20Brickner%20Award

9. In memoriam: Philip W. Brickner, MD. National Health Care for the Homeless Council. Accessed September 16, 2019. https://nhchc.org/in-memoriam-philip-w-brickner-md/

10. 42 USC 254b: public health emergencies. Office of the Law Revision Counsel. Accessed September 5, 2017. http://uscode.house.gov/view.xhtml?edition=prelim&req=42+usc+254b&f=treesort&fq=true&num=20&hl=true

11. America's Health Centers. National Association of Community Health Centers. Accessed September 16, 2019. http://www.nachc.org/wp-content/uploads/2015/06/Americas-Health-Centers-March-2016.pdf

12. Heisler EJ. Federal health centers: an overview. Congressional Research Service. Accessed March 3, 2019. https://fas.org/sgp/crs/misc/R43937.pdf

13. Baggett TP, Hwang SW, O'connell JJ, et al. Mortality among homeless adults in Boston: shifts in causes of death over a 15-year period. *JAMA Intern Med.* 2013;173(3):189-195.

14. Henry M, Watt R, Rosenthal L, et al. US Department of Housing and Urban Development, Office of Community Planning and Development. In The 2016 Annual Homelessness Assessment Report (AHAR) to Congress: Part 1: Point in Time Estimates of Homelessness.2016.

15. Guarino K, Soares P, Konnath K, et al. Trauma-informed organizational toolkit. Center for Mental Health Services, Substance Abuse and Mental Health Administration, and the Daniels Fund, the National Child Traumatic Stress Network and the WK Kellogg Foundation, Rockville, MD. 2009.

16. Clark D. Your career needs many more mentors. Harvard Business Review. Accessed August 13, 2019. https://hbr.org/2017/01/your-career-needs-many-mentors-not-just-one

17. Medical respite care. National Health Care for the Homeless Council. Accessed September 16, 2019. https://www.nhchc.org/resources/clinical/medical-respite/

18. National Healthcare for the Homeless Council. Standards for Medical Respite Care. https://nhchc.org/clinical-practice/medical-respite-care/

19. 2017 DC women's needs assessment report: executive summary. DC.gov. Accessed September 2, 2019. https://ich.dc.gov/sites/default/files/dc/sites/ich/event_content/attachments/2017%20DC%20WNA%20Executive%20Summary.pdf

20. Zaccagnini M, Pechacek JM. *The Doctor of Nursing Practice Essentials: A New Model for Advanced Practice Nursing.* Jones & Bartlett Learning; 2019.

21. Partner with us as a subject matter expert. National Health Care for the Homeless Council. Accessed September 16, 2019. https://nhchc.org/subject-matter-experts-2/

22. Fruit and vegetable prescription program. Wholesome Wave. Accessed September 16, 2019. https://www.wholesomewave.org/sites/default/files/network/resources/files/FVRx%20Placemat_Revised2-22-18.pdf

23. Case study: a transportation solution for rural communities. Center for Care Innovations. Accessed September 16, 2019. https://www.careinnovations.org/resources/case-study-a-transportation-solution-for-rural-communities/

24. Hwang SW, Henderson MJ. Health care utilization in homeless people: translating research into policy and practice. Agency for Healthcare Research and Quality. October 2010. https://meps.ahrq.gov/data_files/publications/workingpapers/wp_10002.pdf

25. Galea S, Tracy M, Hoggatt KJ, DiMaggio C, Karpati A. Estimated deaths attributable to social factors in the united states. *Am J Public Health.* 2011;101(8):1456-1465.

26. Miniño AM, Arias E, Kochanek, KD, Murphy SL, Smith BL. Deaths: final data for 2000. *Natl Vital Stat Rep.* 2002;50(15)1-119.

27. Lantz PM, House JS, Lepkowski JM, Williams DR, Mero RP, Chen J. Socioeconomic factors, health behaviors, and mortality: results from a nationally representative prospective study of US adults. *JAMA.* 1998;279(21):1703-1708.

28. Laio Y, McGee DL, Kaufman JS, Cao G, Coope RS. Socioeconomic status and morbidity in the last years of life. *Am J Public Health.* 1999;89(4):569-572.

29. Marmot M, Shiple M, Brunner, Hemingway H. Relative contribution of early life and adult socioeconomic factors to adult morbidity in the Whitehall II study. *J Epidemiol Community Health.* 2001;55(5):301-307.

30. Marmot MG, Stansfeld S, Patel C, et al. Health inequalities among British civil servants: the Whitehall II study. *Lancet.* 1991;337(8754):1387-1393.

31. Singh GK, Siahpush M. Widening socioeconomic inequalities in US life expectancy, 1980-2000. *Int J Epidemiol.* 2006;35(4):969-979.

32. Booske B, Athens J, Kindig D. County health rankings working paper. County Health Rankings & Roadmaps. Accessed March 3, 2019. https://www.countyhealthrankings.org/sites/default/files/differentPerspectivesForAssigningWeightsToDeterminantsOfHealth.pdf

33. What are social determinants of health? World Health Organization. Accessed August 15, 2019. http://www.who.int/social_determinants/sdh_definition/en/

34. McGinnis JM, Williams-Russo P, Knickman JR. The case for more active policy attention to health promotion. *Health Aff.* 2002;21(2):78-93.

35. Life expectancy & probability of death. Institute for Health Metrics and Evaluation. Accessed March 15, 2019. http://vizhub.health-data.org/le/

36. Cutuli JJ, Desjardins CD, Herbers JE, et al. Academic achievement trajectories of homeless and highly mobile students: resilience in the context of chronic and acute risk. *Child Dev.* 2013;84(3):841-857.

37. Kim P, Evans GW, Angstadt M, et al. Effects of childhood poverty and chronic stress on emotion regulatory brain function in adulthood. *Proc Natl Acad Sci U S A.* 2013;110(46):18442-18447.

38. Laraia BA, Siega-Riz AM, Gundersen C, Dole N. Psychosocial factors and socioeconomic indicators are associated with household food insecurity among pregnant women. *J Nutr.* 2006;136(1):177-182.

39. HR3590: patient protection and affordable care act. Congress. Accessed March 15, 2019. https://www.congress.gov/bill/111th-congress/house-bill/3590

40. Public law 111–5. US Government Publishing Office. Accessed March 15, 2019. https://www.govinfo.gov/content/pkg/PLAW-111publ5/pdf/PLAW-111publ5.pdf

41. Promoting interoperability. HealthIT. https://www.healthit.gov/topic/meaningful-use-and-macra/promoting-interoperability

42. Institute of Medicine. *Capturing Social and Behavioral Domains and Measures in Electronic Health Records*. National Academies Press; 2014.

43. McGinnis JM, Williams-Russo P, Knickman JR. The case for more active policy attention to health promotion. *Health Aff*. 2002;21(2):78-93.

44. Gottlieb L, Sandel M, Adler NE. Collecting and applying data on social determinants of health in health care settings. *JAMA Intern Med*. 2013;173(11):1017-1020.

45. Health center program data. Health Resources & Services. Accessed November 11, 2017. http://bphc.hrsa.gov/uds/datacenter.aspx?q=d&bid=037020&state=DC

46. District of Columbia labor force, employment, unemployment and umeployment rate by ward. DC.gov. Accessed November 11, 2017. https://does.dc.gov/sites/default/files/dc/sites/does/page_content/attachments/2017%20Unemployment%20Rate%20by%20Ward_4.pdf

47. Unemployment rate 2.5 percent for college grads, 7.7 percent for high school dropouts. US Bureau of Labor Statistics. Accessed November 11, 2017. https://www.bls.gov/opub/ted/2017/unemployment-rate-2-point-5-percent-for-college-grads-7-point-7-percent-for-high-school-dropouts-january-2017.htm

48. Health care's blind side. Robert Wood Johnson Foundation. Accessed November 5, 2017. https://www.rwjf.org/en/library/research/2011/12/health-care-s-blind-side.html

49. Rabin RC. 15-minute visit take a toll on the doctor-patient relationship. Kaiser Health News. Accessed November 11, 2017. https://khn.org/news/15-minute-doctor-visits/

50. Bodenheimer T. Coordinating care: a perilous journey through the health care system. *N Engl J Med*. 2008;358:1064-1071.

51. Housing first. National Alliance to End Homelessness. Accessed November 17, 2019. https://endhomelessness.org/resource/housing-first/

52. Henwood BF, Byrne T, Scriber B. Examining mortality among formerly homeless adults enrolled in housing first: an observational study. *BMC Public Health*. 2015;15:1209. doi:10.1186/s12889-015-2552-1

53. Medicaid's role in housing. Medicaid and CHIP Payment and Access Commission. October 2018. Accessed November 17, 2019. https://www.macpac.gov/wp-content/uploads/2018/10/Medicaid%E2%80%99s-Role-in-Housing.pdf

54. Altman SH, Butler AS, Shern L. *Assessing Progress on the Institute of Medicine Report The Future of Nursing*. The National Academies Press; 2016.

# Appendix A
## DIABETES DRIVER DIAGRAM

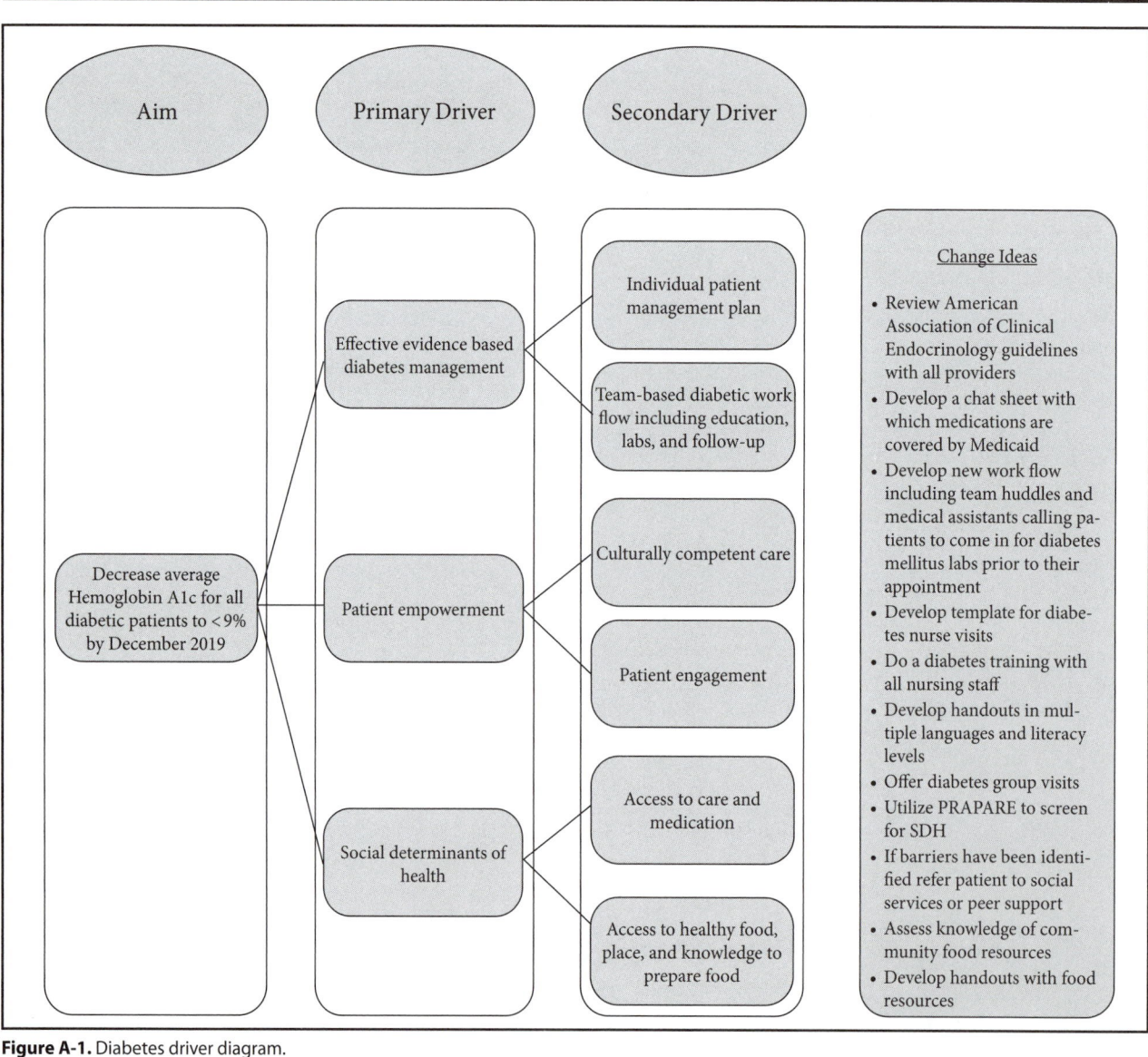

**Figure A-1.** Diabetes driver diagram.

# Appendix B
## Whitehead and Dahlgren Main Determinants of Health Model

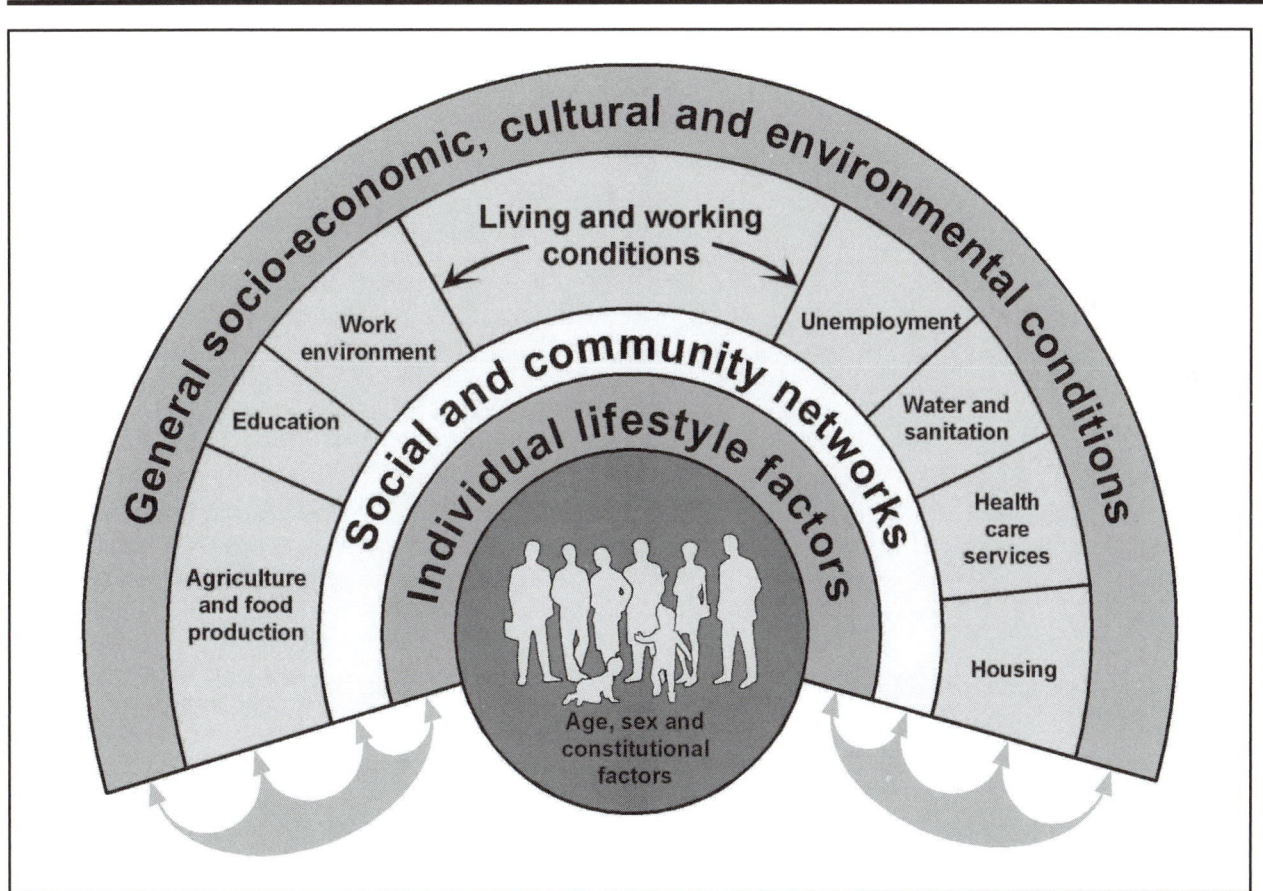

**Figure B-1.** (Reprinted with permission from Dahlgren G, Whitehead M. *Policies and Strategies to Promote Social Equity in Health.* Institute for Futures Studies; 1991.)

# CHAPTER 21

# STRATEGIES FOR INCORPORATING POPULATION HEALTH INTO A DNP PROJECT

*Marcia Johansson, DNP, APRN, ACNP-BC*

## INTRODUCTION

The Doctor of Nursing Practice (DNP) and Doctor of Philosophy (PhD) are the highest degrees that can be completed in nursing. As part of the DNP degree, one of the deliverables is the scholarly project referred to as the DNP project or capstone. This scholarly project involves evaluating evidence-based strategies to improve individual patient and population health outcomes. This chapter focus addresses strategies for incorporating population health into a DNP project that impacts practice.

Healthy People 2020 acknowledged health-associated quality of life and well-being as gauges of population health for the next decade.[1] Population health is defined as "the health outcomes of a group of individuals"[2] and has been identified with increasing frequency as a key element in patient-centered accountable health care delivery. Improving the health of populations is 1 of the 3 key components of the Institute for Healthcare Improvement's (IHI's) Triple Aim framework.[3] The IHI's Triple Aim framework was first developed in 2008 with the goal of improving health system implementation. The Triple Aim highlights on ways to improve the individual patient experience, improve health outcomes for populations of patients, and decrease the cost of health care. Triple Aim has become a fundamental element in the mission of many health care organizations and health systems in the United States, and so has consideration of how to improve population health, which is critical in achieving this undertaking.[3] Population health is an important concept to consider in the development of a DNP project idea. The concept can serve as a basis for a DNP project that can include providing the foundation for clinical prevention, health equity, responsible policy, and practice change.[4]

One of the many issues that need to be addressed prior to project identification and development of a protocol is to ask what is the student's scope of practice based on their master's education and certification. If the education and certification have prepared the nurse practitioner for pediatrics, then a project that concentrates on the older adult/geriatric population is not within the scope and should not be undertaken. Staying within the scope of practice as an advanced practice nurse is one of the key concepts in identifying an appropriate project and developing a protocol. Another consideration is for the students to reflect on their own experiences, both professionally and personally, that can be explored and utilized in the development of a strong scholarly project.

Benson LA, ed. *The DNP Professional:*
*Translating Value From Classroom to Practice* (pp 231-237).
© 2021 SLACK Incorporated.

# Project: How to Decide on a Project and Develop a Protocol

Development of the DNP project is not a straightforward process but involves the student identifying a phenomena of interest, exploring a variety of strategies to develop the project, and identifying areas of need and appropriate outcome measures specific to the population.[5] Identifying a phenomena of interest will take time, and the student should have ample opportunity to explore all options that they find important. Consulting with both the site and project faculty to explore options is the first step in this process. A DNP project needs to be driven by sites or organizations within which the student has access to practice, a contract to practice, and support of that institution, as well as the university.[5] Populations can be defined based on various characteristics and can include age, payer group, primary care provider, geographic region, and disease. When considering population health as a possible focus, the student needs to understand all of these influences and be able to implement an intervention that is appropriate to improve the health of the population.[3]

Another aspect to consider is whether there will be a financial requirement to implement the proposal and if there is financial support for the project. Grants can be obtained through Sigma Theta Tau, American Association of Critical-Care Nurses, American Association of Colleges of Nursing, and disease-specific associations like the American Heart Association or American Diabetes Association. It is important to consider the cost for the patient and family and if the cost would limit their ability to participate in the project.

## Description of the Project to Include Practice Setting and Development of the Proposal

The population health focus chosen for this DNP project was an all-inclusive organization for seniors in the Tampa Bay area. It is a nonprofit integrated network of care that supported those challenged by chronic and advanced illness. They provide support and care for seniors facing chronic illnesses and aging. The goal of the organization was to assist the members to achieve a healthy quality of life, stay active and socially connected, and live safely and independently at home and in the community. Services include primary care, therapies, skilled care, social and emotional support, day care at the day center, in-home care and support, transportation to and from the center, and other approved specialists. With the implementation of the Patient Protection and Affordable Care Act (ACA) in 2010, health care agencies like the one described were charged with controlling health care costs and improving the health care delivery system.[6] Their population included those with diabetes, chronic obstructive

pulmonary disease (COPD), coronary artery disease, dementia, Alzheimer's disease, and heart failure (HF), to name a few of the chronic diseases that are managed at this site. They reported having a higher than the national average of readmissions for HF and were subject to penalties under ACA reform. Medicare created the Hospital Readmissions Reduction Program (HRRP) that contained penalty assessments for 30-day readmissions of HF patients. They had limited funding and these penalties impacted the services that they could provide to the other members. They sought to find ways to improve the care of members with HF and reached out to collaborate with the University of South Florida College of Nursing faculty and students for support in this process.

A literature review was completed and it was noted that, although no single intervention has proven completely effective when implemented by itself, there is significant evidence in the literature that supports the implementation of technology using structured telephone support (STS) as well as mobile messaging (MM) as components of a HF management program to improve outcomes. The proposal was based on the Information, Motivation, and Behavior (IMB) model that guides complex health behaviors pertaining to patient adherence.[7] Information is the basic knowledge about a medical condition that might include how HF develops, its expected course, and effective strategies for its management. Motivation encompasses personal attitudes toward the adherence behavior and perceived social support for such behavior. Behavioral skills include ensuring that the patient has the specific behavioral tools or strategies necessary to perform behaviors such as daily weighing, HF symptom assessment and recognition, and adherence to medication, diet, and exercise.[7] Interventions based on the IMB model have been effective in influencing behavioral change across a variety of clinical applications.[8-10]

The IMB model validates that information is a prerequisite for changing behavior, but in itself is insufficient to achieve the desired behavior change.[11] Motivation is a critical determinant and works largely through engagement in behavioral skills to affect the desired behavior change.[7,8] However, when the behavioral skills are unfamiliar or overly complex, information and motivation can have improved effects on behavior. Engagement is an emerging motivational variable needed for behavior change, and a lack of patient engagement is a risk factor for negative health care outcomes.[12] Health education embedded into a mobile phone application has shown improvement in health outcomes for HF patients.[13]

The Institute for Patient and Family-Centered Care includes several examples of hospitals and health systems that have achieved a culture that embraced patients and families as partners.[14] Thus, the IMB model served as a framework in the implementation of a dual-pronged intervention using STS and MM to bridge the gap in meeting self-care and to promote improvement in HF self-care, knowledge, medication adherence, and quality of life, thereby potentially reducing the costly HF-related readmissions.

Based on the literature review and collaboration with the site management personnel, a proposal was developed that used a pre-post design and data collected at baseline and at 30-days on patients with HF. The technology-based 2-prong self-management intervention included STS and MM. All participants received STS 3 times weekly by the doctoral student. The daily MM included self-care tips regarding diet, exercise, and reminders for medication, symptom identification, and management. Short messages on these topics were programmed into the computer to automatically send every day for 30 days. Participants were given a mobile phone for the duration of the study. Weighing scales and/or sphygmomanometers were also provided if the patients did not own them. The project was approved by the University of South Florida's Institutional Review Board (IRB).

## SETTING: CHOOSING A PRACTICE SITE AND SWOT ANALYSIS

There are many practice sites that are interested in collaborating with a doctoral student to help improve the health of the population. Developing a relationship with the practice site was key to the success of this project. Understanding the challenges that the site faces in the management of these patients with chronic diseases, limited funding, and providing an evidence-based intervention helped to strengthen the relationship with the staff and the patients. Initial interactions included meeting with the staff and having informal meetings to explain the project and project requirements. Questions were answered and families were invited to come and participate in any of the scheduled meetings with the doctoral student. Management was very supportive of the project and gave the doctoral student access to the patient records that were specific to those with the diagnosis of HF. The staff was helpful to identify the patients and let the doctoral student know when the patients arrived at the site so they could be interviewed.

Strengths or successes of this project include the fact that the patients were required to come to the day center on a routine basis. All of their care was provided by one site, which included medication administration, diet counseling, social services, and home care support. Threats or barriers include limited education level of the participants, advanced age, advanced disease, decreased interest in participating in the study, and lack of support at home.

## DNP ESSENTIAL: CLINICAL SCHOLARSHIP AND ANALYTICAL METHODS FOR EVIDENCE-BASED PRACTICE AS INCORPORATED INTO A CLINICAL PROJECT

STS demonstrated improved self-care monitoring and knowledge after discharge.[15] The current practice guidelines recommend telephone follow-up within 3 days of hospital discharge and a follow-up visit within 7 to 14 days after an index HF admission.[16] A systematic review of 49 studies reported improvement after STS on HF knowledge and self-care, particularly regarding sodium reduction, medication adherence, weight monitoring, and physical activity.[17] Similarly, a meta-analysis of 9 randomized controlled trials (RCT) found that individuals who received STS had a significantly lower risk of HF readmission than controls over 6 months (relative risk, 0.74; 95% confidence interval, 0.61 to 0.90).[18] This was further supported in a large, systematic review of 16 RCTs (N = 5613) that exclusively implemented STS in reducing HF-related hospitalization (RR 0.77; 95% CI; 0.68 to 0.87; $P < .0001$) and improved quality of life (RR 0.66; 95% CI; 0.54 to 0.81; $P < .0001$).[19]

Similar to STS, interactive mobile health (mHealth) technology is suggested as an appropriate venue to overcome the long-term barrier to self-care management.[20] Among 60 patients with HF, daily mobile messages from an interactive voice response system (IVRS) using a MP3 player with self-care management tips showed greater than a 50% reduction in the 30-day readmission rate.[21] Similarly, a pre-post pilot study of patients with HF (n = 15) reported that the MM was easy to use (83%), and showed reduced pills missed (66%), and decreased salt intake (66%) with improved self-care maintenance (mean composite score increased from 49 to 78, $P = .003$) and self-care management (increased from 57 to 86, $P = .002$) at 4 weeks.[22]

However, evidence supports that facilities that implemented complementary strategies had significantly improved HF outcomes and lower readmission rates with an average reduction of 0.34-percentage points for each additional strategy utilized.[23] Therefore, this evidence-based quality improvement project used STS and MM intervention strategy to improve HF outcomes among participants enrolled.

When developing the DNP project, it can be helpful to search for reliable and valid surveys and tools that may be modified for use. The use of validated surveys is an integral part of the DNP project. Measurements used for this population health project included:

- Self-care behavior was assessed using the valid and reliable Self-Care of Heart Failure Index (ScHFi) questionnaire comprised of 15 items, rated on a 4-point response scale, and has 3 sub-scales.[24] Reliability of the Self-Care Maintenance subscale was r = .56, Self-Care Management was r = .70 and Self-Care Self-Confidence was r = .82.[24] Multiple studies have tested this scale on persons with HF.[25,26]

- HF knowledge was measured using the Atlanta Heart Failure Knowledge Test (A-HFKT). This standardized, validated instrument has been widely utilized both in research and clinical settings.[27] The A-HFKT has 30 questions with a possible 0 to 30 score. Content validity ratings on relevance and clarity were tested in patients and family members that ranged from 0.55 to 1.0, with 81% of the items rated from 0.88 to 1.0. Cronbach's alpha was .84 for patients and .75 for family members.[27]

- Medication adherence was assessed utilizing the 8-item, self-administered Morisky Medication Adherence Scale (MMAS). The MMAS has a Cronbach's alpha of 0.83, and demonstrated a sensitivity of 95% and a specificity of 53% at a cut-off point less than 6.[28] The MMAS has a total score of 10 and higher scores indicate worse adherence.[28] This tool has been utilized successfully in HF patients with improved medication adherence noted.[29]

- Physical and mental health was assessed using the Short-Form 12 (SF-12) questionnaire.[30] The SF-12 was compared with SF-36 among cardiac participants and found to be valid with a correlation coefficient of physical component summary (r = 0.96, $P < .001$) and mental component summary (r = 0.96, $P < .001$).[31] Similarly, change scores between baseline and 12 months were highly correlated for physical components (r = 0.94, $P < .001$) and mental components (r = 0.95, $P < .001$). Therefore, to reduce patient burden, we used the SF-12 questionnaire.

- The Duke-UNC Functional Social Support Questionnaire (FSSQ) was utilized to assess social support. The short-version FSSQ has 8 items in a 5-point Likert scale (1 = much less than I would like and 5 = as much as I would like) with internal consistency ranged from .50 for useful advice to .85 for help around the house.[32] The higher average score indicates greater perceived social support. Evaluating social support is necessary in the management of individuals with HF as there is current evidence that suggests that low levels of support for these individuals is associated with poor health outcomes.[33]

Demographic variables including age, gender, race, and living status were completed by participants once consented.

# DATA MINING: WHERE DOES THE DATA COME FROM?

Data mining is the process of looking at large data banks of information to generate new information. There are many database platforms to choose from when data are ready to be entered into a database. When choosing a database, look for one that is easy to use and provides tutorials for beginners but can be utilized no matter the experience of the student. For this project, the Statistical Package for the Social Sciences (SPSS) platform was used as it offers advanced statistical analysis and predictive analytics that are necessary for the DNP project.

Data from 51 participants who completed the baseline and 30-day follow-up was entered into a database. The mean age of the participants was 77.39 (SD = 9.34) years, 90% were ≥ 65 years of age, 65% were women, 71% were White, and 24% were Black. One-half of the participants lived alone and 23.5% lived in an independent or assisted-living facility. The data were analyzed using SPSS for Windows (version 21.0, SPSS, Inc.). Descriptive statistics with frequency and percentage for categorical variables such as gender, race, and living status, and mean and standard deviation for the continuous variable of age and the outcome variables, were computed on all data. Difference in distribution of basic measures was computed using a chi-square test and Fisher's exact test. The results demonstrated that STS and MM significantly improved HF self-care maintenance, self-care management, self-care confidence, knowledge, medication adherence, and physical and mental health after 30-days with a $P$ value of < .05.

There was a noted reduction in readmission rates during this project. Data from the previous 3 months were reviewed for hospital readmissions for those patients with HF and there was a 12% readmission rate. For the data collected prospectively during the project, the readmission rate decreased to 4%, which was a significant improvement. Decreased readmissions not only affected the reimbursement rate, but the hospital was not penalized for the readmission. Overall, this was a cost savings for the hospital as well as for the organization.

# BUSINESS PLAN

For those organizations or schools that are interested in pursuing this quality improvement model, there are specific considerations that need to be identified. Program of All-inclusive Care for the Elderly (PACE) patients did not have concerns about the financial cost of the medications, physician or nurse visits, or transportation, as those services were provided by the organization.

The first financial consideration addresses funding for the project. Are there resources such as government grants or special interest groups that have grants to help the organization set up a telephone triage? For this project, Sigma Theta Tau and the American Association of Critical-Care Nurses provided support that was used to purchase weighing scales, sphygmomanometers, and mobile phones for those patients that did not have them. There may also be resources that can be distributed by the agency, like PACE, to assist with the care of the HF patient to improve care and decrease readmissions.

The second consideration involves education of patients and families regarding the symptoms of HF, dietary restrictions, and overall management. For this project, the patients and families underwent evaluation of their knowledge and symptom education during the initial interview process and at subsequent visits. When the project was completed, both patients and families were noted to be very knowledgeable about the symptoms and management of HF.

The third and final consideration was the time it would take to set up the preprogrammed mobile messages and making the telephone calls 3 times per week to the patients. Once the messages were programmed into the computer, they could be scheduled to repeat every 3 to 4 weeks as new patients would be added to the list after hospital discharge. Utilizing the home care nurses would help with continuity of care and would also alert them if the patient was becoming more symptomatic and needed intervention sooner than scheduled. The intervention could begin immediately to prevent readmission.

# DNP Essential: Interprofessional Collaboration for Improving Patient and Population Health Outcomes

In the current role of an assistant professor who is responsible for multiple concentrations there is a lot of interprofessional collaboration for DNP projects and coursework in order to manage the business of the college. Participation in committees for the College of Nursing and for the University of South Florida (as they impact both the undergraduate and graduate programs) is required.

Interprofessional collaboration was required for this DNP project as well as the multiple specialty groups that impact the care of the patients at this site. For this population health project, there was interaction with participants, families, physicians, nurses, social workers, dietitians, administrative professionals, university faculty, and fellow students. Communication with the team regarding how the patients were progressing was extremely important for the DNP project, especially when patients were readmitted or had any change in their physical health and geographic status due to HF. Providing contact information and being involved in the setting was helpful to gain the confidence of many of the staff and of the patients. A flyer was created to be posted in different areas to make patients and families aware of the project and ability to participate. Showing commitment to the organization and not just using the site for the project was extremely important for the advancement of population health at this site. Routine meetings with administrators to keep them informed of the progress of the project are also necessary for a successful DNP project.

# Professionalism

Results of this DNP project were disseminated to the site administrators and stakeholders of the all-inclusive organization for seniors to help improve the care of the patients at that site. Recommendations for possibly incorporating this project into the care of the HF population were discussed, as well as ideas for sustainability of this project at the site including cost and personnel needs. The results could help the administrators of agencies such as the all-inclusive organizations for seniors, home care agencies, and independent living facilities to incorporate self-management interventions with STS and MM into patients' daily treatment plan to prevent physical, psychological, and social problems that negatively affect patients' ability to care for themselves with other chronic diseases.

This DNP project was also presented to the university community in a DNP poster presentation event and presented to the College of Nursing faculty in a podium presentation. It was well received at both events and highlighted the continued need for population health projects by DNP students, especially in the development of community partners and how the student can be an integral part of the relationship.

The project results were also disseminated as a podium presentation at a local Sigma Theta Tau conference, a podium presentation via webinar for the American Association of Critical-Care Nurses, and a poster presentation at an International Conference on Clinical & Experimental Cardiology. It was also published in 2 different journals.

Having a DNP degree and being willing to share the results with others has provided multiple opportunities for leadership on committees locally, nationally, and globally. Opportunities for publications, writing book chapters, and speaking at conferences have become available as the DNP continues as an expert in the phenomena of interest. Collaborating with others in different institutions has also been a wonderful opportunity since obtaining a DNP degree.

## Pearls/Takeaways

Recommendations for DNP students as they advance their education and seek to obtain a DNP degree include picking a project topic that they have some knowledge about and a passion to study. Students should make sure it is within the scope of practice and look for sites and mentors to collaborate with. Having a mentor and project team to include faculty, content expert, and data support are some of the most important factors for success when working with a site and navigating the DNP degree. Continuing to foster a good relationship with the site and keeping administrators informed of the results and possible barriers to the project is paramount as the project is ongoing. Population health projects are keys to the future of health care and will have an impact on both quality and cost outcomes.

## Conclusion: Impact of the DNP Degree

As a result of obtaining my DNP degree, I was able to understand the process of working with a vulnerable patient population with HF and develop a process for other patients with chronic diseases that are part of PACE. HF management remains a burden to the health care system and organizations are required to implement programs to improve the health of their participants and decrease readmission rates. I was fortunate to have grants that provided funds to afford participants a mobile phone with service and weighing scale, and/or sphygmomanometer if they did not have access to one. Funds were provided from the American Association of Critical-Care Nurses and Sigma Theta Tau who supported this project. The initial cost of offering mobile services, setting up the computer to send mobile messages, and calls 3 times a week is offset by the savings over time from avoidance of readmissions and incurred penalties.

Facilities such as the PACE may need to develop creative ways to tap into resources available for older adults, who may live alone, and educate them on ways to improve their health. HF symptom recognition and management are the mainstays of HF treatment and interventions need to be tailored to improve self-care, knowledge, and quality of life. Based on the results of this project, self-care management interventions involving STS and MM have effectively improved outcomes for HF patients and organizations with a clinically and financially significant reduction in readmissions.

Completing a project in population health is important for the DNP student, community partner, and the population of focus. For the DNP student, they are able to establish a relationship with the community partner and seek to find solutions for issues with specific diseases or processes that will satisfy the requirements of the DNP degree. Exploring and addressing the needs of the community partner is important when working to develop a DNP project and can be translated to other projects over time. With the limitations that health care organizations face financially and with few resources, the DNP student is able to help bridge the gap in a cost-effective manner. Through the relationship that was established with PACE through this project, I was able to provide more opportunities for DNP students and work to improve the health of those patients with HF. Working to improve the health of a population impacts the health care costs and improves both quality and quantity of life for the patient.

## Acknowledgments

I would like to thank Dr. Ponrathi Athilingam for her guidance and support in my DNP journey and exposure to population health. My biggest supporter in this process has been my husband, John Marquardt. His unconditional love and support makes me strive to do the very best in all of my endeavors.

## References

1. Barile JP, Reeve BB, Smith AW, et al. Monitoring population health for healthy people 2020: evaluation of the NIH PROMIS global health, CDC healthy days, and satisfaction with life instruments. *Qual Life Res*. 2013;22(6):1201-1211.

2. Kindig D, Stoddart G. What is population health? *Am J Public Health*. 2003;93(3):380-383.

3. Swarthout M, Bishop MA. Population health management: review of concepts and definitions. *Am J Health Syst Pharm*. 2017;74(18):1405-1411.

4. McKinney SH, Herman J, Nkwonta CA. Transformative learning in an online doctor of nursing practice population health course. *J Nurs Educ*. 2019;58(8):481-484.

5. Moran K, Burson R, Conrad D. *The Doctor of Nursing Practice Project: A Framework for Success*. Jones & Bartlett Learning; 2020.

6. Lavigne JE, Brown J, Matzke GR. Population health and medicine: policy and financial drivers. *Am J Health Syst Pharm*. 2017;74(18):1413-1421.

7. Fisher WA, Fisher JD, Harman J. The information-motivation-behavioral skills model: a general social psychological approach to understanding and promoting health behavior. In: Suls J, Wallston KA, eds. *Social Psychological Foundations of Health and Illness*. Blackwell Publishing; 2003:82-106.

8. Bahrami Z, Zarani F. Application of the information-motivation and behavioral skills (IMB) model in risky sexual behaviors amongst male students. *J Infect Public Health*. 2015;8(2):207-213.

9. Fisher JD, Fisher WA. Changing AIDS-risk behavior. *Psychol Bull*. 1992;11(3):455-474.

10. Walsh JL, Senn TE, Scott-Sheldon LA, Vanable PA, Carey MP. Predicting condom use using the Information-Motivation-Behavioral Skills (IMB) model: a multivariate latent growth curve analysis. *Ann Behav Med*. 2011;42(2):235-244.

11. Mazzuca SA. Does patient education in chronic disease have therapeutic value? *J Chronic Dis*. 1982;35(7):521-9

12. Simmons LA, Wolever RQ, Bechard EM, Snyderman R. Patient engagement as a risk factor in personalized health care: a systematic review of the literature on chronic disease. *Genome Med*. 2014;6(2):16.

13. Athilingam P, Osorio RE, Kaplan H, Oliver D, O'Neachtain T, Rogal PJ. Embedding patient education in mobile platform for patients with heart failure: theory-based development and beta testing. *Comput Inform Nurs.* 2016;34(2):92-98.

14. Johnson B. *Profiles of Change.* Institute for Patient and Family-Centered Care; 2015.

15. Albert NM, Barnason S, Deswal A. Transitions of care in heart failure: a scientific statement from the american heart association. *Circ Heart Fail.* 2015;8(2):384-409.

16. Yancy CW, Jessup M, Bozkurt B, et al. ACCF/AHA guideline for the management of heart failure: a report of the american college of cardiology foundation/american heart association task force on practice guidelines. *J Am Coll Cardiol.* 2013;128(16):e240-327.

17. Clark AM, Spaling M, Harkness K, et al. Determinants of effective heart failure self-care: a systematic review of patients' and caregivers' perceptions. *Heart.* 2014;100(9):716-721.

18. Feltner C, Jones CD, Cene CW, et al. *AHRQ Comparative Effectiveness Reviews: Transitional Care Interventions to Prevent Readmissions for People With Heart Failure.* Agency for Healthcare Research and Quality; 2014.

19. Inglis SC, Clark RA, McAlister FA, et al. Structured telephone support or telemonitoring programmes for patients with chronic heart failure. *Cochrane Database Syst Rev.* 2010(8):Cd007228.

20. Oosterom-Calo R, Te Velde SJ, Stut W, Brug J. Development of Motivate4Change using the intervention mapping protocol: an interactive technology physical activity and medication adherence promotion program for hospitalized heart failure patients. *JMIR Res Protoc.* 2015;4(3):e88.

21. Austin LS, Landis CO, Hanger KH. Extending the continuum of care in congestive heart failure: an interactive technology self-management solution. *J Nurs Adm.* 2012;42(9):442-446.

22. Nundy S, Razi RR, Dick JJ, et al. A text messaging intervention to improve heart failure self-management after hospital discharge in a largely African-American population: before-after study. *J Med Internet Res.* 2013;15(3):e53.

23. Bradley EH, Curry L, Horwitz LI, et al. Hospital strategies associated with 30-day readmission rates for patients with heart failure. *Circ Cardiovasc Qual Outcomes.* 2013;6(4):444-450.

24. Riegel B, Carlson B, Moser DK, Sebern M, Hicks FD, Roland V. Psychometric testing of the self-care of heart failure index. *J Card Fail.* 2004;10(4):350-360

25. Buck HG, Lee CS, Moser DK, et al. Relationship between self-care and health-related quality of life in older adults with moderate to advanced heart failure. *J Cardiovasc Nurs.* 2012;27(1):8-15.

26. Moser DK, Lee KS, Wu JR, et al. Identification of symptom clusters among patients with heart failure: an international observational study. *Int J Nurs Stud.* 2014;51(10):1366-1372.

27. Reilly CM, Higgins M, Smith A, et al. Development, psychometric testing, and revision of the atlanta heart failure knowledge test. *J Cardiovasc Nurs.* 2009;24(6):500-509.

28. Morisky DE, Green LW, Levine DM. Concurrent and predictive validity of a self-reported measure of medication adherence. *Med Care.* 1986;24(1):67-74.

29. Granger BB, Ekman I, Hernandez AF, et al. Results of the Chronic Heart Failure Intervention to Improve MEdication Adherence study: a randomized intervention in high-risk patients. *Am Heart J.* 2015;169(4):539-548.

30. Gandek B, Ware JE, Aaronson NK, et al. Cross-validation of item selection and scoring for the SF-12 health survey in nine countries: results from the IQOLA project: International Quality of Life Assessment. *J Clin Epidemiol.* 1998;51(11):1171-1178.

31. Muller-Nordhorn J, Roll S, Willich SN. Comparison of the short form (SF)-12 health status instrument with the SF-36 in patients with coronary heart disease. *Heart.* 2004;90(5):523-527.

32. Broadhead WE, Gehlbach SH, de Gruy FV, Kaplan BH. The Duke-UNC functional social support questionnaire: measurement of social support in family medicine patients. *Med Care.* 1988;26(7):709-723.

33. Moser DK, Arslanian-Engoren C, Biddle MJ, et al. Psychological aspects of heart failure. *Curr Cardiol Rep.* 2016;18(12):119.

# SECTION IX

## INFORMATICS EXEMPLARS

# CHAPTER 22

# A DNP-Prepared Director of Nursing Informatics Transforms Sepsis Recognition and Improves Sepsis Outcomes

*Deborah Chasco, DNP, CCRN, APRN, CNS*

## Introduction

Nurses can improve health care outcomes as leaders who advocate for their communities while contributing to the promotion of global health through a Doctor of Nursing Practice (DNP) program. With DNP preparation and skill sets, nurses influence and guide the quality of health care through communication, collaboration, and coordination with multidisciplinary stakeholders. DNP-prepared nurses improve patient safety and quality across the health care continuum by transforming the delivery of care via data analytics, research, information, and knowledge. Technology and other sciences are utilized to improve health while containing costs and analyzing better methods of moving the pendulum of health care from illness to wellness. As a health care leader, sepsis recognition in a southwest safety-net community hospital needed improvement. In addition, a team approach was necessary to improve sepsis outcomes utilizing the electronic health care system to identify discrete data elements that lead to reliable, valid actionable data to improve sepsis outcomes. Modification of data elements within the electronic health care record lead toward improved documentation and measurable data to improve sepsis outcomes. Challenges continue with changing definitions and required time frames to meet regulatory requirements. Synthesizing literature review results and analyzing findings leads to positive patient outcomes. DNP-prepared nurses can also develop the foundation for health data interoperability and propel health care outcomes that tie into care coordination, operational and administrative financial stability, innovation in data analytics, and population health. DNP graduates can lead organizations toward a successful health care roadmap.

## Practice Setting

This chapter outlines the importance of DNP preparation with the support of a practice setting where research, patient safety, quality care, and patient care outcomes are weaved into the mission and vision of the organization. University Medical Center of El Paso, a safety-net community, academic health care center is home to health care consumers within a 250-mile radius requiring trauma services. It is a Level 1 trauma, stroke, and cardiac center providing

Benson LA, ed. *The DNP Professional:*
*Translating Value From Classroom to Practice* (pp 241-251).
© 2021 SLACK Incorporated.

services to all regardless of ability to pay. Quality and patient safety is at the forefront of all services provided as evident by the hospital's quality ratings. University Medical Center of El Paso received a Leapfrog rating of "A." In addition, the organization is embarking on a Baldrige Journey leading toward sustained quality transformation. Such a practice setting makes a rich environment that fosters evidence-based practice and research, setting the stage for transformational leaders to flourish.

Culture, practice setting, and community, along with the mission and vision of any organization, impacts how a DNP-prepared nurse grows and succeeds in leading change management, engages in evidence-based research, and blends technology and other sciences with the art and science of nursing. The mission of University Medical Center of El Paso is to "Heal. Serve and Educate."[1] Three simple words foster the desire to learn, the ability to heal, and the desire to serve and care for the most vulnerable. The University Medical Center of El Paso is a mecca of learning with many local and national affiliations in the field of education, science, medicine, nursing, technology, research, and the perfect setting for any DNP-prepared nurse.

A DNP program is the beginning of life-long learning in its most active and fundamental state. It reflects professionalism through sharing of ideas, assimilation of practice roles, and active transformation of research in caring for humanity. A DNP program sets the foundation for active engagement in finding solutions to clinical dilemmas with the use of technology and other sciences while sharing clinical data for the improvement of patient care outcomes. It challenges nurses to think globally. Sepsis, population health, regulatory agency requirements for interoperability, value-based care initiatives, and social determinants of health are only a few national issues where tracking trends and synthesis of evidence and knowledge transformation are urgently needed to address and improve patient outcomes.

## ROLE DEVELOPMENT

The opportunity to expand the role of director of nursing informatics was the start of a journey that continues on the roadmap to data analysis, research, hardwiring, and standardizing documentation for nursing and non-nursing health care services. Role development for creating and expanding the department of nursing informatics was inevitable in a rapidly growing southwest safety-net community health care organization. Business plans with detailed return on investment (ROI), proposals for budget planning encompassing citations from peer-reviewed journals related to nursing informatics, and productivity measures benchmarked with other like organizations pathed the way for expanding the department of nursing informatics. The once 2-member team led to the current 8-member team encompassing nursing informatics specialists and analysts for interoperability, a physician educator, and data analyst. The

team is also responsible for the Joint Commission core measures and patient-related measures. The team will continue to grow and lead hospital-wide initiatives related to quality of care and safety through data. It is integral to include nursing informatics in health care planning to link problems, interventions, and outcomes utilizing data that are identifiable and retrievable in an aggregated format used in databases. Organizations are at a disadvantage for improvement related to outcomes without data. Databases mapped appropriately will lead to valid and measurable conclusions. This function becomes important as health care organizations move from the care of one patient to the care of high-risk populations and population health outcomes. Organizations need accurate and complete databases linked to the source of truth (eg, the electronic health care record) regardless of the system or integrated systems and interfaces in place. All organizations have a multitude of data. In many cases, there is an abundance of data coming from different systems measuring different outcomes. Data are linked, mapped, and validated to measure outcomes. Data can be queried appropriately to capture identifiable nursing-sensitive data coming from specific fields in the electronic health care record.

## NURSING INFORMATICS AND DATA ANALYSIS

Nursing informatics specialists utilize data for identifying patterns of data elements. Pattern identification of data is data mining.[2] Coding for many databases comes from structured query language (SQL) databases.[3] The American National Standards Institute (ANSI) develops standard computer language for retrieving and updating data in databases and SQL is an ANSI standard.[3] In order to support major queries and comply with the ANSI standards, "select," "update," "delete," "insert," "where," and other keywords to show code when executing queries is required.[4] Results should be tested, validated, reviewed, and compared to data present in a database for outcomes data presentation. If organizations are looking at predictive analytics, this is the foundation and beginning step necessary to implement. This is a form of research as aggregation of data with specific data elements leading to a result and conclusion related to specific measurable outcomes that are valid, reliable, and replicated for evidence-based nursing practice.

## NURSING INFORMATICS, RESEARCH, AND EVIDENCE-BASED PRACTICE

The knowledge and skills developed and refined with a DNP preparation are extensive and in preparation toward a journey with multiple avenues to include evidence-based practice and research. As with any journey, preparation includes studying and mapping the road, utilizing tools to navigate through the road ahead, stopping to review, replenish, and continue the journey. The journey never ends with evidence-based practice and research related to practice improvement in the clinical setting if outcome improvement is the goal. The journey had many untraveled roads to explore as health care organizations expand their services and invest in technology to aggregate data for specific populations to include high-risk populations and social determinants of health.

The effectiveness of case studies in providing examples of decision trees in formatting how disciplines synthesize research, evidence-based practice, and best practice literature is an essential element in beginning the quest for outcomes data. The development of any scholarly work is to query several questions and to inquire how best to approach each question while finding actionable solutions. How various health care arenas receive and communicate information and share information; how providers and end-users receive and review the information (including patients); how information is stored in various devices, interfaces, existing databases, and patient portals; and how to map each element to make it usable, reliable, and valid to address outcomes is challenging. In today's health care systems, several challenges continue to delay progression of data queries as guidelines and protocols are still in development. Figure 22-1 depicts the utilization of research in any nursing informatics setting to answer unanswerable or unexplored questions. Case studies related to regulatory requirements and the electronic health care record are necessary to focus on outlining outcomes. The utilization of data to include data privacy and security are essential in moving toward the next step necessary for accurate and reliable data specific to individual and population-specific health care data when researching high-risk populations or specific diseases to find solutions to unanswered questions and improve outcome measures. In addition, education of the public and consumer is also necessary as research and evidence-based nursing research related to patient access to health care data in a useful and understandable.

# ROLE TRANSFORMATION

In today's ever-changing health care environment, organizations not focusing on mission-critical priorities to include financial stability face challenges in meeting regulatory agency requirements and payer regulations. An analysis of documentation, integration systems, and upgrades to the admission, discharge, and transfer system (ADT) with regulation checks and balances is necessary for organizations to keep closely on the radar. Clinical information systems and ancillary systems to include documentation, computerized provider order entry (CPOE), and the ability to aggregate data at all levels by reviewing global collection of data for useful data reflecting best practices and evidence-based care can transform organizations. Directors of nursing informatics must be in the know and at every planning meeting to fully integrate systems to provide usable data geared toward measurable outcome data. Systems thinking combined with critical thinking and a combination of theory-based thinking is necessary to integrate services. Change theories are more complex as even a simple change in an organization can lead to major resistance. Leaders must assess the differences in individual perceptions of change. Not all individuals embrace change or view change management as a positive means to a positive outcome. Roger's diffusion of innovations theory focuses on the patterns of acceptance that innovations follow as they move across the continuum of populations and examines decision-making processes that occur in individuals when deciding to adopt an innovation.[3] This theory focuses on global and individual changes through various stages. Roger's diffusion of innovations theory lends itself to organizational change management and alignment of departments within a large organization. Alignment and acceptance is the foundation of leading innovation forward and implementing initiatives that integrate multidisciplinary teams toward a common cause—patient quality care. Aligning information technology services, physician and care provider services, nursing services, case management, social workers, ancillary services, and community services to integrate care and provide services to all community members is continuous. Organizations cannot lose focus on the importance of establishing relationships that improve patient care. Innovation in nursing informatics is about connecting people and groups with tools necessary to provide solutions that are efficient and timely.

A DNP-prepared nurse synthesizes evidence and knowledge, tracks trends, and recommends and develops policies that lead toward other innovative systems and methods of providing care. As a leader, DNP-prepared nurses address national policy issues and advocate for policy change. Alignment of services within organizations that build upon quality, safety, and positive outcomes for patients are focused on evidence-based management practices. Clinical research with vulnerable populations, review of innovation in technology, and collaboration focusing on achieving organizational goals that are patient-care centered are the principles necessary to transform organizations from ordinary to extraordinary health care systems. Figure 22-2 incorporates the essence of nursing informatics leading change and change management principles toward excellence in patient care and global health care. It is through innovation, collaboration, communication, and integration of health care systems where nursing informatics can transform health care.

DNP-prepared nurses can incorporate theory into practice by leading health care teams and advocating for individuals and communities. In providing culturally appropriate health care education and services while actively participating in research, the DNP-prepared nurse can proactively lead transformational teams and impact policy for the improvement of health.

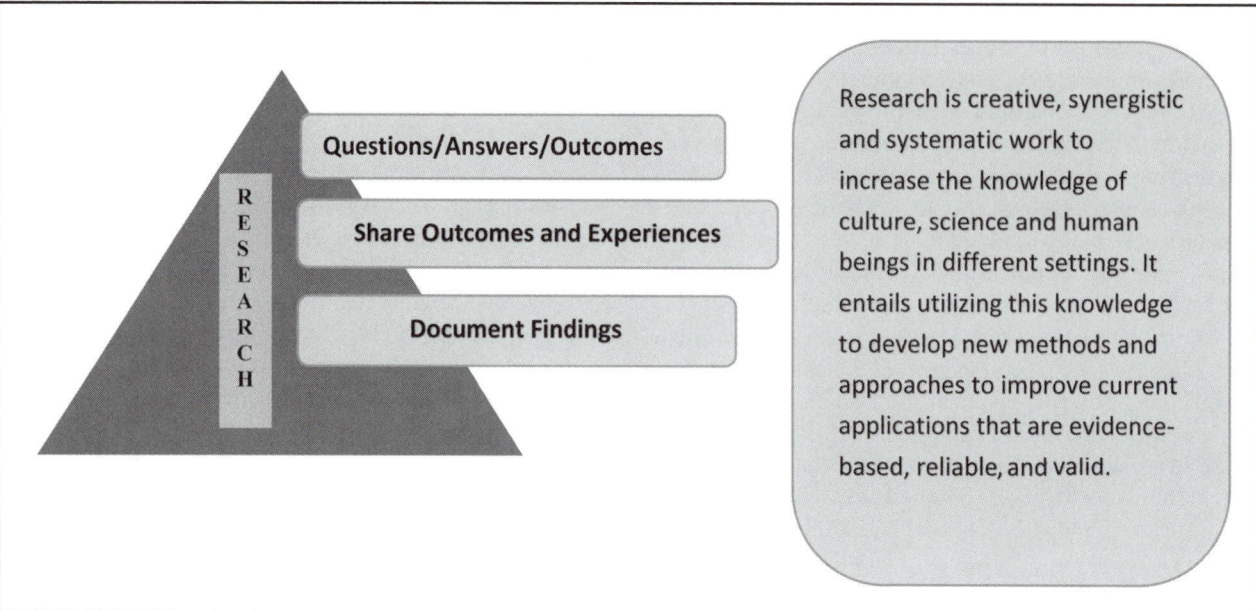

**Figure 22-1.** Utilization of research principles.

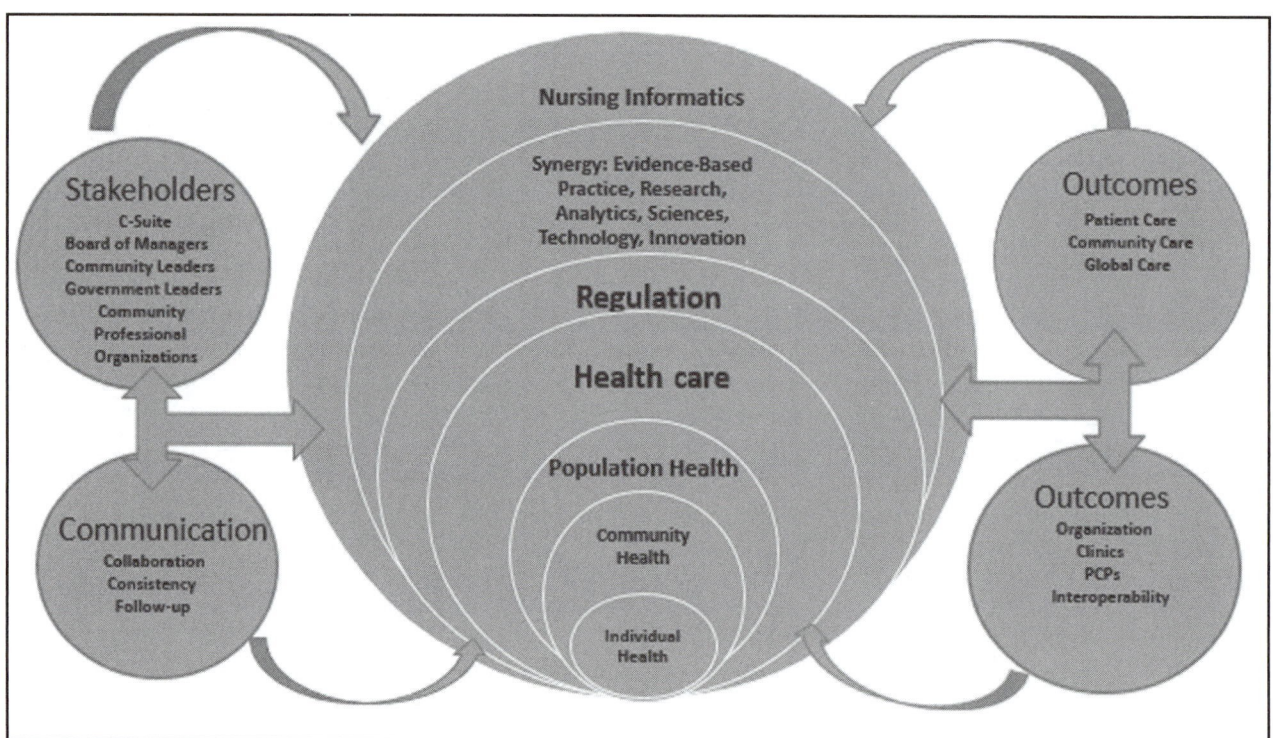

**Figure 22-2.** Nursing informatics synergy model.

# DNP Essentials

The American Association of Colleges of Nursing developed the elements necessary in DNP programs. Required by the Commission on Collegiate Nursing Education for universities seeking accreditation for DNP programs, the DNP Essentials[5] outline the foundational competencies that are core to all advanced nursing practice roles. There are 8 elements outlining criteria necessary for university-level accreditation. These elements include critical values necessary for nursing informatics and focus on successful and sustainable goals that lead toward measurable, valid, and actionable outcomes data. This document introduced in 2006 continues as the basis of DNP program accreditation. Currently, a work group is developing updates focusing on the next decade of health care delivery, measurable competencies, standardization of practice, and research-focused core courses, incorporation of simulation in curriculum content, and the next 10 years of practice community expectations of DNP graduates.[6] This DNP framework served as the basis for the nursing informatics department and the director of nursing informatics competencies in a growing safety-net, Level 1 trauma center.

## Science and Practice Initiatives

The DNP-prepared director of nursing informatics must utilize all sciences to include genetics, biomedical, ethical, biophysical, psychosocial, analytical, change management, and organizational sciences as the basis for health maintenance and health care delivery while evaluating actionable and measurable outcomes for all populations served. The development and evaluation of new practice approaches, new technology, and electronic tools that will decrease and improve clinical documentation based on best practice principles and research with proven results is an essential competency. Documenting results and sharing data are necessary in the quest to answer questions needing resolution for actionable quality outcome measures.

## Systems Thinking: Operational and Clinical Leadership and Quality Improvement

Systems thinking, critical thinking, and global thinking principles are competencies necessary to lead teams toward quality and safety initiatives, to eliminate health disparities and social determinants of health, and to prepare for global population health initiatives that are patient focused. In addition, competency in policy and regulatory knowledge of community-based and global population health care initiatives are necessary as policy change and continued assessment to sustain positive outcomes utilizing actionable data is necessary in all leadership competencies. Identification of organizational risk, vulnerability, and the ability to lead teams to change current practices impacting patient care and quality by utilizing business management, financial data, productivity measures to develop valid, consistent, and reliable data in addressing patient quality and safety are skills that cannot be ignored in organizations. The development of research-based data and ROI with implemented processes is scarce in the literature. The DNP-prepared director of nursing informatics must have the fundamental elements necessary to evaluate and analyze cost-effective and efficient strategies necessary to concentrate on the improvement of outcomes related to patient care and organizational sustainability.

## Evidence-Based Practice and Analytical Approaches to Outcome Measures

Identifying complex clinical and practice situations and addressing solutions to complex issues requires knowledge and understanding of several theories and evidence-based practice principles to address translating research into practice and to find solutions to complex diseases that affect mind, body, spirit, and the genetic and biological make-up of human beings in various settings. A DNP-prepared director of nursing informatics must translate this knowledge into actionable interventions that are best practice principles and have positive outcome results.

This principle directly integrates with effective, efficient, and safe quality care for all populations served. The data must be benchmarked, proven effective, and the DNP-prepared director of nursing informatics must analyze and map the data to transform health care. Sharing of the methods utilized to achieve transformation, gain knowledge of best practices throughout the nation, and communication of regulatory agency requirements that are integral to the sustainability of results and the ability to keep up with constant change are skills necessary for improvement and change management success. In addition, the ability to design databases that generate actionable and meaningful data that can transform current practices, predict, and analyze outcomes is essential for all health care organizations concentrating efforts to improve complex issues related to population health. The ability to identify gaps in data and gaps in mapping databases is critical to approaching measurable and meaningful data affecting individual, group, community, and global health care outcomes efficiently. It is equally important to collaborate and communicate findings to improve health care outcomes and to document evidence-based best practice findings and research related to health care in vulnerable high-risk populations.

## Information Systems and Technology: Transforming Health Care

The distinguishing factor identified in a DNP-prepared nurse from other nurses is the ability to transform knowledge of systems, utilize technology to improve data and patient care outcomes, and integrate organizational structure to transform patient care at the bedside. Technology is an ally and a means to gain and apply new knowledge in the quest for reliable, actionable, and valid data. The DNP-prepared nurse can transform documentation systems with innovative tools aimed at decreasing the burden of documentation while streamlining health care services and improving patient care outcomes.

The timeliness of identifying critical, complex conditions such as sepsis that require multifocal analysis and multidisciplinary teams utilizing technology is an example of utilizing the use of information technology, communication systems, and patient care technology to improve sepsis outcomes. Meeting protocols and guidelines, regulatory requirements with best practice, and research findings while utilizing the electronic health care system as the conduit to guide teams in early identification of sepsis with discrete coded elements to aggregate, measure, and validate is an example of actionable data utilized to transform sepsis recognition and improve sepsis outcomes. The complexity of sepsis is impacted by the changing definitions and regulatory guidelines utilized to measure results. Furthermore, sepsis coding as a principle International Classification of Diseases, Tenth Revision, Clinical Modification (ICD-10-CM) diagnosis is not always clear-cut and absolute. Patients present with other signs and symptoms.[10] Documentation is critical to the early identification and final diagnosis for sepsis. The DNP-prepared nurse must assess and analyze coding requirements and perform a deep dive in validating documentation and information related to sepsis diagnosis. Certain sepsis conditions have an underlying cause with multiple body system medical presentations due to the underlying cause for sepsis making the definition of sepsis difficult to identify and code. For such complex conditions, ICD-10-CM has a coding convention that requires the underlying cause or condition to be sequenced first, followed by the manifestation of the condition.[8]

The mapping of such codes adds to the complexity of documentation in the electronic health care record. Identification of each data element, aggregation, and validation of transparent actionable data to improve sepsis outcomes, and sharing of findings with multiple stakeholders to include physicians, health care leaders, board members, nursing, and non-nursing teams, becomes problematic and challenging for organizations not focused on transformational principles that lead toward change.

## Health Care Advocacy

Health care policy focusing on ethical, equitable access to care for all individuals, groups, and communities is essential for DNP-prepared leaders. The ability to utilize data to improve outcomes and change policy or change guidelines that lead toward positive patient care is a value necessary in transformational leaders. Active participation in national professional organizations, presentations at national conferences that enable sharing of data and results, documentation of research findings in peer-reviewed professional journals, and participation in national organizations focused on health care advocacy and the improvement of patient care demonstrate actionable leadership. Advocating for vulnerable populations to improve services is fundamental in transforming health care with data.

## Patient and Population Health Collaboration and Improvement

Nursing informatics is the dynamic driving force of communication, collaboration, and consistency integrating nursing science and nursing process with informational, analytical, biomedical, and transformational sciences to create synergistic innovation that formulates data, information, knowledge, and wisdom for the delivery of quality and safe care to every patient/family/community during every encounter, every opportunity, every day.[9]

Without synergistic interaction with people, fluid and flexible multifocal teams focused on patient care needs will not succeed in identifying the complexities of population health. Epidemiologists, biomedical informaticists, data analysts, physicians, case managers, social workers, psychologists, psychiatrists, specialty physicians, generalists, hospitalists, and nurses at all levels are necessary to address population health issues. The sharing of data via a health care information exchange that integrates care with vital data elements for comprehensive care services is necessary for the success of interoperability and transitions of care. The ability to digitalize access to care is challenging and complex.

## Improving and Impacting National Population Health

The focus on health promotion and prevention of illness with the reduction of illness for individuals, communities, and vulnerable populations at risk is the goal of improving health care nationally. Finding cost-effective and efficient processes that make a positive impact on patient care outcomes is critical to the concept of improving national statistics and transforming the delivery of patient care utilizing prevention of illness models. The United States continues to fall behind in comparison to other nations when comparing health care spending. On average, other countries spend half as much in the delivery of health care services than the United States.[10]

Sepsis data aggregation is problematic based on measurable data elements necessary to address regulatory requirements. The Centers for Medicare & Medicaid Services (CMS) implemented "SEP-1" as part of its Hospital Inpatient Quality Reporting Program (IQRP) in October 2015 to measure sepsis quality outcomes. This requires hospitals to report compliance with 3- and 6-hour sepsis treatment and resuscitation bundle protocols for patients identified with sepsis. Antibiotic and fluid administration, blood culture, lactate measurement, the use of vasopressors for fluid-refractory hypotension, and the bedside evaluation of a patient's response to treatment are required elements of measurement and analysis specific to the care and outcomes measures for septic patients. Challenges continue with identifying sepsis rapidly and coordinating care within the health care continuum with the end goal of keeping populations healthy.

## *Advanced Nursing Practice*

The conceptualization of analyzing skills necessary to specialize in providing evidence-based best practice initiatives to vulnerable populations, groups, and individuals is complex. Specializing in advanced nursing practice leads to the exploration of various sciences that incorporate multifactorial concepts in the care of diversified global health. Research questions related to how to improve health care efficiently and effectively with the use of data-driven results that formulate improvements in patient care are the fundamental basis of advanced practice skills resonating in collaborative efforts with other disciplines. The development of innovative models of care within various practice settings will improve patient care outcomes for years to come.

# BUSINESS PLAN TO INSTITUTIONALIZE THE DNP-PREPARED LEADER

The internal motivating factor to serve others, to facilitate healing based on patient goals and preferences, and to include palliative care and the right to death and dying with dignity stems from culture, beliefs, and caring. The value of research in finding evidence-based solutions for complex care issues and sharing knowledge with others on improving health care outcomes is the locus of control for DNP-prepared nurses and leaders in health care who utilize transformational leadership principles. Systematic change management is critical in today's health care systems. Transformational leaders provide the basis for rapid and fluid systematic change that leads toward effective outcomes. Convincing health care organizations to invest in leadership roles to improve services utilizing data analysis and business principles is challenging. Facilitating measurable ROI through data governance, clinical content review while utilizing evidence-based practice in health care settings is not frequent. Structuring change management in electronic health care system(s) selection is dependent on a business plan that builds on positive results and proven success.

Calculating the ROI provides a comparison of net gain to net costs and is a measure of profitability.[11] The ROI is calculated as the return (net gain) due to an action divided by the cost of the act.[11] An ROI for a DNP-prepared registered nurse hired for $120 000 per year including benefits to work on improving sepsis mortality in 90 days adds a social element to the ROI. The mean cost per sepsis readmission within 30 days of discharge is $16 852.[12] Utilizing the ROI calculation, if there are 2 sepsis readmissions yearly, the ROI in hiring a DNP-prepared registered nurse is 28%. A full ROI for employing a DNP graduate occurs after only 8 sepsis readmissions are prevented. This speaks to both the clinical and cost-effectiveness of hiring a DNP-prepared nurse. A ROI within 90 days and 365 days is the same. However, for an organization whose focus is on patient safety and quality care, decreasing readmissions in 90 days is viewed in more positive terms than waiting a year (ie, 365 days).

The ROI for future role expansion for nursing informatics team members and expanding roles in nursing informatics has led to yearly budget meetings with detailed business plans. Expanding roles and investing in people has led to innovation. Future goals were to hire another team member in 2019 with plans to hire another nursing informatics specialist in 2020. The expansion of systems analysts and data analysts has been positive. Strategic initiatives aligned with departmental initiatives lead to the development of a data governance team with plans to expand into a data governance committee throughout the organization focused on quality and safety, actionable data, validity and transparency, and business planning with knowledge management for high performance and positive outcomes.

# RESEARCH: SEPSIS

Research related to best practices in identification, treatment, long-term effects of exposure to sepsis, biomedical, and immunologic factors continues. Sepsis is one of the most difficult conditions to identify early and treat. In addition, coordination of care post-discharge is equally important. Although statistics focused on sepsis survival indicate decreased mortality rates, hospitals continue to struggle with early identification of sepsis, adherence to protocols for sepsis prevention, and documentation in the electronic health care record. The goal for University Medical Center of El Paso to address this global concern was to facilitate sepsis recognition early and improve sepsis outcomes. Efforts to treat sepsis based on recognized sepsis as identified by laboratory results, signs and symptoms, and presenting clinical findings without early intervention proved ineffective. Collaborative meetings with several teams focused on improving sepsis outcomes with actionable and measurable data. An analysis of the number of patients identified with sepsis and mortality rate presentations at all hospital community meetings took place. Early identification, treatment plans, selection of antibiotics with antimicrobial stewardship guidelines imbedded in electronic order sets, time frames for each intervention from cultures, to lab work, to assessments documented in the electronic health record at each critical phase of sepsis SEP-1 standards identified areas of improvement. Strategies included electronic health care documentation review, workflow analysis, and process mapping utilizing Plan Do Study Act cycles to address gaps and modify build in the electronic health care record. Modifications to orders in the emergency, critical care, and inpatient departments with provider input, testing, and validation proved positive.

Next steps focused on methods of alerting providers, nurses, and quality team members to sepsis alerts without the addition of false negatives into information sent from the electronic medical record to clinical staff for the purpose of identifying and flagging patients needing follow-up based on sepsis triggers. Discern alerts in the system worked well when clinical staff were in electronic systems documenting patient care. When not directly in the electronic medical record, nursing informatics worked with information management teams to send email alerts and information via phone and pager to sepsis clinical teams. This allowed for early identification with review and assessment of patients requiring additional monitoring based on sepsis triggers. The addition of notifying clinical care teams improved outcome data. The time of implementation correlated to improved identification of sepsis and improved patient care outcomes.

The research on sepsis identified a marked improvement in recognizing sepsis early. Data prior to implementation of early recognition processes and the development of a roadmap for clinicians to communicate findings electronically identified sepsis recognition at 14% with all measures. Post-implementation of early identification and electronic documentation led to 58% recognition of sepsis. Physician orders were modified to include antimicrobial guidelines. In addition, fluid volume guidelines were added to the order sets. Areas of deficiency in documentation were outlined and communicated at physician driven committees with targeted goals to meet regulatory guidelines and improve patient care outcomes. Change in practice took place with a reduction in sepsis mortality. There were 2 deaths related to sepsis at the beginning of 2018. By March 2019, no deaths were attributed to sepsis. Documentation in the electronic medical record continues to improve with sepsis order sets review. Challenges related to sepsis coding were identified. Change management team meetings continue to identify opportunities with concurrent review. Waiting for coding upon discharge poses a challenge with documentation and improvement measures. Weekly review of data with drilldown to each patient's experience continues. The battle to eradicate sepsis continues. Researchers are turning toward biomedical sciences to develop new assays that will identify and predict the affinity for developing sepsis with biomedical markers that can identify patients at low, medium, and high risk utilizing predictive analytics.[13]

# Research: Procalcitonin

Reviewing research results presented at the American Nursing Informatics Association Conference in 2018 allowed for additional questions related to sepsis and sepsis outcomes. The addition of procalcitonin levels to the sepsis bundle order sets at University Medical Center of El Paso generated further research. Would procalcitonin levels identify antibiotic therapy for continued use for patients and also identify patients prone to sepsis earlier than utilizing lactic acid levels? This question triggered the need for further investigation of data. Reports generated from the electronic medical record identifying the use of sepsis order sets along with ordering procalcitonin levels identified all patients with

sepsis with appropriate antibiotic therapy consistently. Levels above 2.0 ng/mL are highly suggestive of systemic bacterial infection/sepsis and severe localized bacterial infection to include severe pneumonia, meningitis, or peritonitis.[13] Levels can also occur after severe noninfectious inflammatory stimuli such as major burns, severe trauma, acute multiorgan failure, or major abdominal or cardiothoracic surgery.[13] In cases of noninfectious elevations, procalcitonin levels should begin to fall after 24 to 48 hours.[13]

DNP-prepared nurses search for answers utilizing evidence-based practice principles to improve outcomes. Data included time of patient registration to the time sepsis was identified utilizing lactic acid levels and procalcitonin levels for 643 patients from January 1, 2019 to October 31, 2019. Sepsis codes were utilized for identifying patients with sepsis. Fifty-nine patients were identified with sepsis based on coding data. Lactic acid results ranged from 0.8 to 16.8. Thirteen of these patients had elevated lactic acid levels caused by dehydration vs sepsis. Time from admission and registration to identification of sepsis was 0.07 to 1.83 in this group of patients. The odds ratio of sepsis resulted as 3.927244582 in this aggregate group.

In comparison, 46 patients had procalcitonin levels ordered. Time frames from registration to identification of sepsis ranged from 0.07 to 1.63 in 277 patients. Procalcitonin levels ranged from 0.27 to 89.83 based on coding for sepsis with an odds ratio of sepsis at 3.811428571. Procalcitonin levels with the order sets for sepsis identification are optional and not part of the sepsis bundle requirements. Procalcitonin levels continue to be discussed and evaluated. Sepsis coding was identified as a process improvement measure to facilitate the actual diagnosis of sepsis and its source. There was a positive correlation between lactic acid and procalcitonin levels as indicated in the following diagrams. Figure 22-3 compares lactic acid results to procalcitonin results based on identified true positives.[14]

The question is whether procalcitonin will prove to be the best marker to identify sepsis and assist with antibiotic therapy for the treatment of sepsis in all patients. More research is needed in the early identification and treatment of sepsis.

# Pearls/Takeaways

The DNP-prepared nurse has the ability to collaborate with health care leaders by sharing research findings, transforming health care organizations with systems thinking, and mentoring nursing students on the principles of advanced practice nursing. Communication principles in a collaborative, consistent, and cohesive manner allows for the success of others. Developing partnerships in solving today's complex challenges allows for more manageable and creative ways of maintaining positive relationships. It is through community health care partnerships where solid decisions can lead to change.

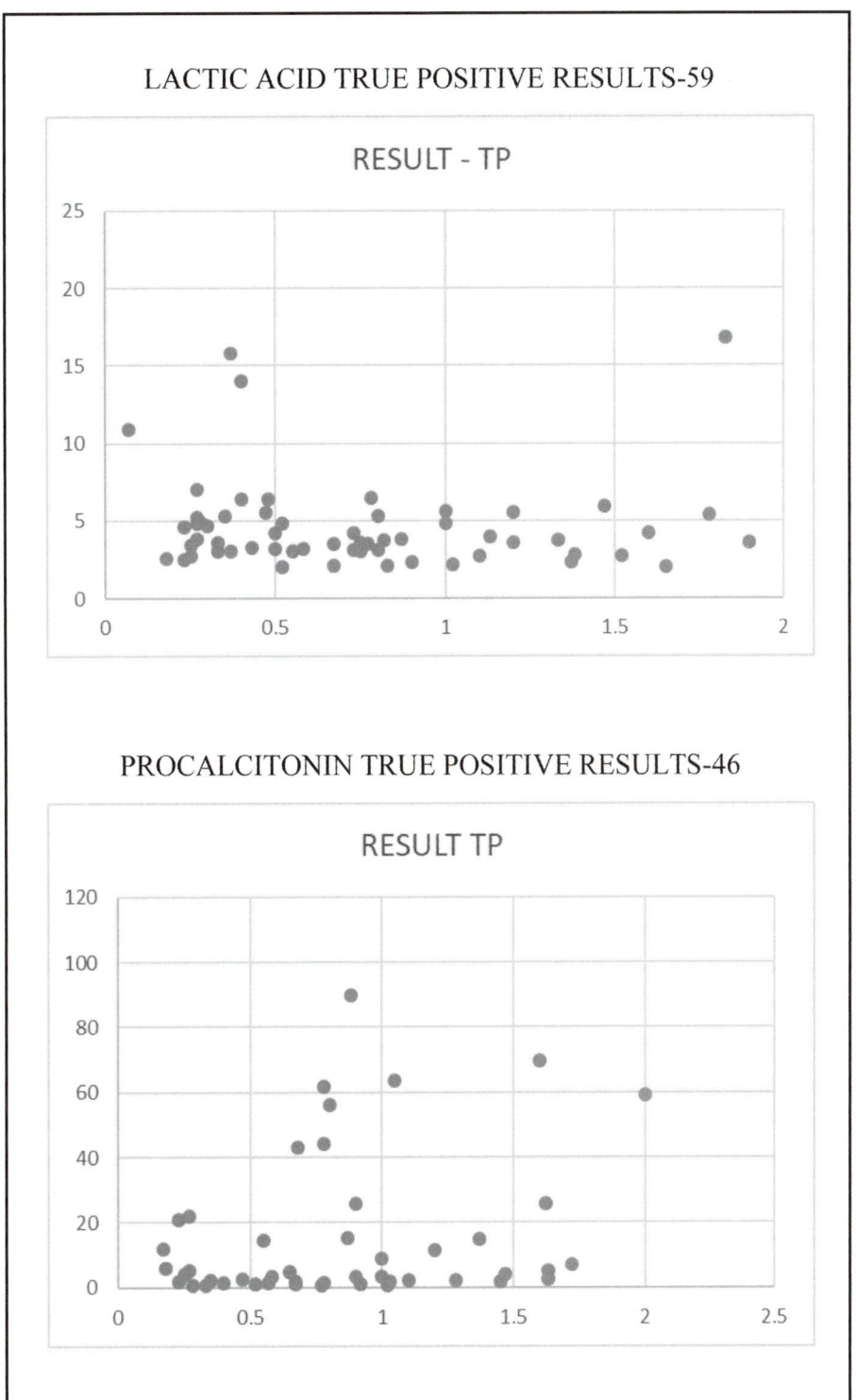

**Figure 22-3.** Comparison of lactic acid and procalcitonin levels.

DNP programs prepare nurses for leading new, efficient, effective, and valued care outcomes throughout the continuum of care. Complex interactions are managed through the values of high-reliability organizations that include team work, and empowerment of individuals to identify and implement corrective action. The concept of addressing gaps within organizations and recognizing them as process improvement opportunities, empowering teams to bridge gaps with actionable interventions with proven results, and valuing people are concepts inherent to DNP-prepared nurses in a complex health care environment.

The ability to share with other nurses by teaching in the university setting, presenting research at conferences and sharing ideas for further research, implementing change in the electronic medical record for positive patient outcomes, leading committees within health care organizations, and developing nursing informatics theories with powerful actionable data with the use of data analytics that transcends from descriptive analytics to predictive analytics and prescriptive analytics will change health care and sustain positive health care outcomes.

# Conclusion: Impact of the DNP Degree

As a result of obtaining my DNP degree, I gained knowledge beyond the classroom. I first envisioned furthering my education while still working full-time as an administrator of a free-standing children's hospital. I have always valued higher education. I did not expect to gain a whole new perspective and a new role as an administrator of a nursing informatics department at a rapidly growing university medical center. Nursing has brought a multitude of gifts as a profession in my experience as a nurse: the gift of caring, helping others in need at their most vulnerable time, and teaching families to better care for their loved ones and themselves and a richer sense of purpose. My DNP degree has prepared me to collaborate with health care teams and organizations to better manage patient care and facilitate cohesive, coordinated care with successful patient outcomes. I have gained insight to the researcher, the specialist, the communicator, the educator, and the author with my DNP degree. The dedication to pursue informatics, technology, genetics, genomics, telehealth, and telemedicine to cultivate making a difference in the lives of many was cultivated from the knowledge I gained with my DNP degree. I was able to continue to ask the question, "Why?" and to pursue answers beyond imagination with a global perspective.

A person's knowledge is only as good as how the knowledge is shared, implemented, and tested within other settings and by other researchers. Obtaining a DNP degree facilitated sharing. Health care abounds with examples of high-reliability organizations where care is efficient and effective for all patients seeking care. Health care also has many examples where care delivery systems are broken and need innovative

and effective ways of implementing quality safe care. DNP programs offer nurses the ability to lead and use information systems, program evaluation, and evidence-based research. DNP-prepared nurses can enhance and transform health care with active engagement in health care reform, policy development and policy change, and developing, evaluating and improving health care delivery for individuals, groups, and communities. For example, utilizing validation of statistics and formulating predictive analytic processes while organizing a data governance committee within a safety net hospital is an example of leading an organization toward positive patient care outcomes with actionable data to make a difference in the delivery of patient care.

In addition, utilizing predictive analytics in improving care for patients identified with chronic health care needs has brought acute care and ambulatory health care teams together to review data and identify ways of delivering care while focusing on social determinants of health triggers for positive patient care outcomes. The ability to participate in research that can lead to evidence-based practice outcomes while changing how we identify sepsis to improve mortality rates is priceless.

# Acknowledgments

To the patients and families at University Medical Center of El Paso who teach us humility and complete love of family.

# References

1.  About us. University Medical Center of El Paso. https://www.umcelpaso.org/about-us

2.  Beal A, Hamlin B. Research approaches for real-world evidence generation. AcademyHealth. Accessed August 19, 2019. https://www.academyhealth.org/blog/2018-05/research-approaches-real-world-evidence-generation

3.  Sewell J. Informatics and nursing: opportunities and challenges. Chegg Books. Accessed September 2, 2019. https://www.chegg.com/textbooks/informatics-and-nursing-5th-edition-9781451193206-1451193203

4.  Chasco D. Nursing informatics synergy model. Presented at: Summer Institute Nursing Informatics Conference; July 19, 2019; Baltimore, Maryland.

5.  The essentials of doctoral nursing education for advanced nursing practice. American Association of Colleges of Nursing. October 2006. Accessed October 3, 2019. https://nursing.lsuhsc.edu/Docs/Quality/AACN%20Essentials%20of%20Doctoral%20Education%20for%20Adv%20Nsg%20Practice%20(2006).pdf

6.  Doctor of nursing practice (DNP) toolkit. American Association of Colleges of Nursing. Accessed November 1, 2019. https://www.aacnnursing.org/DNP/Tool-Kit

7.  ICD-10-CM official guidelines for coding and reporting FY 2018. Centers for Medicare & Medicaid Services. Accessed November 2, 2019. https://www.cms.gov/Medicare/Coding/ICD10/Downloads/2018-ICD-10-CM-Coding-Guidelines.pdf

8.  ICD-10-CM diagnosis code A41: other sepsis. ICD10 Data. Accessed November 2, 2019. https://www.icd10data.com/ICD10CM/Codes/A00-B99/A30-A49/A41-/A41

9.  Chasco D. Language, culture, disparities of care. Presented at: UMSON; May 7-8, 2018; Baltimore, Maryland.

10.   Sawyer B, Cox S. How does spending in the US compare to other countries? Peterson Center on Healthcare. Accessed November 2, 2019. https://www.healthsystemtracker.org/chart-collection/health-spending-u-s-compare-countries/#item-start

11.   Schmidt M. Return on investment ROI metric measures profitability. Solution Matrix Limited. Accessed November 2, 2019. https://www.business-case-analysis.com/return-on-investment.html

12.   Cheney C. Cost of sepsis readmissions estimated at more than $16,000 per patient. HealthLeaders. Accessed November 2, 2019. https://www.healthleadersmedia.com/clinical-care/cost-sepsis-readmissions-estimated-more-16000-patient?webSyncID=a4b0eec5-00a2-74cb-0116-b989c3e68574&sessionGUID=93a50a aa-81ee-0b8c-83a2-64c118971481

13.   Test ID PCT. Mayo Clinic Laboratories. Accessed November 3, 2019. https://www.mayocliniclabs.com/test-catalog/Clinical+and+Interpretive/83169

14.   Chasco D. Comparison of lactic acid and procalcitonin levels. Data results presented at: American Nursing Informatics Association Conference; August 18, 2020.

# CHAPTER 23

# APPLYING DNP ESSENTIALS WITHIN THE FIELD OF NURSING INFORMATICS TO IMPACT PATIENT CARE AND TRANSFORM HEALTH CARE PROVISION

*Carol Shade, DNP, MS, RN, CPHIMS, FHIMSS and Mary Field, DNP, MBA, RN, CPHON*

## INTRODUCTION

The combination of nursing informatics and the 8 Doctor of Nursing Practice (DNP) Essentials allows for the true and full expression of both subject areas. Nursing informaticists are called to critically apply information sciences with technology systems to generate solutions. Through incorporating the DNP Essentials, nursing informaticists can enact change at either a population or systems level, as opposed to at an individual patient level. These DNP Essentials will help clinicians create meaningful business cases, support evidence-based care, and practice interprofessional collaboration, among others. While the field of information technology (IT) is expanding at a rapid pace, a DNP-prepared nurse can take IT evidence and translate it into tactical practice changes at the bedside. This can be achieved through academic dissemination or organization-wide systems dissemination. The presence of big data, predictive analytics, and data mining create an ideal environment for a DNP-prepared nurse to express the 8 Essentials to propel nursing care forward. While the 8 Essentials are expressed in every field of nursing, they are particularly meaningful in the field of nursing

informatics. This field is a relatively new form of nursing, however, the academic institution of DNP Essentials combined with this ever-evolving profession provides the rigor needed to gain widespread adoption of the field of nursing informatics to meaningfully impact patient care.

## SETTING

The field of nursing informatics integrates nursing science with information and analytical sciences to identify, define, manage, and communicate data, information, knowledge, and wisdom in nursing practice.[1] The combination of our roles as director of nursing informatics, training, and technology and clinical practice manager (CPM) have established a collaboration that blends Carol's experience as a clinical informaticist with Mary's role as a clinical nursing expert in pediatric oncology. Our years of professional collaboration have allowed us to bring many innovative informatics solutions to fruition. We have applied concepts present within the DNP program for health care leadership to translate information science evidence into meaningful practice changes. This is in direct result to our close alignment with

Benson LA, ed. *The DNP Professional: Translating Value From Classroom to Practice* (pp 253-260).

clinical practice and professional collaboration. This chapter represents the expression of our many years of professional nursing collaboration at Seattle Children's Hospital (SCH). For context, this is a 407-bed academic hospital with approximately 1600 registered nurses serving patients from a 4-state WAMI region (Washington, Alaska, Montana, and Idaho).[2] The hospital is known for its fundamental belief in the organizational mission: to provide hope, care, and cure for every child, promoting the healthiest and most fulfilling life possible. In all the work we do together, our goal is to propel this mission forward by leveraging information science combined with nursing practice. Much of our work is enhanced by incorporated Essentials from the DNP framework.

In addition to our professional relationship within the workplace, we have developed a strong academic partnership. Over the past few years, we have published a peer-reviewed article, given a podium and multiple poster presentations, and taught a doctorate-level health care informatics 10-week course together. As a DNP herself, Carol has mentored Mary throughout these projects, ultimately encouraging her to enroll in a doctorate program. Subsequently, Mary has successfully completed her DNP program. Her capstone project involved surveying clinical nurses for satisfaction in using the electronic health record (EHR). It is this blend of professional and academic collaboration that allows for the full expression of the DNP Essentials, including but not limited to organizational and systems leadership.

# CREATION AND EXPANSION OF ROLES

## Carol's Role

As the director of nursing informatics, training, and technology, Carol directs the necessary training for technology systems at an organizational level for all clinical nurses. In this role, Carol interfaces closely with other team members to provide strategic guidance for the EHR and other technology and informatics initiatives. Currently, SCH is adopting a new EHR, so much of Carol's time is spent partnering with the chief medical informatics officer (CMIO) and transformational leadership council to ensure the EHR project is progressing along the strategic timeline. In addition, Carol received delegation directly from the chief nursing officer (CNO) to oversee all EHR aspects for nursing, as well as other clinical areas reporting through the CNO. Carol holds the responsibility to ensure nursing and other allied health areas like social work and behavioral health medicine are clearly and thoughtfully integrated across the EHR implementation

project. Carol's role provides an ideal opportunity to advocate for multidisciplinary representation helping to meet the design needs of a patient- or family-centered EHR. Carol also serves as the organizational leader for the Super User training support program, a crucial at-the-elbow support program for every successful implementation or "go live."

Specifically with the EHR project, Carol defines, establishes, and maintains structure around nursing representation within the project by guiding all global communications for nursing and ensuring critical care aspects for the design of the EHR are not missed. Carol is working with the CMIO and hospital leadership to develop a long-term Super User program that will ensure ongoing clinical support when new enhancements within the EHR are deployed. Carol also has oversight for the vision and redesign of the clinical informatics council that falls under the umbrella of nursing shared governance. She ensures council representation from acute care, critical care, peri-operative, and ambulatory nursing, guiding members to work on specific EHR projects that impact nursing. Carol aims to develop informatics competencies for both nursing leaders and clinical staff as there is literature to support the significance of such competencies.[3] The DNP Essentials have provided Carol with the skills and resources to support nursing through this large-scale transformational project.

## Mary's Role

As the CPM on the inpatient hematology, oncology, and bone marrow transplant unit, Mary directly oversees the 200 nurses and certified nursing assistants staffed on the unit. While at the same time, she coordinates daily operations and regulatory compliance. In addition, approximately half her time is dedicated to unit-level quality improvement projects and continuous process improvement. Throughout Mary's time as a manager, she obtained a master's degree in business administration with an emphasis in health care informatics. Mary has used this formal academic training frequently for partnership with Carol and her team. Mary's role within our current EHR redesign is to provide divisional-level oversight and guidance for the oncology division. Her work spans both inpatient and outpatient, and crosses many disciplines such as medical doctors, advanced registered nurse practitioners, pharmacy, occupational therapy, physical therapy, nutrition, and child life to name a few. Much of her informatics work is focused specifically within the oncology division, while Carol oversees hospital-wide informatics. Throughout the EHR project, Mary will practice using the DNP Essentials with Carol as her mentor. It is this mentorship that will ensure the ultimate success in the hospital's integrated EHR project.

# INCORPORATION OF DNP ESSENTIALS

## DNP Essential: Organizational and Systems Leadership for Quality Improvement and Systems Thinking

Effective systems leadership of information systems requires a multidisciplinary organizational approach. As the director of nursing informatics, Carol has set the direction and tone for nursing informatics at a systems level. To do this, Carol finds herself relying on her strong foundational leadership skills. Carol has also recognized one of the key attributes for a nursing informatics leader is to have a strong educational foundation, such as a team that places emphasis on obtaining a graduate degree and specialty certification. This allows them to serve as experts in technology applicable to nursing practice. There is an established link between nursing informatics competencies and transformational leadership for nursing leaders. This link can help support safe, integrated, high-quality care delivery.[4] However, transformational leadership is a skill grown from solid, foundational nursing leadership skills.

To gain leadership skills, Carol took a progressive approach to her nursing career. After graduating with a bachelor's degree in nursing, she worked as a clinical staff nurse for 5 years in a pediatric hospital until she received a promotion to the role of unit educator, which led her to pursue a master's degree in nursing. This opened the door to more projects and leadership opportunities, such as serving as chair for a variety of hospital-wide committees like policies, regulatory requirements, forms, and serving as the lead nurse in the selection of an EHR vendor.

Carol later worked in roles allowing her to do analyst builds in the EHR systems and helping her define organizational strategy for evidence-based pathway development within the EHR. She then served in the role of the first nursing informatics specialist within her organization, helping lead a number of large EHR nursing projects. For her to have a greater impact on health care, a doctorate-level degree was the right path. The DNP degree provided Carol the perfect blend of graduate-level nursing theory and further development of continued leadership skills. Examples of leadership skills included advocating and receiving approval of a business case for the integration of central line bloodstream infection (CLABSI) bundle elements into the EHR. Carol has been able to incorporate the 8 DNP Essentials in all aspects as she has grown both a nursing and clinical informatics team. In addition, she has been able to assess organizational systems' issues to facilitate organizational-wide changes.

Mary is still building her foundational nursing leadership skills. She has been in a formal nursing leadership role for the past 3 years. In that time, she has progressively taken on more responsibility within her oncology division. While this professional and academic training has been extremely beneficial, the act of enrolling in the DNP program and selecting a DNP scholarly project has helped Mary gain the most leadership skills. This program has helped foster Mary's ability to communicate clearly to stakeholders to gain support for quality improvement projects. For example, in her quality improvement class, Mary presented a final project regarding the importance of nursing huddles. This project included a gap analysis, evaluation, and implementation plan using quality improvement methodologies. Mary shared this project with her senior nursing leaders and has now been asked to lead this project on the inpatient oncology unit. It is this intersection of doctorate-level academic work that is propelling Mary's professional leadership skills forward. Mary will continue to use the communication and project management skills gained in her DNP program throughout the integrated EHR project.

## DNP Essential: Clinical Scholarship and Analytical Methods for Evidence-Based Practice

While scholarship is often synonymous with research, we have found a much deeper meaning within our roles as nurses and clinical informaticists, and we have applied this use of scholarship to a variety of evidence-based projects. Scholars can give context and meanings to facts to establish connections across disciplines.[5] One example of a collaborative clinical scholarship activity is our application of clinical decision support within the EHR. In part of our sepsis identification work, nursing informatics recognized a gap in early sepsis identification. To address this, a multidisciplinary sepsis workgroup was formed. This group included nursing informatics, clinical nursing, pharmacy, and providers, among others. Carol was able to apply this group's recommendations to the EHR. Specifically, visual indicators were identified to automatically identify low blood pressures, clear icons for patients on the sepsis pathway were added, and automatic mean arterial pressure calculations were included. Another example of clinical scholarship was Mary's DNP scholarly project. With Carol's mentorship, Mary assessed nursing's needs and current satisfaction in order to achieve optimal user satisfaction with future EHRs. There are many reliable and valid tools that evaluate multidisciplinary user satisfaction; however, there are currently no best practices surrounding nursing's unique EHR needs.

## DNP Essential: Information Systems/Technology and Patient Care Technology for the Improvement and Transformation of Health Care

Our true calling is combining our professional expertise in information science with our passion for improving health care in the pediatric setting. This combination provides the backbone for many of our clinical initiatives. DNP graduates are called to use information systems to improve patient care and health care systems, as well as to manage individual and population-level information contained within the EHR.[6] One of the greatest examples of our combination of all things informatics with patient outcomes is our patient-centric model. Our patient-centric model, also fondly referred to as "customer-obsessed" model, allows us to use patient outcomes as the guiding principle and common denominator for many of our projects. For example, in one recent project we were challenged to improve our quality and frequency of patient education. While we could have asked our clinical nurse specialists (CNS) or CPMs to partner with clinical nurses to improve education, we decided to focus upstream on information system solutions. After conducting many information gathering meetings with patient advisory councils and clinical nurses, a solution was found that allowed clinical nurses to order educational videos for the family within the EHR. This video then pops up on the family's television or tablet within the patient room. Once the video is watched by the patient or family, a completion note is automatically documented via an interface within the patient's EHR. While this has not replaced 1:1 nursing education, it has become an adjunct teaching method that has assisted many families. From a technology perspective, it eliminates the additional step of the nurse needing to remember to document that the video was viewed, and this also gave more time back to the nurses that could be used for direct patient care. Another benefit for use of this technology solution is that it ensures documentation was done, which can be of such significant value when following up with patients on future visits. The ideal clinical workflow is assigning the video to a family a day or 2 before assigned nursing teaching. Six months after implementation of this functionality, families on Mary's unit are successfully watching educational videos assigned by their care team and the organizational completion rate goal has been met. In October 2018, we had almost 650 videos watched by inpatient families! By using an information science solution, we added no additional work time to the clinical nurse, but were able to improve the breadth and depth of education offered to patients and families. Future optimization of this project incorporates a third-party education content for written materials, as well as the ability of families to view information post-discharge or even assigning education videos via an application.

## DNP Essential: Interprofessional Collaboration for Improving Patient and Population Health Outcomes

One of the most effective ways to improve patient outcomes is to embrace a multidisciplinary team approach. In fact, the delivery of effective, high-quality clinical care depends upon interprofessional collaboration, often established with shared interprofessional education.[7] This collaborative approach is modeled at the organizational level by a combination of physician, nursing, pharmacy, and administration personnel comprising many of the transformational governance committees. At a divisional level, we also have multidisciplinary work groups tasked with ensuring the delivery of high-quality clinical care. For example, in Mary's oncology division, there is a chemotherapy safety committee that is comprised of physicians, nurses, administrators, pharmacists, and quality specialists. This committee is ultimately responsible for ensuring our ordering, checking, and administration of chemotherapy within the EHR is safe and effective.

We have also embraced a strong support of interprofessional collaboration within the nursing chain. We frequently consult with CNSs, practice managers, and associate chief nurses when soliciting useful feedback for our EHR and new project initiatives. However, perhaps the closest example of interprofessional collaboration is our professional alignment. By combining our shared love of informatics with our organization's strategic plan, we are able to improve the system that supports nursing care and practice throughout the hospital.

# BUSINESS PLAN

Any new program deployed within an organization needs a general business case or justification at some level. This holds true for core technology solutions as well as the use of new operational constructs that use technology to achieve goals. A DNP-prepared nurse specializing in nursing informatics can utilize the 8 DNP Essentials in order to provide foundational groundwork for how to recognize what is needed in a business plan and to assist in making it a successful selling point. What issue are you trying to solve? What is the target you are trying to achieve? How will you measure this? What data do you have to indicate what the industry standard is or what the benchmarking comparisons are? How are patients affected or benefited in both the short- and long-term? All of these questions need to be addressed in a good business plan. For technology solutions, you must also think beyond the initial cost: what will the maintenance or support of any new solution cost and how will it be resourced?

One of the recent projects Carol has been involved in was to develop a milk management system where breast milk is centralized within a Milk Lab. Evidence has shown that a centralized inventory system ensures milk integrity as well as safety of administration (ie, right milk product to the right patient).[8] By combining this strong evidence with a well-thought-out business case, Carol was able to achieve senior leadership's approval to implement this project. A business case is a proposal that assists organizations and executives in presenting and understanding the need for change, organizational impact, and financial impact.[9] For this project, the business case included data specific to lost milk, patient errors with potential harm occurring as a result of wrong breast milk, or formula administration. An advanced degree in nursing practice helps a nurse leader identify all these aspects needed for approval of a business plan specific to a technology solution. A well-formulated business plan can help achieve early support from senior leadership.

Another example of a business case Carol helped contribute to involved evaluating which technology solution best met the needs for the hospital's external critical care transport team. As part of this work, Carol partnered with the nursing leader for the transport team and IT leadership to help defend why the transport team met criteria for a best-of-breed solution. Best-of-breed refers to an industry product that provides a specific technology solution for an identified need. When deciding between best-of-breed and a larger core system, the 80/20 rule is often applied weighing the benefits of selecting a specialized solution that surpasses the challenges associated with the core vendor. To reach this conclusion, we asked a variety of questions. What system do peer organizations use? What are the pros and cons of the transport-specific solution vs the core EHR vendor? What interface work is required? Which system impedes or supports quick access to patient information when needed most? Will one of the systems provide more discrete data that can then be used to determine improvement opportunities, such as safer care, quality outcomes, or increased efficiency? Collaboration with IT experts, transport leadership, as well as frontline staff and other organizational roles was needed to make a good business plan.

# Cost Savings/Revenue Generation

Efficiency and cost-effective elements are vital to validate a return on investment (ROI) when implementing new strategies. One program Carol developed soon after graduating with a DNP in health care leadership was to restructure the EHR training approach for clinical staff nurses from an in-person classroom method of instruction to web-based eLearnings. Carol ensured the training team had the proper equipment and software to develop the web-based modules and hired new staff with experience in this area of work. Literature was reviewed on different approaches to providing EHR training. There is value in allowing people to learn at their own pace,[10] and therefore a proposal of switching to

an eLearning approach was investigated. According to Dale's cone of experience, people generally remember 10% of what they hear regarding a task, and 90% of what they do as they perform a task.[11] Capturing cost savings as well as end-user satisfaction with the new training approach were important elements of this proposal. While the overall time-saving varies slightly by specialty, an average of 3.5 hours of instruction was saved for each inpatient nurse hired. This represents a time-saving for both the trainer and new nurses. All 5 instructors could be redeployed to support training or technology needs elsewhere. In this case, they were able to shift their role to become curriculum developers for the newly integrated EHR system. Another benefit to web-based learnings is the ability of clinical staff to repeat viewings of the training if needed.

# Outcomes and Incorporation of Evidence-Based Practice

As technology solutions continue to evolve within health care, the need for DNP nursing informaticists also expands. Numerous nurse quality indicators are monitored with the intention to prevent patient harm or identify patients at risk. Examples include nurses completing falls risk assessments or skin breakdown scoring in an effort to determine if a patient is at a higher risk of a fall or pressure injury. Many EHRs are now capable of triggering alerts based on scoring outcomes of various risk tools helping to bring awareness to action items such as adding components to the patient care plan, ordering specialty consults, or implementing patient care interventions.

One specific project we were able to collaborate with IT staff to develop was a unit-based electronic visibility board (EVB; Figure 23-1).[12] This project had a focused objective to provide visibility to those high-risk items noted through evidence-based practice or nurse quality indicators. We were able to help each unit or team identify the specific elements that should be included on the EVB for a given unit or team. This included items like a restraint order nearing expiration, interpreter order needed based on language identified, central line presence, high-risk medications, or other significant precautions. A DNP-prepared nurse is the ideal person to work collaboratively with IT specialists and frontline clinical staff to capture actionable patient safety or quality items for the EVBs. Another dashboard that was developed at our organization is used by a group of our intensive care unit (ICU) nurses known as *risk nurses*. These nurses use a risk dashboard as a tool to track patients who may be at risk of decompensating, requiring a need to transfer to critical care. The objective of the risk nurse program is for the nurse to monitor the patients closely, providing guidance to other nurses, and recommending relative interventions. This risk nurse dashboard not only provides an electronic solution for

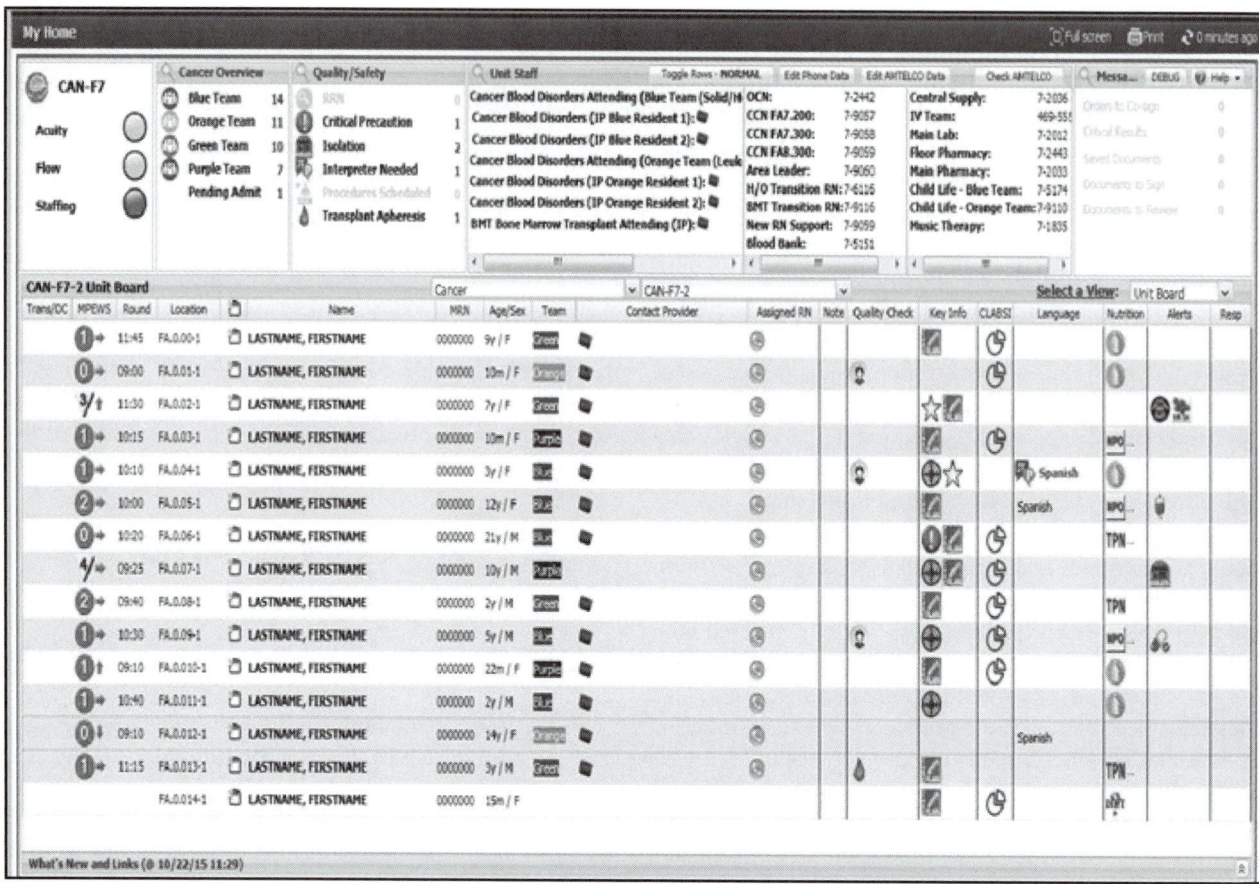

**Figure 23-1.** A unit-based electronic visibility board. (Reprinted with permission from Field M, Fong K, Shade C. Use of electronic visibility boards to improve patient care, quality, safety, and flow on inpatient pediatric acute care units. *J Pediatr Nurs*. 2018;41:69-76. doi:https://doi.org/10.1016/j.pedn.2018.01.015)

tracking all patients deemed at risk, but it also includes time triggers for reassessing patients. Patients can also auto-populate the risk dashboard based on acuity or modified pediatric early warning scores.

# DATA MINING AND PRACTICE OUTCOMES

One of the most valuable aspects of information systems within health care is the ability to use logic and rules within the constructs of the system to trigger recommended practice. The use of technology and a language that uses rules to analyze data is referred to as *clinical decision support*. Nurses having completed a DNP program with a focus in informatics are looking to apply clinical expertise with processes such as clinical decision support to have an impact on patient outcomes and improving the health for entire populations.

Capturing discrete data is the foundation upon which clinical decision support is built. Examples we have been able to utilize include designing a dashboard to capture barcode scanning compliance for medications and breast milk. The data captured for a single barcode-scanned medication includes the nurse performing the task, the patient involved, the medication scanned, exact time scanned, any errors or

alerts that fired, and the action taken by the nurse when the alert fired. All this data can be compiled into a dashboard that can be manipulated by unit managers and pharmacy to identify problem areas, trends, and staff noncompliance. This dashboard allows unit level leaders to individually follow up with nurses to discuss their medication administration practices. The use of such proactive monitoring has grown in recent years to help pull data from multiple systems into a single enterprise warehouse.

One aspect that cannot be underestimated is the value of clinicians, such as a graduate-level nursing leader, to help both interpret the reports generated as well as to serve as a liaison between IT staff and clinical care. As DNP-prepared informaticist leaders, we have been able to contribute to strategy for how our organization develops data-based reports aimed at measuring patient outcomes. One example is the creation of a dashboard that uses predictive analytics to identify patients at highest risk for a CLABSI. Understanding how the EHR is built, including where and how nurses document within it, is essential to validate a report for accuracy. By using CLABSI data on various dashboards along with predictive analytics for those patients most at risk, we have made actionable information visible to the care team. The team can then use this information to guide clinical decision making. For example, clinicians may begin to ask new questions such: Are the labs truly needed? Can labs be bundled? Can intravenous medications transition to oral?

Another example is design of a multidisciplinary discharge readiness tool within the EHR. As our organization looked at delays in discharges impacting the ability to admit patients needing care and even potential diverted patients, it was imperative to look at innovative ways to identify waste, gaps in communication, and missed opportunities to use the data captured within the EHR to help streamline and drive discharge care aspects. We worked with physicians, care coordination, and IT staff to design a custom web-based tool within the EHR to capture patient education, discharge medications, transportation needs, and other coordination of care. Logic built within the page displayed orders and needs at a patient level, and then once completed, the page visually showed this step as completed. This allowed all members of the care team to log into the EHR at any time and see the status of discharge tasks both completed as well as those outstanding. Some of the outstanding patient discharge needs could then also be rolled up to a unit-based dashboard for visibility across a unit (see Figure 23-1). Other new processes were created within the EHR such as the ability of nurses to enter an "anticipated discharge order," which also created visibility on unit-based dashboards as well as within a single patient chart. Many of the Essentials of a DNP program, such as Organizational and Systems Leadership for Quality Improvement and Systems Thinking and Interprofessional Collaboration for Improving Patient and Population Health Outcomes, helped make innovations like this a success.

## PROFESSIONALISM

We feel extremely fortunate to work for an organization that both expects and encourages professional practice from the nursing team. In fact, organizational culture has direct impact on nursing professionalism and patient outcomes.[13] Our entire professional and academic relationship is a direct reflection of our promotion of the nursing profession. Through our work together we have disseminated evidence and information through presentations, posters, publications, and co-teaching a nursing informatics class. However, perhaps the most powerful expression of professionalism is Carol's mentoring of Mary throughout this process. We first met 12 years ago when Mary was a junior inpatient bedside nurse. Since that time Mary has received a graduate degree and been promoted to a nursing leader. Carol's mentorship had a direct positive impact on Mary's career trajectory, inspiring her to pursue and ultimately attain a DNP degree. Carol continued mentoring Mary throughout her capstone project, with the ultimate goal of publishing the findings.

## PEARLS/TAKEAWAYS

If we could offer the reader one piece of advice, it would be this: The best outcomes are achieved through multidisciplinary collaboration with a spirit of continuous innovation. We feel strongly that this is true in any care setting: inpatient, outpatient, peri-operative, rural health care, etc. This is most effectively realized when your professional values align directly with your employer or organization's mission, vision, and values. Our calling as nurses is to provide the best possible care to our patients and families. As advanced practice nurses, we must take a systematic approach to population health. One of the most effective ways to do this is by leveraging the information systems we use every day in clinical care. We are practicing nursing in an exciting time, and technology will only continue to improve and refine itself. Keeping an inquisitive mind and an open heart will allow you to embrace your EHR and technology systems to improve patient outcomes.

## CONCLUSION: IMPACT OF THE DNP DEGREE

As a result of the DNP degree, we have been able to advocate for and represent the field of nursing informatics at the systems level. Acknowledgment of the value of nursing informatics at the executive level happened slowly over time, with diligent advocacy, combined with technological advancements. At a high level, we gathered recognition and support through decreasing training costs while maintaining efficacy and value of training, conducting a nursing satisfaction with the EMR research study, partnering with multidisciplinary peers in a variety of quality improvement projects, and academically disseminating our findings.

Having earned the DNP degree, we were prepared to design, implement, and evaluate systems-level initiatives. This program design and evaluation skill set has allowed us to meaningfully present our outcomes with strong data support. For example, we have evaluated nursing satisfaction at a systems level and stratified satisfaction by a variety of demographics (eg, tenure, age, unit of work, nursing role). This data allow us to provide targeted enhancement and training interventions to the demographic groups with the lowest satisfaction rating. The ability to target these interventions is an efficient use of organizational time and resources.

Ultimately, the DNP degree gave us the skills necessary to represent the value of nursing informatics at the highest executive level. We are thrilled that the combination of this degree and our passion for the field gives us the ability to champion projects that improve the care delivery for nursing throughout the entire health system.

# Acknowledgments

We would like to genuinely thank all the professional and academic mentors we have worked with both at SCH and the Seattle University College of Nursing. There are too many names to list, but we would be remiss for not acknowledging Debra Ridling, PhD, RN; Karen Thomas, PhD, RN; and Bonnie Bowie, PhD, MBA, RN. These 3 expert nurses continue to inspire our nursing practice every day. We would also like to acknowledge the strong collaboration between the nursing informatics and IT teams. Thank you for helping us fully express the DNP Essentials in our everyday work.

# References

1.  American Nurses Association. *Scope and Standards of Practice: Nursing Informatics.* 2nd ed. American Nurses Association; 2015.

2.  2017 facts and stats. Seattle Children's Hospital. Accessed March 29, 2019. https://www.seattlechildrens.org/about/facts-and-stats/

3.  Strudwick G, Nagle L, Kasam I, Pahma M, Sequeira L. Informatics competencies for nurse leaders: a scoping review. *J Nurs Adm.* 2019;49(6):323-330.

4.  Remus S, Kennedy MA. Innovation in transformative nursing leadership: nursing informatics competencies and roles. *Nurs Leadersh (Tor Ont).* 2012;25(4):14-26.

5.  Boyer EL. *Scholarship Reconsidered: Priorities of the Rrofessoriate.* Jossey-Bass; 1997.

6.  America Association of Colleges of Nursing. *The Essentials of Doctoral Education for Advanced Nursing Practice.* American Association of Colleges of Nursing; 2006.

7.  Reeves S, Perrier L, Goldman J, Freeth D, Zwarenstein M. Interprofessional education: effects on professional practice and healthcare outcomes. *Cochrane Database Syst Rev.* 2013;2013(3):CD002213.

8.  Gabrielski L, Lessen R. Centralized model of human milk preparation and storage in a state-of-the-art human milk lab. *Infant Child Adolesc Nutr.* 2011;3(4):225-232.

9.  Drenkard K. The business case for magnet. *J Nurs Adm.* 2010;40(6):263-271.

10. Koch J, Andrew S, Salamonson Y, Everett B, Davidson P. Nursing students' perception of a web-based intervention to support learning. *Nurse Educ Today.* 2010;30(6):584-590.

11. Davis B, Summers M. Applying Dale's Cone of Experience to increase learning and retention: a study of student learning in a foundational leadership course. Paper presented at: Engineering Leaders Conference; 2014.

12. Field M, Fong K, Shade C. Use of electronic visibility boards to improve patient care, quality, safety, and flow on inpatient pediatric acute care units. *J Pediatr Nurs.* 2018;41:69-76. doi:https://doi.org/10.1016/j.pedn.2018.01.015

13. Manojlovich M, Ketefian S. The effects of organizational culture on nursing professionalism: implications for health resource planning. *Can J Nurs Res.* 2002;33(4):15-34.

# SECTION X

## LEGISLATIVE ACTIVITY EXEMPLAR

# CHAPTER 24

# ADVOCATING FOR POLICY CHANGE THROUGH DNP LEADERSHIP

*Robert Metzger, DNP, APRN, FNP-BC*

## INTRODUCTION

Before I explain how leadership can assist Doctor of Nursing Practice (DNP) graduates in advocating for policy change, I would like to state how my work and professional endeavors relate to this topic. I performed many nursing leadership roles throughout my career. First, in undergraduate school, I served as the president and previous treasurer of my student nurses' association. I learned early on the value of nursing organizations and their ability to provide us with a common voice, especially as we become leaders advocating for change. Later, after finishing my master's degree as a family nurse practitioner (FNP), I served twice as the president of our local nurse practitioner (NP) organization, which has more than 750 members, and am currently the group's administrator. Statewide, I held multiple committee and chair positions and various board positions, the last as president of our state NP organization, with more than 5000 members. Nationally, I currently serve as a volunteer member of one NP organizational committee and as an elected member and chair of another committee.

My main employment is at a large, metropolitan academic teaching hospital with more than 600 advanced practice providers (APPs). Initially hired there to manage and treat patients as a clinician within a specialized clinic, career advancements placed me in an administrative role. I am currently the surgical services APP manager supervising 53 APPs employed in surgical clinics and inpatient critical care units. One personal goal in obtaining my DNP degree was to open possible avenues toward a future academic pathway. Immediately upon graduating, I accepted an adjunct faculty position with an esteemed university, where I teach the advanced practice roles course, helping bachelor-prepared nurses (ie, registered nurses) to learn their new roles as advanced practice registered nurses (APRNs). Utilizing the general concepts of advanced practice nursing, I instruct these soon-to-be APRNs regarding the importance of leadership and advocacy for health policy and organizational change.

Although active in leadership roles prior to my DNP degree, I knew that it would provide multiple opportunities to affect systems and health policy change, not only within the nursing profession but within general organizational and legislative arenas as well. Through my various academic,

Benson LA, ed. *The DNP Professional:*
*Translating Value From Classroom to Practice* (pp 263-271).
© 2021 SLACK Incorporated.

practice, and organizational roles, I have utilized my DNP degree to personally encourage and strengthen me to achieve these tasks. In doing so, I grew professionally, and I enjoy mentoring others to do the same. Therefore, that is my goal with this chapter: to influence DNP graduates and students to utilize the Essentials in order to improve their profession through leadership and advocacy for change.

# IMPORTANCE OF LEADERSHIP AND ADVOCACY

So why is leadership and advocacy so important for a DNP-prepared nurse? Leadership occurs when individuals use their attributes and skills to effect change at all organizational and policy levels to attain a commonly defined goal.[1] Similarly, advocacy is the ability of an individual to argue or persuade others of needed change in a positive manner.[1] The main reason leadership and advocacy are so important is that our profession has received an astounding call to action from multiple organizations, including the Institute of Medicine, currently renamed the National Academy of Medicine, in their "The Future of Nursing" report to increase our participation as dynamic leaders in changing today's complex health care system.[2] In fact, for APRNs, leadership is listed as one of Hamric's Core Competencies, and both health policy and organizational structure and culture are listed as critical environmental elements affecting advanced practice nursing.[3]

DNP graduates should be at the forefront leading changes in health care. Through our educational training in the DNP Essentials, we are provided the skills to serve as change agents. It is up to DNP nurses to evaluate the effectiveness of organizations and/or their policies, while also looking at state and/or national policy development on a broader scale. In fact, the redesign of our health care system relies on doctoral-prepared leaders to not only guide these changes but sustain them for the future. Eighty-one percent of participants in a survey regarding the perception of the DNP degree agreed that these nurses are prepared to successfully influence change in health care systems, policy, and interprofessional collaboration.[4] The following are some key examples as to how DNP-prepared nurses can utilize leadership, as well as other DNP Essentials to assist in their professional development as a leader capable of influencing systems and policy change.

# DNP ESSENTIALS II, V AND VI: ADVOCATING FOR HEALTH POLICY CHANGE

Health policy is typically defined as decisions that can direct or influence the actions and behavior of others affecting health law, rules, and regulations.[1] Policy has an extensive impact on the practice of nursing. As nurses, we must follow these laws, rules, and regulations in order to perform our professional duties. Therefore, it is vital that we assist in determining what they dictate and how they are to be implemented. After all, our ability to care for patients is regulated by our state nursing practice acts. If we are not active participants in affecting the laws that govern our practice, then we are allowing others to decide the fate of our profession.

Nearly all health care policy follows the triad of cost, quality, and access. With nurses being the largest population of health care providers, it is valuable that we engage in policy discussions to help ensure that our patients have access to the quality care they deserve. Additionally, with the variety of types of nursing available today, joining the fight toward policy change can have impacts in an array of areas, such as bedside care, health promotion, population health, informatics, and health care administration. Due to these growing roles, it remains crucial that nurses be involved in expanding nurse practice acts.

As nurses continue to pursue more advanced roles, further implications may result from other policy changes. APRNs may not be able to prescribe certain medications, order radiological images, or sign certain forms due to changes in law. If we remain silent as non-participative partners in health, there are many others who would happily determine what we can, but more than likely cannot do. These restrictions do not only hinder us as practitioners, but they also hinder our patients' ability to obtain high-quality, cost-effective health care.

Nursing's influence on policy dates back historically to key figures, such as Florence Nightingale, and includes the formation of important nursing organizations, such as the National League for Nursing, the American Nurses Association, and more recently the American Association of Nurse Practitioners. These leaders and organizations helped formalize the profession and provided uniformity so nursing would have a collective voice to help govern itself. In fact, it was nursing that spearheaded changes to the US public health care practice and policies through the actions of Lillian Wald, Mary Brewster, and Margaret Sanger.

Following in the footsteps of these dynamic leaders, DNP-prepared nurses can play important roles in changing health policy by utilizing the 8 DNP Essentials taught in their programs. As well, due to the ever-changing US health care system, a new demand has been implemented requiring highly educated nursing leaders, who can strategize and use political savvy, to assist in making fair and wise decisions.

Essentials that are important in policy decision making include DNP Essentials II, V, and VI. In fact, DNP Essential V is specifically entitled Health Care Policy for Advocacy in Health Care.[5] Since DNP Essential V is all about health policy, it lays out the importance of DNP-prepared nurses' involvement in instituting change. DNP Essential II is related to organizational and systems leadership and systems thinking, which can assist DNP-prepared nurses in determining how to evaluate the current US health care system and figure out ways to improve upon, remove, and add policies in order to affect change. DNP Essential VI relates to interprofessional collaboration. Vital to all professions is our ability to work together to solve problems. DNP-prepared nurses are key leaders through our ability to work collaboratively with other professions in order to evaluate care provided to our patients and determine appropriate changes, which may require policy changes, institutionally or legislatively, to impact quality outcomes.

An effective way that I personally utilized my DNP education was to serve as a leader and advocate impacting policy change. Despite being knowledgeable about policy before my DNP degree, I lacked the courage to discuss health care policies openly with fellow colleagues or legislators. I felt physicians might look at me as though I did not know what I was talking about or lacked the appropriate education to be a stakeholder in the conversation. However, through developing the leadership and policy skills instructed in DNP programs, these doubts were removed and replaced with confidence. I understand as a DNP-prepared nurse that I had an obligation to personally discuss with my peers, physicians, and other stakeholders the importance of policies and their proposed changes. However, by also being a valuable stakeholder, I could recommend changes to health care policies that I deemed necessary to improve practice.

So, what are ways that nurses can advocate for health policy? Joining your professional organization is one of the easiest and best ways to help influence policy change. In fact, membership should not only be an expectation of all DNP graduates but a requirement, most importantly at the state and national levels. As mentioned earlier, the importance of membership within professional organizations is that together our numbers provide a unified political voice. We are not only advocating for our profession but also for our patients.

Within their organizations, nurses can partake in grassroots efforts to assist with policy advocacy. For APRNs, limitations on our abilities to practice to the full extent of our education and to perform duties such as prescribing certain medications, signing patient forms, ordering diabetic shoes, or ordering home health remain present in many states and federally. Currently, 22 states, the District of Columbia, and 2 territories in the United States have full practice authority removing these limitations.[6] By participating in grassroots efforts, DNP nurses can learn about the policy issues at hand and actively visit with their legislators to discuss these items. It is through this communication that legislators become informed of the importance of health care topics as they relate

to the nursing profession and to our patients. DNP nurses can even serve as content experts on health care issues providing education on these topics to legislators and their staff as they arise or when needed. DNP nurses may even be called upon to be expert witnesses to provide oral testimonies at legislative hearings on bills regarding important health care policies. Another way that DNP nurses could improve the future of politics is to see an increase in the number of nurses running for legislative seats.

There are other ways to contribute to health care policy without having to visit your legislator. DNP-prepared nurses can apply to participate in specialized fellowship programs for health policy where they can expand on their general knowledge learned in school. Through these programs, DNP-prepared nurses can use their knowledge and communication skills to assist with the development of policy agendas and the drafting of legislation. Their knowledge on political issues can also be important in disseminating policy information through editorials, published articles, or continuing education seminars.

If DNP-prepared nurses do not feel they are able to assist in either of the previous scenarios, then their efforts can be utilized in coalition building, which involves networking with other organizations or individuals to provide a network of support for legislative items. They can be active in the political action committees (PACs) of their organization, which assist with donations to political candidates, through voluntary participation or by monetary contributions.

Success is one of the most encouraging paths toward involvement in changing health policy. Although not always to the desired degree, nurses are gaining ground in improving our profession and access to patient care. DNP-prepared nurses provided grassroots efforts to make multiple visits to their legislators locally, statewide, and even nationally. I have seen changes made to the rules and regulations within my home state from these actions. Nationally, through the advocacy efforts of DNP nurses and others, changes continued with more states providing full practice authority for their APRNs.

APRNs in Texas helped make some legislative changes recently to improve advanced practice nursing. Working with key legislators supportive of our practice, APRNs were able to pass Texas HB 278/SB 311 allowing our ability to sign workers' compensation forms. Additionally, we obtained support from one of our physician legislators in improving our required communication for our prescriptive practice agreements. With Texas HB 278/SB 311, APRNs are now able to complete our monthly face-to-face visits via virtual means rather than in person. Both bills improved our ability to provide care to patients, especially in rural communities.

There have been multiple past successes as well. An NP colleague, who also has her DNP degree, worked diligently with her legislators to advocate for palliative care. Due to her efforts in 2017, Texas SB 919 passed allowing the ability of APRNs within hospice or palliative care settings the ability to sign death certificates. Through the collaborative efforts of many of our NPs in Texas, and the joining of the professional organizations for the 4 advanced practice roles and the Texas Nurses Organization into an APRN Alliance, nursing was finally able to change our regulations through the passage of Texas SB 406 to remove site-based prescriptive authority and replace it with new prescriptive practice agreements, which removed mileage stipulations between collaborating physicians and the APRNs that worked with them. Another advantage of this bill is that it provided the provision for APRNs that work within inpatient units the ability to prescribe Schedule II medications upon discharge for patients, as well as within hospice and palliative care settings. Through the efforts of the APRN Alliance, our nursing organizations were able to join forces with other organizations to form a coalition in support of full practice authority for APRNs in Texas.

Over the past 2 legislative sessions, this coalition worked hard to educated legislators and the public regarding improved access to care by removing barriers to practice for APRNs. With these efforts and our advocacy, our bill toward barrier reductions was finally heard in both the Texas House of Representatives and Senate chambers. Unfortunately, it did not move past committee. Although bills are not always successful in passing the legislature, the ability of DNP-prepared nurses to advocate for change is clearly demonstrated.

Another major benefit and DNP Essential is our ability to collaborate with other colleagues to find common goals to improve patient care. This is very beneficial when advocating for legislative change. One of my biggest successes as the Texas Nurse Practitioners president, was to work together with the president of the Texas Association of Physician's Assistants. Coming together for common goals, we helped improve our stature within the Texas legislature. Additionally, it demonstrated to medicine that we were willing to stand up for issues that affected our practice and the care we provide to patients. Together, our organizations introduced 2 bills: HB 2250/SB 1308, which would expand Schedule II prescriptive authority to all APPs, and HB 3128, which would allow the evaluation of concussion patients and the signing of their return-to-play forms. Both efforts would have improved patient care by reducing barriers facing patients in obtaining access to services.

Our state professional organization has seen a significant rise in the number of active participants in grassroots efforts with DNP-prepared nurses providing wonderful expert testimony for our legislative bills. The PAC was developed with many DNP-prepared nurses serving as liaisons, as well as monetary contributors, and has sustained significant growth over the past several years to be considered a stakeholder in political arenas. Nationally, the health policy conference attendance has continued to increase yearly as more and more nurses become politically active.

Despite successes, barriers must still be overcome. The number one barrier faced by nurses involved in policy change is typically physicians. Large medical associations continue to fight bills implemented by nursing organizations.

Other groups remain opposed to the ability to write for diabetic shoes, a cost-effective preventative measure, or order home health care services to provide quality care for patients at home after discharge from the hospital. When faced with these barriers, DNP-prepared nurses, based on our training, are influential and well positioned to perform interdisciplinary collaboration to find feasible solutions.

# DNP ESSENTIALS II AND VI: ADVOCATING FOR ORGANIZATIONAL POLICY CHANGE AND SYSTEMS THINKING

Health care, like many other professions, consists of multiple integrated systems, with the overall entity known as the US health care system. The services provided by these systems range from preventative care to treating diseases and illnesses. In any system, there are many integral stakeholders. Therefore, due to the various disciplines that operate in a health care system, multidisciplinary collaboration is key. Physicians and nurses are important in helping the system run and work to improve access to services for patients, enhance the quality of care they receive, and maintain appropriate cost utilization. However, even in the best operating systems, there are needs for improvement.

In order to enact change within an organization, it is critical that DNP-prepared nurses be knowledgeable in organizational structure and systems theory. There are many different types of theories that can be utilized. Some of the most important for consideration include Ludwig von Bertalanffy's *General System Theory* and Kurt Lewin's "Change Theory". Each theory describes a system as a collection of interacting parts for which the changing of one part typically has a counter effect on the other parts and the whole system in general. Health care organizations are complex systems with multiple competing, collaborating, and conflicting multidisciplinary parts. DNP-prepared nurses must identify areas for improvement and develop appropriate strategies to institute change with the least side effects on the whole system.

The most important DNP Essential for organizational policy change is DNP Essential II: Organizational and Systems Leadership for Quality Improvement and Systems Thinking.[5] Within this Essential, DNP nurses are able to use scientific findings from their own profession, and those of others, to evaluate health care delivery methods and develop changes within these practice models to improve their functionality and facilitation of care. Another important DNP Essential is DNP Essential VI: Interprofessional Collaboration for Improving Patient and Population Health Outcomes. Without DNP-prepared nurses' ability to collaborate with other professionals, developing and implementing organizational changes would be difficult. As the US health care system continues to evolve, DNP graduates will be needed to not only provide clinical care but to use systems thinking to evaluate, develop, and lead innovative practice models of care.[2]

Using a few personal examples, I will demonstrate how DNP-prepared nurses can affect organizational change. When I started my current career, there were a variety of reporting structures in place for our APRNs. Some were reporting to fellow APRNs, while others reported to registered nurses, social workers, or business staff. Working collaboratively with a fellow DNP-prepared nurse, we used systems thinking techniques, taught within our DNP programs, to evaluate the organizational structure for APRNs. Many issues arose from this analysis. First, APRNs were reporting to people who lacked similar clinical knowledge or understanding of an APRN's scope of practice. Second, APRNs felt disengaged from the system due to their manager not understanding their role and how best to evaluate their performance. Finally, many APRNs were hired into the system with poorly defined roles, while others had issues relating to credentialing and privileging. Overall, there seemed to be a lack of standardization for practice. As a result, these various items can lead to poor job satisfaction, low job retention, and decreased job accountability.[7]

We then determined that we needed to develop strategies to reorganize the organizational model for APRNs within our institution, while guiding others who desired to follow our example in the future. Looking at the various departments where APRNs were employed, we developed a new organizational leadership model instituting APRN managers over all the APRNs employed within the institution. Additionally, we created a chief of advanced practice position with equal power and oversight as the chief medical officer and chief nursing officer (CNO). We presented our ideas to the APRN Council, which is a shared governance group for all APRNs employed at our institution, who voted on and approved the recommended changes. The next step was to introduce our idea to the CNO. Although understanding the necessity for this organizational reform, the CNO did not agree with the proposed model. Unfortunately, our developed strategies were placed on hold.

Another organizational change that I worked on was a position statement regarding the use of the title "doctor" by nurses with terminal doctoral degrees. Once again, as the DNP Essentials stated, collaboration was of utmost importance. I met with a fellow DNP graduate and the 2 of us researched our institutional policies, along with state rules and regulations. In the end, we found that occupational code existed that allowed the use of the title "doctor" by anyone completing a terminal degree of doctorate. The recommendation continued that all doctoral-prepared professionals must identify themselves by their given profession, such as nurse practitioner, physician, pharmacist, physical therapist, psychologist, optometrist, etc. Our recommendations in the finalized version of this position statement indicated that a nurse with a doctoral degree (eg, DNP or PhD) could identify themselves as "doctor," if they also clearly stated to the patient their specific role in the institution, such as NP or certified nurse-midwife.

Like before, this position statement was voted on and approved by our APRN Council. It was taken to the nursing operations council, which helps determine nursing practice issues within our institution, for their review. It was approved and signed off by our CNO. However, this statement met opposition from physicians, who refused to hear our position statement within the medical executive committee. Therefore, the position statement, although shared with our APRNs, was never formally adopted by the institution.

As seen in the previous examples, barriers are expected when instituting change at the organizational level. Ironically, one barrier faced in making organizational change was from fellow nurses within our own profession. As DNP-prepared nurses work to change how our organizations function in providing care to our patients, other nurses may be the largest hurdle to overcome. Much of baccalaureate nursing education involves caring for individualized patients and not having to address system-wide issues. Therefore, trying to change what seems to be working for them may cause conflict. Physicians once again remain a barrier to organizational change. Historically, physicians were placed at the top step in a social hierarchical model. With organizational changes and future recommendations, this loss of position can cause some backlash from physicians against proposed changes, especially if instituted by nursing professionals. Conflict may arise at any level due to interpersonal disagreements regarding foresight of how the organization should be managed.

Although both personal endeavors listed previously failed to be fully implemented, changes did occur within our institution as a result of their introduction, which makes them successful to a degree. One such success, related to the endeavor of our APRN organizational leadership model, was that my colleague and I published our work in a professional nursing journal (*The Journal for Nurse Practitioners*). This provided DNP-prepared nurses with an example of how their degree can assist in organizational restructuring and professional development, which will be addressed in the next section.

After a few years, my employer decided to reevaluate the idea of restructuring the organizational model for our APPs. Surveyors were hired to evaluate the needs of our APPs. Their results informed our administrators that a need for change was identified. They provided suggestions and recommendations for restructuring advanced practice within the institution. To assist in these changes, a group of APPs were organized into an advanced practice advisory council to work collaboratively to find solutions for these recommendations. Further development occurred, utilizing the concepts from my published article. Today, we have an APP organizational leadership structure at my institution where I currently serve as one of these APP managers. Although a chief of advanced practice was not included, we did create several director of advanced practice positions that report directly to both our CNO and chief medical officer.

Likewise, although the doctor title position statement did not get formal approval, it did not prevent doctoral-prepared APRNs from utilizing this information and appropriately calling themselves "doctor" while identifying themselves as their professional role (NP, nurse anesthetist, nurse-midwife, etc). As the number of registered nurses and APRNs completing their DNP degrees has increased at our institution, perhaps this position statement may serve a further purpose. One way that it provided some success was benefiting our professional APRN organizations with information regarding title usage within our state. Similarly, this position statement could be utilized by other professions, such as pharmacists, physical therapists, and even physician assistants to assist them in their same battles over terminal degree title recognition.

# DNP Essentials II, III, V, VI, and VIII: Advocating for Professionalism

In order to perform the previous tasks, a DNP-prepared nurse must first understand what it truly means to have this degree. How does the DNP degree make you a leader and a professional in the field of nursing? How does this degree allow you to advocate for health policy and organizational change? Before you can do these things, you must first believe in yourself as a true leader and then you must work to improve and strengthen the nursing profession.

Lisa Chism described a study performed by Elizabeth Joyce in 2002 regarding leadership perception among nurse practitioners.[8] In this study, the themes of visionist, facilitator, role model, and professional were identified. It further went on to describe the professional as someone who is capable of inspiring and enabling others toward achieving improved standards and higher outcomes.[8] Certain attributes were identified for a professional, which included possession of time management skills, confidence, good judgment, resourcefulness, accountability, competency, and the ablilty to set standards and demonstrate integrity.[8] Similarly, Hamric identified 3 characteristics for nurse leaders, which included mentoring, innovation, and activism.[3] For some DNP-prepared nurses, leadership may come naturally, while others may have to spend some time in developing leadership skills. But no matter how it is obtained, leadership is not an option, it is an expectation of DNP-prepared nurses.

One of the easiest ways for DNP-prepared nurses to influence change is through professional leadership. Active participation in professional organizations allows multiple opportunities for involvement. DNP nurses can serve on or chair organizational committees, deliver presentations that follow evidence-based practice (EBP) guidelines, or even hold officer or director positions within organizations. No matter what tasks the DNP-prepared nurse performs, the result of this membership is that it works to unify the voice of the nursing profession. With a unified front and increasing numbers, nursing can then become a larger stakeholder in changing not only our profession but also the US health care system.

So, what DNP Essentials help develop professionalism and leadership within nursing? Although different authors may state differing opinions, DNP Essentials II, III, V, VI, and VIII are all very important for DNP-prepared nurses to utilize to improve their own, and others professionalism. Within DNP Essential II, DNP-prepared nurses are prepared to promote excellence in practice through organizational changes that improve delivery approaches for care leading to quality improvements. Using DNP Essential III, DNP-prepared nurses will work collaboratively with other nurses, as well as other professions, to evaluate, translate, integrate, and apply EBP into our profession. This helps to generate new knowledge for the nursing profession while also working to improve patient outcomes. DNP Essential V is important because when DNP-prepared nurses evaluate our profession, we may have to actively participate in changing some rules, regulations, or policies, at all levels, from institutional to national, that affect our practice, making us a better profession.

As typical, no efforts to improve professionally can be done alone. Therefore, collaboration remains essential to improving our profession. Hence, Essential VI is once again of vital importance for DNP nurses. Lastly, DNP Essential VIII: Advanced Nursing Practice, states its purpose up front. DNP-prepared nurses are to work through their advanced nursing education to assist other nurses in advancing our profession. Whether their skills are within a certain specialty or just general overall mentoring, DNP-prepared nurses can work with others to maintain the excellence within the nursing profession and work toward continued improvements. By serving as mentors and preceptors, DNP-prepared nurses can demonstrate their advanced critical thinking and decision-making skills, which leads to improved patient outcomes.

Throughout my nursing career, I worked diligently to help advance the nursing profession. Advantages obtained from the DNP degree, utilizing the DNP Essentials described previously, assisted me in improving my skills as a professional. Although some organizational structures were previously in place when I started my current position, such as a shared governance committee known as the APRN Council, many of these lacked appropriate structure. Through participation, even prior to my DNP degree, I collaborated with my colleagues to improve the functionality of our group and make it more effective in meeting the needs of the APRNs employed at my institution. Stepping up as president of this council for 2 years provided me the opportunity to inspire and enable other APRNs to speak up regarding practice concerns or professional challenges that affected us personally as employees, how we practiced, and even our patient care itself. These issues would be evaluated and discussed with final recommended changes to policies presented to higher administrators for consideration. Successes included a change in our reimbursement for continuing education hours, improved representation of APRNs on key committees within the institution, and even a seat on the medical executive committee for our directors of advanced practice.

Following DNP Essential III, an advantage of the DNP degree is the existential exposure to EBP, as well as some research. DNP-prepared nurses should collaborate with their PhD nurse colleagues to generate new knowledge and implement evidence into practice to improve patient outcomes. Primarily clinical leaders, DNP-prepared nurses have hands-on patient experiences to develop practical questions affecting patient care. A major advantage of DNP-prepared nurses is our vast knowledge in EBP. Working collaboratively with some of the other doctoral nurses at my institution, we developed the Nursing Research and Best Practice Committee, which today is one of our shared governance committees. Building from the ground up, this group of doctoral nurses worked together, developed, and strengthened the committee by encouraging and involving other nurses to participate in our efforts. Through the work of this committee, nursing at my institution saw an evaluation and critique of several EBP models, finally choosing the IOWA Model for nursing EBP. Several other nurses were encouraged to participate in the Texas Christian University Evidence-Based Practice Fellowship program. Several DNP and PhD nurses served as mentors for those registered nurses who were selected. Throughout this time, our institution has seen more than 40 nursing research projects started and/or completed. Work continues to improve how EBP is instituted throughout the hospital in all nursing areas, especially at the bedside. Without DNP-prepared nurses, a lot of this enthusiasm for change would be lacking.

Another example of a DNP-inspired initiative within my employer was the Consortium for Interdisciplinary Collaboration and Professional Development. This committee was developed by a DNP colleague to improve collaboration at our institution and encourage professionalism among all employees. As a DNP leader, when my colleague left the institution, I accepted the chair position and steered this committee toward the direction it has arrived at today. The main advantage of this committee is that it follows the recommendation of the IOM "The Future of Nursing" report. This committee encourages a multidisciplinary approach toward improving collaboration and personal development skills for all 12 000-plus employees at our institution. Much of this work is completed through active participation in learning workshops and presentations, which are geared toward developing professional skills in others. Examples of our successes include improved professional speaking skills, encouraging publication of multidisciplinary EBP projects enhancing diversity and inclusion as it relates to fellow employees and our patients, and working collaboratively to achieve healthier outcomes for our patients.

As stated in the previous paragraphs, one of the easiest ways to get involved to enhance professionalism is through active participation in professional organizations. Much of my work career is dedicated to the advancement of our profession. As with many other DNP nurses, these efforts began at a more local level. I had the pleasure of serving as the president of the North Texas Nurse Practitioners for two, 1-year terms. While doing so, I worked with the board members to help institute a more professional outlook and strategies for our organization. Rather than just being a venue for educational dinner meetings, I helped strengthen our group to become one of the best affiliate groups in Texas, as well as within the American Association of Nurse Practitioners. Our organization grew from around 400 members to now close to 800 members. We increased our student scholarships from 4 to 6 annually, which are available for members obtaining their bachelor to DNP and post-master's DNP degrees as well. Additionally, we participated in grassroots legislative efforts visiting our legislators locally to educate them on health policies that affect our practice. To help advance and promote our profession, we also offered philanthropic grants to local organizations that assist patients and performed community outreach projects to help vulnerable populations demonstrating our belief in improving care for others.

As many leaders grow, so did I. I utilized my skills as a DNP leader and ran for state committees and eventually served as the president of the Texas Nurse Practitioners. In these committees, I worked to help increase our membership growth and advocate for health policy change to advance our profession. Throughout my tenure as a board member, Texas Nurse Practitioners saw our membership grow to more than 5000 nurse practitioners. Working with the chief executive officer, we improved our organization through professional endeavors, such as revising our bylaws, enhancing our internal policies and procedures, and working to develop a program for other state leaders to work collaboratively together on issues faced across the nation. Legislatively, our organization has become a key stakeholder in health care issues within our state. We have seen an increase in the number of legislative bills introduced each session, several being successful in passing. As mentioned earlier, our PAC has increased in its numbers and impact as well.

Skills learned at the institutional, local, and state level allowed me to advance my commitment to the profession to the national level. If you, as a DNP-prepared nurse, wish to improve your leadership skills, one of the easiest ways is by attending a leadership program. I was lucky enough to participate in the American Association of Nurse Practitioners leadership program during its second cohort. Taking the DNP Essentials taught in the DNP program, I realized how using the skills taught in the leadership program would enhance the DNP Essentials and improve my ability to promote our profession to others more effectively.

Another advantage of the leadership program was that it allowed me to work collaboratively with fellow DNP nurses to use systems thinking in evaluating current diversity initiatives within the organization and offer recommendations for improvement. We were able to identify areas for improvement and provided an appropriate action plan for consideration by the organization's board members. We were excited that the board appreciated our presentation and incorporated a diversity and inclusion committee to continue work on the development and improvement of these policies within the organization. I currently sit on this committee. Additionally, I was elected by the American Association of Nurse Practitioners membership for the nomination council, where I assist in recruiting, evaluating, interviewing, and choosing appropriate candidates for leadership election for our organization.

Barriers remain for DNP-prepared nurses working to improve professionalism. As mentioned, although my institution improved practice for APRNs with the addition of representation at the medical executive committee, this position is a non-voting position. Physician resistance remains a key issue toward advancing the nursing profession. Lack of involvement in the profession by other nurses exists as well. Many view nursing not as a profession but simply a job that pays their bills. DNP-prepared nurses will have to work hard to demonstrate professionalism that might help change the mindset of these nurses.

## Pearls/Takeaways

As you can see from all these examples provided, despite personal involvement as a DNP leader, success involved collaboration. Think of leadership as 2 words: leader and ship. If you took the "I" out of the word ship, it would not be a ship and it would sink. So, think of the "I" as the leader of that ship. Thinking in this manner, it is best for DNP-prepared nurses to consider themselves as the Is, or captains (leaders), of the ship. Standing at the helm of the ship, they inspire and enable the other crew members, such as fellow nurses or multidisciplinary professionals, to participate in the tasks at hand to achieve the stated goals. Using this metaphor, it is clear to see how important DNP Essential VI (Interprofessional Collaboration for Improving Patient and Population Health Outcomes) truly is within our profession. It may in fact be one of the most vital DNP Essentials in helping us make change. For without the "team" in teamwork, you, and you alone, would have work.

Be motivated and develop confidence in yourself. I mentioned earlier that my DNP degree inspired me to become more active and do things that I typically would not have felt comfortable doing before. That is my best advice to you as a DNP graduate or a student looking to obtain your DNP degree. Being self-motivated and developing self-confidence are instrumental to your success as a DNP-prepared nurse. These endeavors will shine through and demonstrate to others your belief that change is needed and that your voice should be heard. With these endeavors, you will be a strong advocate, not only for the profession, but for patients as well.

Be active. The last (and most important) pearl is that you must become active in your professional organizations.

Membership in professional organizations has multiple benefits as previously listed. DNP-prepared nurses are true leaders essential to the continuation, advancement, and promotion of the nursing profession. DNP-prepared nurses should be officers leading organizations toward future changes. They can also be advocates helping the association fight legislative battles. No matter what degree of participation they choose, it is essential that DNP-prepared nurses be at the forefront of political and organizational change.

## Conclusion: Impact of the DNP Degree

As a result of obtaining my DNP degree, I expanded my understanding regarding the importance of leadership and advocacy of DNP-prepared nurses. Through this growth, I was personally able to strengthen my ability to serve as a change agent for improved outcomes for our profession.

The DNP coursework, especially health care policy, helped emphasize advocacy and its importance. Serving as president of our state organization, I utilized these skills and confidently spoke with my legislators on important issues affecting our practice that included lack of full practice authority, the inability to write for Schedule II drugs, and the inability to write for home health orders. Part of these efforts paid off with the achievement of ordering home health within the CARES Act on a federal level. Although not passing in our state legislature, the other 2 items made significant progress.

I influenced others in following this lead and taking their own initiatives toward continued change in their states and our US health care system. It is important to remember that as DNP-prepared nurses who are politically active, we are advocating not only for ourselves but for our patients as well. Any professional advancements we make typically help to improve patient access to care.

Utilizing systems thinking, I was able to evaluate existing organizational structures and recommend practice changes. I helped our institution develop an organizational leadership structure so that all APPs could report to another APP manager. This led to improved provider satisfaction and retention while still providing efficient, if not improved, quality health care and patient outcomes. This work was published so that other institutions could also work toward achieving this goal.

Additionally, I was able to help gain the recognition and respect for the work we do and the title we earned by obtaining this degree. The DNP helped me to think of nursing more professionally and to teach others to do so as well. In doing so, I encouraged nurses to come together and work collaboratively, as discussed in the IOM's "The Future of Nursing" report, to change health policy and improve practice.

Although already possessing leadership and advocacy skills prior to the DNP, having earned this degree solidified these competencies within my practice allowing me to be more self-confident. With this confidence, I was then able to make the changes described above to help improve health policy and organizational structure, in turn improving practice and advancing our profession. As we demonstrate how the DNP degree impacts our practice, nursing will be seen as the strong profession that it is, and the importance of the DNP as our terminal degree will be recognized.

## Acknowledgments

I would like to acknowledge my mentors for the guidance they provided me to become a great nursing leader. Most importantly, I would like to thank my mother and father who encouraged and supported my education and ambitions, which allowed me to be who I am today.

## References

1. Shillam C, Maclean L. Leadership influence. *Nurs Adm Q.* 2018;42(2):150-153. doi:10.1097/naq.0000000000000276

2. Tran A, Nevidjon B, Derouin A, Weaver S, Bzdak M. Reshaping nursing workforce development by strengthening the leadership skills of advanced practice nurses. *J Nurses Prof Dev.* 2019;35(3):152-159. doi:10.1097/nnd.0000000000000534

3. Tracy MF, O'Grady ET. *Hamric and Hanson's Advanced Practice Nursing: An Integrative Approach.* 6th ed. Elsevier; 2019.

4. Udlis K, Mancuso J. Perceptions of the role of the doctor of nursing practice-prepared nurse: Clarity or confusion. *J Prof Nurs.* 2015;31(4):274-283. doi:10.1016/j.profnurs.2015.01.004

5. The essentials of doctoral education for advanced nursing practice. American Association of Colleges of Nursing. Accessed August 7, 2019. https://www.aacnnursing.org/Portals/42/Publications/DNPEssentials.pdf

6. State practice environment. American Association of Nurse Practitioners. Accessed August 7, 2019. https://www.aanp.org/advocacy/state/state-practice-environment

7. Metzger R, Rivers C. Advanced practice nursing organizational leadership model. *J Nurse Pract.* 2014;10(5):337-343. doi:10.1016/j.nurpra.2014.02.015

8. Chism L. *The Doctor of Nursing Practice: A Guidebook for Role Development and Professional Issues.* Jones & Bartlett Learning; 2010.

# Conclusion and Future Essentials

This book contains a diverse collection of DNP success stories with several common themes. The chapter authors were able to describe how the DNP degree enhanced their practices and how the DNP Essentials produced improved patient outcomes when implemented. As this textbook was being submitted for publication, the American Association of Colleges of Nursing had completed a revision to the original Essentials crafted in 2006, and a new DRAFT Domains and Descriptors was presented in November 2019.[1] These new DRAFT Domains and Descriptors were finalized in 2020, and while there is no decision at this time as to the format or number of documents, curricular recommendations will be developed for baccalaureate, master's, and DNP programs.[2] Knowing that this is the course of the future, focusing on the domains seemed necessary for the conclusion of this textbook.

## Domain 1: Knowledge for Nursing Practice

Several of the authors participated in evolutionary changes in practice. On the clinical practice side, there were innovative care delivery models such as DNP-prepared nurse practitioners who managed a free clinic to an underserved vulnerable population and a mobile clinic that delivered high-end health care to the home setting. Medical respite for the homeless was a focus for another nurse practitioner who implemented successful models in different states. Genetic counseling in a pediatric practice served as another cutting-edge practice depicted by one of the authors.

With the nurse executives, several novel approaches were taken for advanced practice registered nurse (APRN) growth opportunities in fellowship development, e-hospital, and distance health roles and expansion of international APRN services. Another executive decreased the nurse manager span of control which in turn impacted patient

Benson LA, ed. *The DNP Professional:*
*Translating Value From Classroom to Practice* (pp 273-276).
© 2021 SLACK Incorporated.

engagement, patient safety, team member engagement, and registered nurse turnover. With interprofessional education in mind, one nurse executive supported the collaboration that gave rise to an interprofessional education unit serving students, not only in nursing but physical therapy, occupational therap, speech-language pathology, and physician assistant studies as well.

## DOMAIN 2: PERSON-CENTERED CARE

While many of the authors described population or aggregate patient care, a prime example of patient-centered care based on evidence was provided by one of the nurse-midwife authors. During a delivery, she was able to convince a father who wanted an episiotomy performed on the mother to avoid a fourth-degree laceration that episiotomies were not evidenced as best practice. She was able to show this on her phone and quickly print the current practice bulletin from the professional organization.

One of the certified registered nurse anesthetist (CRNA) authors describes a patient-centric quality approach to one of the most basic, but sometimes not mastered, procedures—establishing intravenous access. After initial chloro-preparation, topical application of a local anesthesia and massaging the infiltration into the skin for 60 seconds is performed while speaking to the patient and family. Then, additional chloro-preparation of the skin is completed, allowing the vein to fill optimally with blood. While still speaking with the patient and family, the insertion of a short 20-gauge intravenous catheter is inserted.

Patient-centric care was also described in the chapter by the tobacco cessation specialist. An individualized plan of care was developed through active listening for each one of the clients. By developing services that include a high degree of convenience and flexibility, such as brief telephone follow-up, services delivered via secure messaging, and video chat options, the program has achieved higher cessation rates than benchmark.

## DOMAIN 3: POPULATION HEALTH

Specific population health initiatives were shared by various authors with detailed, full-length chapters on initiatives for the heart failure and homeless populations being described in detail. Considerations for DNP students when planning their capstone projects around a population health initiative were described.

Population health often involves embracing the principle of equity and partnering with community stakeholders to improve health care for a given population. Health care as depicted by several authors needs to be both affordable and accessible. Strategies described by the authors were put into place to ensure that patients could adhere financially to their prescribed treatment regimens.

The authors depicted working with local, state, and federal representativeness to raise awareness of population needs. Itemized business plans have been provided for replication of these efforts.

## DOMAIN 4: SCHOLARSHIP FOR NURSING PRACTICE

Across the board, the authors have described the impact of the DNP Essentials on patient health. Establishment of practice underpinned in science and evidence has resulted in opioid reduction, maternal substance abuse strategies, and disease readmission prevention.

For the diabetic patient population, one author described educational efforts for both staff and patients. To improve nursing scholarship, core training that received interprofessional input and utilized a case study approach was depicted. Training for patients involved usage of an electronic medical record program.

The DNP program directors who served as authors for the academic chapters are all DNP-prepared. Unique topics on transformational leadership programs, incorporation of telehealth into DNP curricula, and a DNP study abroad program were all presented. Another chapter discusses the possible addition of genetics into DNP education and practice.

## DOMAIN 5: QUALITY AND SAFETY

Multiple authors reported that they were employed by facilities that had achieved Magnet designation. Magnet hospitals not only practice to meet exemplar definitions but must demonstrate data that are better than benchmark performance in the various nursing-sensitive safety indicators. Doctoral-educated nurses spearheaded the system-wide performances in quality that led to these designations.

Many of the authors also referred to the Institute of Medicine's (IOM) definition for quality as encompassing safety, timeliness, effectiveness, efficiency, equity, and patient-centeredness.[3] One nurse specialist partnered with her chief nursing officer, who were both DNP-prepared, to develop a nursing strategic plan that was based on the IOM model. Authors described metrics and interventions in the safety domain that contributed to reductions in hospital-acquired pressure injuries, falls with injury, catheter-associated urinary tract infections, and central line associated bloodstream infections.

Several of the CRNA authors described implementation of early recovery after surgery (ERAS) in which one of the featured elements is an opioid-sparing philosophy post-operatively.[4] The DNP-prepared CRNA authors were able to utilize scientific, evidence-based practice to demonstrate improvements in quality of care such as reductions in respiratory depression, nausea and vomiting, length of stays, and an ultimate cost savings.

## DOMAIN 6: INTERPROFESSIONAL PARTNERSHIPS

DNPs are educated on performance improvement strategies and tools. DNP-led initiatives typically involve having key stakeholders involved in the improvement process, which is vital to the success of the change. Evidence of interprofessional collaboration and partnership were pervasive throughout. Outcome improvement and DNP impact were demonstrated as a result. Associated cost savings were generated with sepsis initiatives including DNP return on investment, promotion of skin-to-skin contact following caesarean section births, video monitoring, and changes to nursing education involving e-learnings.

## DOMAIN 7: SYSTEMS-BASED PRACTICE

Chapters on nurse executive leadership and academia emphasized the unique contributions of the DNP-prepared professional. The chief nurse executives served as role models and change agents for their organizations/systems, aligned nursing strategic priorities with those of the organization, and promoted obtaining doctoral education for their nursing leadership teams.

A collaborative effort between 2 DNP-prepared co-authors depicted multidisciplinary efforts to implement best practices across hospital systems, particularly as it pertains to critical care standards and sepsis best practice. Shared decision making and performance improvement councils served as the framework for change.

## DOMAIN 8: INFORMATICS AND HEALTH CARE TECHNOLOGIES

Health care technology can be leveraged to yield data that, in turn, is utilized by nursing management and staff to transform and improve practice. Informatics serves as the linchpin providing the information on which to build and change practice. Many of our authors described data-mining techniques and dissemination to evoke data-centric practice change.

In addition, 2 separate chapters were written by DNP directors of informatics. Both were able to leverage the electronic medical record in shaping patient care. Development of risk dashboards to enhance safety, scorecards to drive care across systems and organizations, and predictive analytics for acute and chronic illnesses in both inpatient and ambulatory care settings were described.

## DOMAINS 9 AND 10: PROFESSIONALISM AND PERSONAL, PROFESSIONAL, AND LEADERSHIP DEVELOPMENT

Professionalism and advocacy were strong themes carried across the chapters. Authors not only promoted their respective professional organizations, but many of the authors were in leadership positions within their professional organizations. Across the board, authors discussed pushing your professional course outside of your comfort zone. Establishing mentors and partnerships with interprofessional partners was a common takeaway. Legislative activism and advocacy for policy change were described in several chapters with examples of assisting state senators in reviewing health care related legislation to one author's political campaign for office. One chapter was entirely devoted to policy change through DNP leadership by focusing on both individual alliances and organizational involvement. Many authors were active to advance the ability of their professional role to practice to the full extent of their education. The DNP skill set enhances the ability to develop, critique, and advocate for policy change. With this advocacy, a few authors mentioned conflict had been encountered that affected their practice or even their employment, but they found support from their professional colleagues. As a profession, we must continue to advocate for full practice and prescriptive authority even in the face of conflict.

As DNPs or DNP students seek to enhance their own professionalism, continuing to take advantage of DNP resources and being active in DNP professional activities is of paramount importance. One such resource is the DNP website that is an online community for professional growth and practice innovation. Highlights include a monthly outcomes newsletter, a DNP project repository, a list of university DNP programs, and an annual DNP professional conference.[5]

As the new Essentials are finalized, this book should serve as a reference on the impact of the DNP professional and the translation of that value from classroom to practice settings.

# REFERENCES

1.    AACN essentials draft domains and descriptors. American Association of Colleges of Nursing. November 2019. Accessed December 20, 2019. https://www.aacnnursing.org/Portals/42/Downloads/Essentials/Essentials-Revision-Domains-Descriptors.pdf

2.    Revisiting AACN's essentials series: re-envisioning nursing education. American Association of Colleges of Nursing. April 2020. Accessed December 20, 2019. https://www.aacnnursing.org/Portals/42/Downloads/Essentials/Essentials-Revision-Frequently-Asked-Questions.pdf

3.    Institute of Medicine Committee on Quality of Health Care in America. *Crossing the Quality Chasm: A New Health System for the 21st Century.* National Academy Press; 2001.

4.    ERAS society guidelines. ERAS Society. http://www.erassociety.org

5.    Home. Doctors of Nursing Practice. Accessed December 29, 2019. https://www.doctorsofnursingpractice.org/

# FINANCIAL DISCLOSURES

*Dr. Mallory Andrzejak* has not disclosed any relevant financial relationships.

*Dr. Tammy Austin-Ketch* has received an advanced nursing education grant.

*Dr. Debbie Barber* has no financial or proprietary interest in the materials presented herein.

*Dr. Rebecca A. Bates* has no financial or proprietary interest in the materials presented herein.

*Dr. Linda A. Benson* has no financial or proprietary interest in the materials presented herein.

*Dr. Garry Brydges* has no financial or proprietary interest in the materials presented herein.

*Dr. Debra A. Burke* has no financial or proprietary interest in the materials presented herein.

*Dr. Deborah Chasco* has no financial or proprietary interest in the materials presented herein.

*Dr. Ileen Craven* has no financial or proprietary interest in the materials presented herein.

*Dr. Janet Hunt Davis* has no financial or proprietary interest in the materials presented herein.

*Dr. Michelle M. Davis* has no financial or proprietary interest in the materials presented herein.

*Dr. Melinda Earle* has no financial or proprietary interest in the materials presented herein.

*Dr. Carol Essenmacher* has no financial or proprietary interest in the materials presented herein.

*Dr. Mary Field* has no financial or proprietary interest in the materials presented herein.

*Dr. Kelly Hancock* has no financial or proprietary interest in the materials presented herein.

*Dr. Marcia Johansson* has not disclosed any relevant financial relationships.

*Dr. Mary C. Loughran* has no financial or proprietary interest in the materials presented herein.

*Dr. Robert Metzger* has no financial or proprietary interest in the materials presented herein.

*Dr. Tracie L. Moore* has no financial or proprietary interest in the materials presented herein.

*Dr. Kara Morgan* has not disclosed any relevant financial relationships.

*Dr. Maria Teresa Palleschi* has no financial or proprietary interest in the materials presented herein.

*Dr. Pamela Paplham* has not disclosed any relevant financial relationships.

*Dr. Courtney Pladsen* has no financial or proprietary interest in the materials presented herein.

*Dr. Dixie Shaheen Rasmussen* has not disclosed any relevant financial relationships.

*Dr. Nancy Renn-Bugai* has received a program grant from Blue Cross Blue Shield and Spectrum Health Foundation for administrative support.

*Dr. Carol Shade* has no financial or proprietary interest in the materials presented herein.

*Dr. Susanna Sirianni* has no financial or proprietary interest in the materials presented herein.

*Dr. Jorge A. Valdes* has no financial or proprietary interest in the materials presented herein.

# INDEX